Drugs Used in Psychiatry

This guide contains color reproductions of some commonly prescribed psychotherapeutic drugs. This guide mainly illustrates tablets and capsules. A † symbol preceding the name of a drug indicates that other doses are available. Check directly with the manufacturer. *(Although the photos are intended as accurate reproductions of the drug, this guide should be used only as a quick identification aid.)*

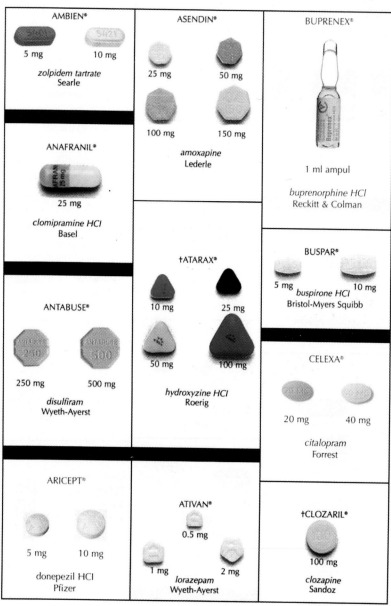

AMBIEN®

5 mg   10 mg

zolpidem tartrate
Searle

ANAFRANIL®

25 mg

clomipramine HCl
Basel

ANTABUSE®

250 mg   500 mg

disulfiram
Wyeth-Ayerst

ARICEPT®

5 mg   10 mg

donepezil HCl
Pfizer

ASENDIN®

25 mg   50 mg

100 mg   150 mg

amoxapine
Lederle

†ATARAX®

10 mg   25 mg

50 mg   100 mg

hydroxyzine HCl
Roerig

ATIVAN®

0.5 mg

1 mg   2 mg

lorazepam
Wyeth-Ayerst

BUPRENEX®

1 ml ampul

buprenorphine HCl
Reckitt & Colman

BUSPAR®

5 mg   10 mg
buspirone HCl
Bristol-Myers Squibb

CELEXA®

20 mg   40 mg

citalopram
Forrest

†CLOZARIL®

100 mg

clozapine
Sandoz

Lippincott Williams & Wilkins

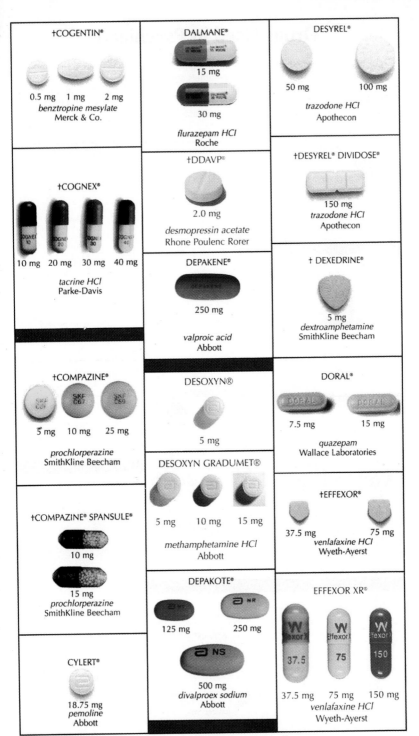

†COGENTIN®

0.5 mg 1 mg 2 mg
benztropine mesylate
Merck & Co.

†COGNEX®

10 mg 20 mg 30 mg 40 mg

tacrine HCl
Parke-Davis

†COMPAZINE®

5 mg 10 mg 25 mg

prochlorperazine
SmithKline Beecham

†COMPAZINE® SPANSULE®

10 mg

15 mg
prochlorperazine
SmithKline Beecham

CYLERT®

18.75 mg
pemoline
Abbott

DALMANE®

15 mg

30 mg

flurazepam HCl
Roche

†DDAVP®

2.0 mg

desmopressin acetate
Rhone Poulenc Rorer

DEPAKENE®

250 mg

valproic acid
Abbott

DESOXYN®

5 mg

DESOXYN GRADUMET®

5 mg 10 mg 15 mg

methamphetamine HCl
Abbott

DEPAKOTE®

125 mg 250 mg

500 mg
divalproex sodium
Abbott

DESYREL®

50 mg 100 mg

trazodone HCl
Apothecon

†DESYREL® DIVIDOSE®

150 mg
trazodone HCl
Apothecon

† DEXEDRINE®

5 mg
dextroamphetamine
SmithKline Beecham

DORAL®

7.5 mg 15 mg

quazepam
Wallace Laboratories

†EFFEXOR®

37.5 mg 75 mg
venlafaxine HCl
Wyeth-Ayerst

EFFEXOR XR®

37.5 mg 75 mg 150 mg
venlafaxine HCl
Wyeth-Ayerst

Lippincott Williams & Wilkins©

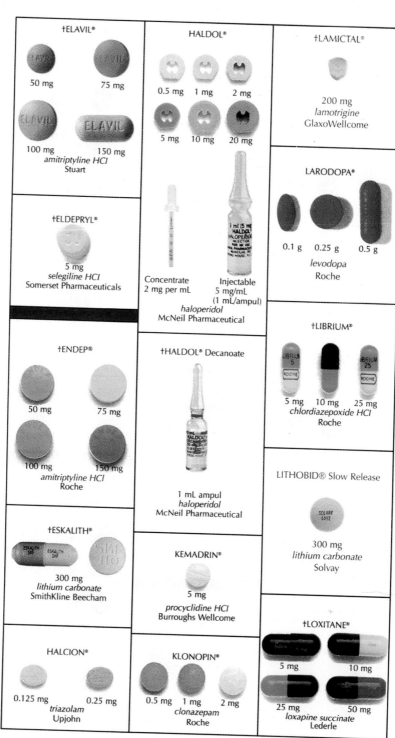

†ELAVIL®

50 mg   75 mg

100 mg   150 mg

amitriptyline HCl
Stuart

†ELDEPRYL®

5 mg
selegiline HCl
Somerset Pharmaceuticals

†ENDEP®

50 mg   75 mg

100 mg   150 mg

amitriptyline HCl
Roche

†ESKALITH®

300 mg
lithium carbonate
SmithKline Beecham

HALCION®

0.125 mg   0.25 mg

triazolam
Upjohn

HALDOL®

0.5 mg   1 mg   2 mg

5 mg   10 mg   20 mg

Concentrate
2 mg per mL

Injectable
5 mg/mL
(1 mL/ampul)

haloperidol
McNeil Pharmaceutical

†HALDOL® Decanoate

1 mL ampul
haloperidol
McNeil Pharmaceutical

KEMADRIN®

5 mg

procyclidine HCl
Burroughs Wellcome

KLONOPIN®

0.5 mg   1 mg   2 mg

clonazepam
Roche

†LAMICTAL®

200 mg
lamotrigine
GlaxoWellcome

LARODOPA®

0.1 g   0.25 g   0.5 g

levodopa
Roche

†LIBRIUM®

5 mg   10 mg   25 mg

chlordiazepoxide HCl
Roche

LITHOBID® Slow Release

300 mg
lithium carbonate
Solvay

†LOXITANE®

5 mg   10 mg

25 mg   50 mg

loxapine succinate
Lederle

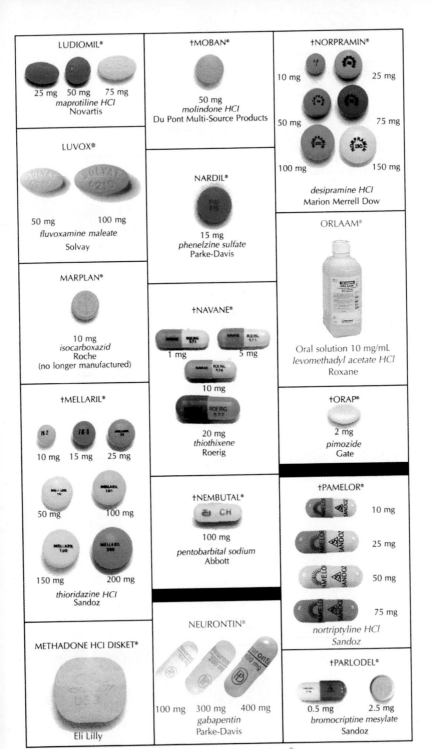

LUDIOMIL®

25 mg 50 mg 75 mg
maprotiline HCl
Novartis

LUVOX®

50 mg 100 mg
fluvoxamine maleate
Solvay

MARPLAN®

10 mg
isocarboxazid
Roche
(no longer manufactured)

†MELLARIL®

10 mg 15 mg 25 mg

50 mg 100 mg

150 mg 200 mg

thioridazine HCl
Sandoz

METHADONE HCl DISKET®

Eli Lilly

†MOBAN®

50 mg
molindone HCl
Du Pont Multi-Source Products

NARDIL®

15 mg
phenelzine sulfate
Parke-Davis

†NAVANE®

1 mg 5 mg

10 mg

20 mg
thiothixene
Roerig

†NEMBUTAL®

100 mg
pentobarbital sodium
Abbott

NEURONTIN®

100 mg 300 mg 400 mg
gabapentin
Parke-Davis

†NORPRAMIN®

10 mg 25 mg

50 mg 75 mg

100 mg 150 mg

desipramine HCl
Marion Merrell Dow

ORLAAM®

Oral solution 10 mg/mL
levomethadyl acetate HCl
Roxane

†ORAP®

2 mg
pimozide
Gate

†PAMELOR®

10 mg

25 mg

50 mg

75 mg

nortriptyline HCl
Sandoz

†PARLODEL®

0.5 mg 2.5 mg
bromocriptine mesylate
Sandoz

Lippincott Williams & Wilkins©

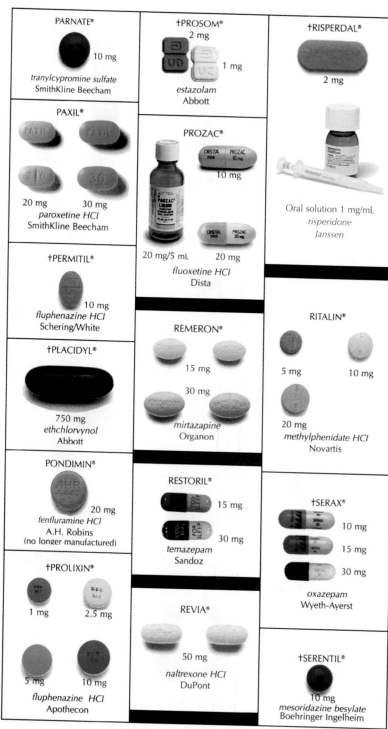

PARNATE®

10 mg

tranylcypromine sulfate
SmithKline Beecham

†PROSOM®
2 mg

1 mg

estazolam
Abbott

†RISPERDAL®

2 mg

Oral solution 1 mg/mL
risperidone
Janssen

PAXIL®

PAXIL

20 mg   30 mg

paroxetine HCl
SmithKline Beecham

PROZAC®

DISTA   PROZAC
3104   10 mg

10 mg

PROZAC
LIQUID

DISTA   PROZAC
3105   20 mg

20 mg/5 mL   20 mg

fluoxetine HCl
Dista

†PERMITIL®

10 mg

fluphenazine HCl
Schering/White

REMERON®

15 mg

30 mg

mirtazapine
Organon

RITALIN®

5 mg   10 mg

20 mg

methylphenidate HCl
Novartis

†PLACIDYL®

750 mg
ethchlorvynol
Abbott

PONDIMIN®

AHR
6447

20 mg

fenfluramine HCl
A.H. Robins
(no longer manufactured)

RESTORIL®

FOR
SLEEP   15 mg

RESTORIL
30 mg   30 mg

temazepam
Sandoz

†SERAX®

10 mg

SERAX
15   15 mg

SERAX
30   30 mg

oxazepam
Wyeth-Ayerst

†PROLIXIN®

PPH
1   PPL
           2.5

1 mg   2.5 mg

PPH   PPH
5 mg   10 mg

fluphenazine HCl
Apothecon

REVIA®

50 mg

naltrexone HCl
DuPont

†SERENTIL®

10 mg
mesoridazine besylate
Boehringer Ingelheim

Lippincott Williams & Wilkins©

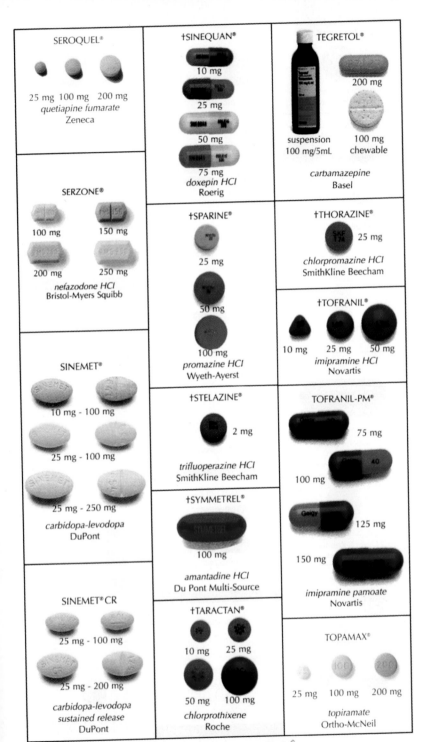

SEROQUEL®

25 mg 100 mg 200 mg
quetiapine fumarate
Zeneca

SERZONE®

100 mg 150 mg

200 mg 250 mg

nefazodone HCl
Bristol-Myers Squibb

SINEMET®

10 mg - 100 mg

25 mg - 100 mg

25 mg - 250 mg

carbidopa-levodopa
DuPont

SINEMET® CR

25 mg - 100 mg

25 mg - 200 mg

*carbidopa-levodopa
sustained release*
DuPont

†SINEQUAN®

10 mg

25 mg

50 mg

75 mg
doxepin HCl
Roerig

†SPARINE®

25 mg

50 mg

100 mg
promazine HCl
Wyeth-Ayerst

†STELAZINE®

2 mg

trifluoperazine HCl
SmithKline Beecham

†SYMMETREL®

100 mg

amantadine HCl
Du Pont Multi-Source

†TARACTAN®

10 mg 25 mg

50 mg 100 mg
chlorprothixene
Roche

TEGRETOL®

200 mg

suspension 100 mg
100 mg/5mL chewable

carbamazepine
Basel

†THORAZINE®

SKF
T74 25 mg

chlorpromazine HCl
SmithKline Beecham

†TOFRANIL®

10 mg 25 mg 50 mg
imipramine HCl
Novartis

TOFRANIL-PM®

75 mg

100 mg 40

Geigy 125 mg

150 mg

imipramine pamoate
Novartis

TOPAMAX®

25 mg 100 mg 200 mg

topiramate
Ortho-McNeil

Lippincott Williams & Wilkins©

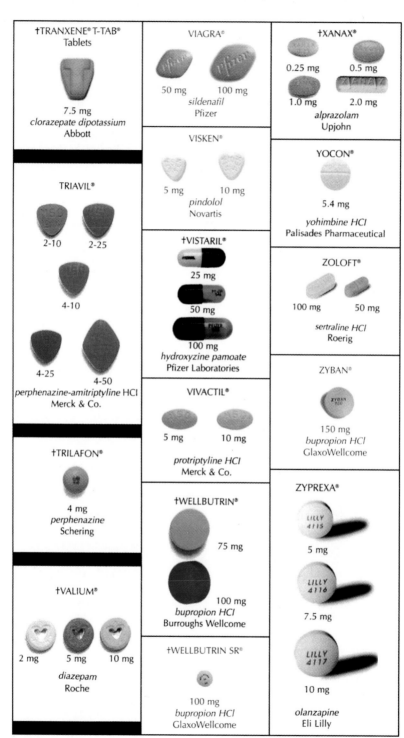

†TRANXENE® T-TAB®
Tablets

7.5 mg
clorazepate dipotassium
Abbott

TRIAVIL®

2-10   2-25

4-10

4-25   4-50
perphenazine-amitriptyline HCl
Merck & Co.

†TRILAFON®

4 mg
perphenazine
Schering

†VALIUM®

2 mg   5 mg   10 mg

diazepam
Roche

VIAGRA®

50 mg   100 mg
sildenafil
Pfizer

VISKEN®

5 mg   10 mg
pindolol
Novartis

†VISTARIL®

25 mg

50 mg

100 mg
hydroxyzine pamoate
Pfizer Laboratories

VIVACTIL®

5 mg   10 mg

protriptyline HCl
Merck & Co.

†WELLBUTRIN®

75 mg

100 mg
bupropion HCl
Burroughs Wellcome

†WELLBUTRIN SR®

100 mg
bupropion HCl
GlaxoWellcome

†XANAX®

0.25 mg   0.5 mg

1.0 mg   2.0 mg
alprazolam
Upjohn

YOCON®

5.4 mg

yohimbine HCl
Palisades Pharmaceutical

ZOLOFT®

100 mg   50 mg

sertraline HCl
Roerig

ZYBAN®

ZYBAN
150

150 mg
bupropion HCl
GlaxoWellcome

ZYPREXA®

LILLY
4115
5 mg

LILLY
4116
7.5 mg

LILLY
4117
10 mg

olanzapine
Eli Lilly

Lippincott Williams & Wilkins©

KAPLAN & SADOCK'S POCKET HANDBOOK OF CLINICAL PSYCHIATRY

Third Edition

Senior Consulting Editor
ROBERT CANCRO, M.D., MED. D.SC.   Lucius N. Littauer Professor and Chairman, Department of Psychiatry, New York University School of Medicine, New York, New York; Director, Department of Psychiatry, Tisch Hospital, New York, New York; Director, Nathan S. Kline Institute for Psychiatric Research, Orangeburg, New York

Contributing Editor
EUGENE RUBIN, M.D.   Assistant Professor of Clinical Psychiatry, Wayne State University School of Medicine, Detroit, Michigan

Collaborating Authors
JAMES C. EDMONDSON, M.D., PH.D.   Clinical Assistant Professor of Psychiatry, New York University School of Medicine, New York, New York

MYRL R. S. MANLEY, M.D.   Associate Professor of Clinical Psychiatry, Director of Medical Student Education in Psychiatry, New York University School of Medicine, New York, New York

RICHARD PERRY, M.D.   Clinical Associate Professor of Psychiatry, Division of Child and Adolescent Psychiatry, New York University School of Medicine; Attending Psychiatrist, Tisch Hospital; Attending Psychiatrist, Bellevue Hospital Center, New York, New York

BARRY REISBURG, M.D.   Professor of Psychiatry, Clinical Director of Aging and Dementia Research Center, New York University School of Medicine, New York, New York

MATTHEW SMITH, M.D.   Clinical Assistant Professor of Psychiatry, New York University School of Medicine; Attending Psychiatrist, Tisch Hospital; Attending Psychiatrist, Bellevue Hospital Center, New York, New York

NORMAN SUSSMAN, M.D.   Clinical Professor of Psychiatry, New York University School of Medicine; Director, Psychopharmacology Research and Consultation Service, Bellevue Hospital Center, New York, New York

KAPLAN & SADOCK'S POCKET HANDBOOK OF CLINICAL PSYCHIATRY

Third Edition

BENJAMIN J. SADOCK, M.D.

Menas S. Gregory Professor of Psychiatry and Vice Chairman,
Department of Psychiatry, New York University School of Medicine;
Attending Psychiatrist, Tisch Hospital;
Attending Psychiatrist, Bellevue Hospital Center;
Consulting Psychiatrist, Lenox Hill Hospital,
New York, New York

VIRGINIA A. SADOCK, M.D.

Clinical Professor of Psychiatry, Department of Psychiatry,
New York University School of Medicine;
Attending Psychiatrist, Tisch Hospital;
Attending Psychiatrist, Bellevue Hospital Center,
New York, New York

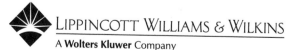

LIPPINCOTT WILLIAMS & WILKINS
A **Wolters Kluwer** Company
Philadelphia · Baltimore · New York · London
Buenos Aires · Hong Kong · Sydney · Tokyo

Acquisitions Editor: Charles W. Mitchell
Developmental Editor: Lisa R. Kairis
Project Editor (New York): Justin A. Hollingsworth
Production Editor: Melanie Bennitt
Manufacturing Manager: Benjamin Rivera
Cover Designer: Christine Jenny
Compositor: Maryland Composition
Printer: R.R. Donnelley–Crawfordsville

© **2001 by LIPPINCOTT WILLIAMS & WILKINS**
530 Walnut Street
Philadelphia, PA 19106 USA
LWW.com

"Kaplan Sadock Psychiatry" with the pyramid logo is a trademark of
Lippincott Williams & Wilkins

Notice. The indications and dosages of all drugs in this book have been recommended in the medical literature and conform to the practices of the general medical community. The medications described do not necessarily have specific approval by the Food and Drug Administration (FDA) for use in the diseases and dosages for which they are recommended. The package insert for each drug should be consulted for use and dosage as approved by the FDA. Because standards for usage change, it is advisable to keep abreast of revised recommendations, particularly those concerning new drugs.

Printed in the USA

First Edition 1993
Second Edition 1996

Library of Congress Cataloging-in-Publication Data

Sadock, Benjamin J.
   Kaplan & Sadock's pocket handbook of clinical psychiatry / Benjamin J. Sadock, Virginia A. Sadock.--3rd ed.
     p. ; cm.
   Rev. ed. of: Pocket handbook of clinical psychiatry / Harold I. Kaplan, Benjamin J. Sadock. 2nd ed. c1996.
   Companion v. to: Kaplan & Sadock's comprehensive textbook of psychiatry / editors, Benjamin J. Sadock, Virginia A. Sadock. 7th ed. 2000.
   Includes bibliographical references and index.
   ISBN 0-7817-2532-1
   1. Psychiatry--Handbooks, manuals, etc. I. Title: Kaplan and Sadock's pocket handbook of clinical psychiatry. II. Title: Pocket handbook of clinical psychiatry. III. Sadock, Virginia A. IV. Kaplan, Harold I., 1927–1998, Pocket handbook of clinical psychiatry. V. Kaplan & Sadock's comprehensive textbook of psychiatry. VI. Title.
   [DNLM: 1. Mental Disorders–Handbooks. WM 34 S126k 2001]
RC456 .K36 2001
616.89--dc21
                                            00-065513

10 9 8 7 6 5 4 3

*Dedicated
to Our
Parents*

Preface

This is the third edition of *Kaplan & Sadock's Pocket Handbook of Clinical Psychiatry* to be published and the first to appear in the new century. Every section has been updated and revised, and all diagnoses conform to the criteria listed in the fourth edition of the American Psychiatric Association's *Diagnostic and Statistical Manual of Mental Disorders* (DSM-IV) and the newly released "text revision" (DSM-IV-TR).

This compact guide covers the entire range of psychiatric disorders and provides a reference to the diagnosis and treatment of mental illness in children and adults. All aspects of both psychological and pharmacological management are discussed, and as in other *Kaplan & Sadock* books, completely up-to-date colored plates of all the major drugs used in psychiatry are included.

The *Pocket Handbook of Clinical Psychiatry* will be of use to medical students, psychiatric residents, and psychiatrists who require an easily-accessible guide to consult in their day-to-day work with patients. Primary care physicians and others who work with the mentally ill, including psychiatric social workers, nurses, and clinical psychologists, have also found this book useful.

The *Pocket Handbook* is the minicompanion to the much larger and more encyclopedic seventh edition of *Comprehensive Textbook of Psychiatry* (CTP/VII), edited by the authors. The *Pocket Handbook* is a distillation in that it provides brief summaries of psychiatric disorders, which include key aspects of etiology, epidemiology, clinical features, and treatment. Psychopharmacological principles and prescribing methods are discussed briefly, but thoroughly. Each chapter ends with references to the more detailed relevant sections in *CTP/VII*. The *Pocket Handbook* cannot substitute for a major textbook of psychiatry, such as *CTP/VII* or its companion, *Kaplan & Sadock's Synopsis of Psychiatry*. It is meant instead to be a ready reference to be used by the busy doctor-in-training or clinical practitioner.

ACKNOWLEDGMENTS

We thank Eugene Rubin, M.D., who served as contributing editor to this edition. With his help we were able to update all sections to keep the book current and completely up-to-date. He is an outstanding psychiatrist who worked with skill and enthusiasm.

We also thank our collaborating authors who were extremely helpful in their respective areas of expertise. They include Richard Perry, M.D., in child psychiatry; Barry Reisburg, M.D. in geriatric psychiatry; James Edmondson, M.D., and Norman Sussman, M.D., in psychopharmacology; and Matthew Smith, M.D., and Myrl Manley, M.D., in clinical psychiatry. We also thank Rebecca Jones, M.D., James C.Y. Chou, M.D., and Henry Weinstein, M.D., for their help in previous editions of this book. Victoria Sadock, M.D. and James Sadock, M.D., provided important information in the area of emergency medicine, their area of expertise. We thank them for their help. We especially acknowledge Jack Grebb, M.D., our valued co-author on the seventh edition of *Synopsis* and contributing editor to *CTP/VII.*

Our staff at NYU, under the able direction of Justin Hollingsworth, who served as project editor, deserves thanks: Peggy Cuzzolino and Yande McMillan. They worked with alacrity and enthusiasm. Finally, the authors thank Robert Cancro, M.D., Professor and Chairman of the Department of Psychiatry who served as Senior Consulting Editor. He is a distinguished clinician, researcher, and educator. We are deeply grateful for his unwavering support and for the support and leadership he provides to the entire NYU Department of Psychiatry. We are proud and honored to have him as our friend and colleague.

Benjamin J. Sadock, M.D.
Virginia A. Sadock, M.D.

New York University Medical Center
New York, New York.

Contents

KAPLAN & SADOCK'S POCKET HANDBOOK OF CLINICAL PSYCHIATRY

Third Edition

1

Clinical Interview: Psychiatric History and Mental Status

I. General introduction

    A. The purpose of a diagnostic interview is to gather information that will help the examiner make a diagnosis. The diagnosis guides treatment and helps predict the patient's future course.

    B. Psychiatric diagnoses are based on descriptive phenomenology: signs, symptoms, and clinical course.

    C. The psychiatric examination consists of two parts: (1) a history, which describes the course of the present and past illnesses and provides family and other personal information (Table 1–1), and (2) a mental status examination, which is a formal assessment of the patient's current thinking, mood, and behavior (Table 1–2). The following outline provides a model for how this information is commonly organized. All topics should be covered, but they need not be followed rigorously.

II. Psychiatric history

    A. Identification

        1. Always—age, sex.

        2. When appropriate—occupation, ethnicity, marital status, religion.

    B. Chief complaint. In the patient's own words, reasons for hospitalization or consultation.

    C. History of present illness (HPI)

        1. When and how current episode began.

        2. How symptoms have progressed over time.

        3. Treatments to date.

            a. Medications—drugs, doses, response, side effects, compliance.

            b. Therapies—modalities, frequency, perceived benefit.

        4. Current drug and alcohol use.

    D. Past psychiatric history

        1. A chronological list of all previous episodes and symptoms (treated or not), starting with the earliest and progressing to the most recent.

        2. Description of symptoms.

        3. Precipitants, if any.

        4. Prior treatments and response, as in the HPI. (The best predictor of future treatment response is past treatment response.)

        5. Hospitalizations: dates of stay, reasons for admission, treatments and response, discharge plans, compliance and follow-up.

E. Medical history

1. Current medical conditions and treatments.
2. Major past illnesses and treatments.
3. Medical hospitalizations.
4. Surgical history.

TABLE 1-1
OUTLINE OF PSYCHIATRIC HISTORY

I. Identification
II. Chief complaint
III. History of present illness
    1. Onset
    2. Precipitating factors
IV. Past illnesses
    A. Psychiatric
    B. Medical
    C. Family
V. Personal history (anamnesis)
    A. Prenatal and perinatal
    B. Early childhood (through age 3)
    C. Middle childhood (ages 3–11)
    D. Late childhood (puberty through adolescence)
    E. Adulthood
        1. Occupational history
        2. Marital and relationship history
        3. Military history
        4. Educational history
        5. Religion
        6. Social activity
        7. Current living situation
        8. Legal history
    F. Sexual history

TABLE 1-2
OUTLINE OF THE MENTAL STATUS EXAMINATION

I. General description
    A. Appearance
    B. Overt behavior and psychomotor activity
    C. Attitude
II. Emotional expression
    A. Mood
    B. Affect
    C. Appropriateness of affect
III. Speech
IV. Thinking and perception
    A. Thought process
    B. Thought content
V. Sensorium
    A. Consciousness
    B. Orientation and memory
    C. Concentration and attention
    D. Reading and writing
    E. Visuospatial ability
    F. Abstract thought
    G. Information and intelligence
VI. Judgment and insight
VII. Reliability

F. Family history
  1. Current family members—ages and sex.
  2. Family members with psychiatric disorders or symptoms—their treatment histories (as above).
G. Personal history. The purpose of the personal history is to (1) describe events of significance during the patient's life—especially those that may cause or exacerbate psychiatric symptoms, and (2) portray changes in functional capacity over time.

It is seldom necessary to describe all of the following for all patients. For example, developmental milestones are seldom important for adults with Axis I disorders, but are always important for children and adolescents. The clinician will make ongoing selections, determining what is diagnostically significant on the basis of information received from the patient.

  1. Birth and infancy—maternal drug use, perinatal complications, temperament, walking, talking.
  2. Childhood—bowel and bladder control, tolerance of separation, friendships, school, extracurricular activities.
  3. Adolescence—onset of puberty, peer relations, dating and sex, drug use, development of career goals, education, work and extracurricular activities.
  4. Adulthood—marriage and other romantic relationships, sexual history, work history, military history, drug and alcohol use, prison experience, avocational interests. It is often useful to have the patient describe the activities of a typical day.

III. Mental status examination (MSE)

The MSE is analogous to the physical examination; it is a formal, systematic format for recording findings about thinking, feeling, and behavior. Observations are objective and noninferential (what you see and hear, not what you think is going on underneath). Only phenomena observed at the time of the interview are recorded in the MSE; other data are put in the histories.

A. Appearance. Dress and hygiene, attitude and behavior, physical signs (e.g., tremor, gait ataxia); particular attention should be paid to abnormalities and eccentricities.
B. Speech. Physical production, not content. Volume, rate, articulation, vocabulary.
C. Emotional expression
  1. Subjective—patient's description of inner emotional state (e.g., "I feel sad").
  2. Objective—emotion communicated through facial expression, body posture, and vocal tone.
  3. "Affect" is commonly used to describe the following:
     a. The objective, observed component of emotion.
     b. The variability of emotion as thoughts change. (In contrast, "mood" describes prevailing, underlying emotional tone.)

D. Thinking and perception

1. Thought form—the way ideas are linked. Are they logical and goal-directed? If not, the patient may have a disorder of thought form, or "formal thought disorder."
2. Thought content. Abnormalities include the following:
   a Delusions—fixed, false beliefs not shared by others.
   b. Ideas of reference—everyday natural occurrences that carry unique personal significance (e.g., a stranger walking by on the street blowing his nose signals impending danger).
   c. Obsessions—unwanted, intrusive thoughts that are often unpleasant (e.g., thoughts of distasteful sex, behaving in socially inappropriate ways) and commonly felt to be beyond the patient's ability to control (ego-dystonic).
   d. Preoccupations—predominant and recurrent thoughts, not felt to be symptomatic or unwanted (ego-syntonic).
   e. Thought insertion—thoughts being implanted by external forces.
   f. Thought withdrawal—thoughts being removed from a person's mind by others.
3. Perception.
   a. Hallucinations—sensory perceptions generated within the central nervous system that are not triggered by external stimuli. Hallucinations may be in any sensory modality, and the modality has no diagnostic significance.
   b. Illusions—a sensory perception triggered by an external stimulus that is misprocessed or misinterpreted (e.g., a patient sees threatening monsters while looking at moving shadows on the wall).

E. Sensorium.

This section includes an assessment of several cognitive functions. Collectively, they help describe the overall intactness of the central nervous system, as different functions are subserved by different brain regions. Abnormalities of the sensorium are seen in delirium and dementia, and they raise the suspicion of an underlying medical or drug-related cause of symptoms.

Much of this information can be acquired by observation during the course of the general interview. Specific tests of cognitive function can be used to describe deficiencies more precisely (Table 1–3).

1. Alertness—degree of wakefulness, constant or fluctuating.
2. Orientation to person (who the patient is, who the examiner is, nature of their interaction), place, and time. If the patient is disoriented, describe the extent; does the patient know the month but not the day of the week? The name of the city but not the hospital?
3. Concentration—the ability to focus and sustain attention.
4. Memory—remote, recent, and immediate recall.
5. Calculations—can the patient do simple arithmetic manipulations in her head?
6. Fund of knowledge—is the patient registering the events of the world to which he is exposed?
7. Abstract reasoning—the ability to shift back and forth between general concepts and specific examples (e.g., fruit—apple).

TABLE 1–3
TESTS OF COGNITIVE FUNCTION USED IN THE SENSORIUM SECTION OF THE MENTAL STATUS EXAMINATION

Function	Questions / Comments
1. Alertness	1. Observe the patient's degree of wakefulness and changes in the level of arousal.
2. Orientation	2. "Do you know where you are? What is this building? Where is it located? Who am I? Why am I talking with you? What is today's date? The day of the week? The month, year, or season? What time of day is it? Is it morning or afternoon?"
3. Concentration	3. "Spell the word *world.* Now spell it backward. Count backward from 100 by 7s. Say the alphabet backward starting with *Z."*
4. Memory	4. Immediate: "Repeat these numbers after me: 7, 3, 1, 8, 6." Recent: "I want you to remember these three things: a cocker spaniel, a red pencil, and a refrigerator. Keep them in mind. I'll ask you to repeat them after a few minutes." "What did you eat for dinner last night? What did you have for breakfast?" Long-term: "What was your address when you were in grade school? Who was your teacher in fifth grade?" **Hint:** Asking overlearned facts such as birthdates or social security numbers does not accurately test long-term memory.
5. Calculations	5. "If you buy something that costs $3.65 and pay with a five dollar bill, how much change should you receive? How much is 19 plus 13? How much is 23 minus 15?" **Hint:** Questions should test only one function at a time; if serial 7s are used to test concentration, these cannot be used to test calculations also.
6. Fund of knowledge	6. "What is the capital of this state? What is the capital of France? How many miles from New York to California? Name the last five presidents of the United States. What topic is currently in the news?" Questions should be shaped by the patient's age, level of education, and interests.
7. Abstract reasoning	7. "How are an apple and an orange alike? What do people mean when they say, 'A bird in the hand is worth two in the bush'? Which item doesn't belong in this series: a rock, a tree, a bird?" **Hint:** Abstract thinking cannot be assessed by asking about differences (e.g., "What is the difference between an apple and an orange?") because the only plausible answers are concrete.

8. Insight—the capacity to recognize and understand one's own symptoms.

9. Judgment—the ability to make good decisions on one's own behalf, behave in socially accepted ways, and cooperate with treatment.

IV. Medical and neurological examination

A complete physical examination, including a neurological evaluation, should be considered in the initial assessment of all psychiatric patients. It is especially advisable in the following situations:

A. The patient is hospitalized.

B. Physical signs are present (e.g., dilated pupils, gait ataxia).

C. The patient has a history of current medical illness.

D. Features in the history or MSE raise the possibility of an underlying medical or drug-related cause.

1. Abrupt onset of psychiatric symptoms with no prior history.

2. History of significant concurrent drug or alcohol use.

3. Physical symptoms (e.g. nausea, cold intolerance).

4. Abnormalities in the sensorium section of the MSE.

V. Techniques for the psychiatric assessment

The clinician tries to establish rapport and create an atmosphere of confidence and trust.

A. The length of the consultation is typically 45 to 60 minutes and should be agreed on in advance.

B. The consultation should take place in a comfortable room with pleasant lighting. The examiner should avoid interruptions, such as routine phone calls.

C. Begin with a general, open-ended question ("How can I help you today?") and allow the patient to talk freely for several minutes. More structured questioning is often necessary as the interview progresses.

D. The interviewer has in mind the categories of information necessary to establish a diagnosis. However, it is seldom necessary to proceed in a rigid, checklist manner.

E. Courteous interruptions are sometimes necessary if a patient rambles or is unfocused. ("Excuse me for interrupting, but I'd like to come back to the point we were discussing a little while ago.")

F. Use both open- and closed-ended questions (Table 1–4).

  1. Open-ended—little structure or organization provided by the examiner. ("Tell me about your growing up.")

   a. Often useful in starting the interview.

   b. Content not limited by examiner's preconceptions.

   c. Formal thought disorders more likely to be revealed.

   d. Patients may be more comfortable telling their story without interruptions.

TABLE 1–4
PROS AND CONS OF OPEN- AND CLOSED-ENDED QUESTIONS

Aspect	Broad, open-ended questions	Narrow, closed-ended questions
Genuineness	*High* They produce spontaneous formulations.	*Low* They lead the patient.
Reliability	*Low* They may lead to nonreproducible answers.	*High* Narrow focus, but they may suggest answers.
Precision	*Low* Intent of question is vague.	*High* Intent of question is clear.
Time of efficiency	*Low* Circumstantial elaborations.	*High* May invite yes/no answers.
Completeness of diagnostic coverage	*Low* Patient selects the topic.	*High* Interviewer selects the topic.
Acceptance by patient	*Varies* Most patients prefer expressing themselves freely; others become guarded and feel insecure.	*Varies* Some patients enjoy clear-cut checks; others hate to be pressed into a yes/no format.

From Othmer E. Othmer SC: *The Clinical Interview Using DSM-IV.* Washington, DC: American Psychiatric Press, 1989:48, with permission.

TABLE 1–5
SUPPORTIVE AND OBSTRUCTIVE INTERVENTIONS

Supportive

1. Encouragement	Patient: "I'm not very good at putting things into words." Doctor: "I think you've described the situation very well."
2. Reassurance	Doctor: "I can understand how frightening those experiences must have been, but I think it's very likely they'll respond to treatment."
3. Acknowledging emotion	Doctor: "Even now it brings tears to your eyes when you talk about your mother."
4. Nonverbal communication	Body posture and facial expression that convey interest, concern, and attentiveness.

Obstructive

1. Compound questions	Doctor: "Have you been hearing voices, and does it seem that people want to hurt you?"
2. Judgmental questions	Doctor: "Have you treated other people as badly as you're treating your wife?"
3. "Why" questions	Doctor: "Why do you feel anxious when you go outdoors?"
4. Not following the patient's lead	Patient: "I have trouble sleeping through the night." Doctor: "Any change in appetite?" Patient: "I keep waking up out of nightmares about my daughter." Doctor: "Do you have less energy than usual?"
5. Minimization or dismissal	Patient: "I'm not able to keep my checkbook balanced the way I need to." Doctor: "Oh, I wouldn't worry about it. Lots of people don't even try."
6. Premature advice	Patient: "Work is almost unbearable. My supervisor watches me like a hawk and criticizes the tiniest little mistake I make." Doctor: "Why not write her a memo and outline your grievances?"
7. Nonverbal communication	Yawning, checking one's watch. Patients can often detect an interviewer's inattention by the absence of facial expression or body movement.

    2. Closed-ended—ask for factual responses to specific questions. ("How far did you go in school?")
      a. Useful in clarifying information and gathering factual data.
      b. Necessary to describe pertinent negatives. (Patients seldom spontaneously describe what they are not experiencing.)
      c. Increase interview efficiency.
      d. May be necessary for patients who are psychotic, paranoid, or depressed.
  G. Supportive and obstructive interventions. In addition to gathering information, the examiner provides feedback, offers reassurance, and responds empathetically to what the patient is saying. The examiner's body posture, and facial expression convey information. Interventions are classified as "supportive" or "obstructive" to the extent that they increase the flow of information and increase or diminish rapport. Examples are provided in Table 1–5.
  H. A session should never be recorded without the patient's consent. Keep note taking to a minimum.

VI. Special interview situations

    Certain interview situations require a modification of techniques or emphasis. These are summarized in Table 1–6.

TABLE 1–6
SPECIAL INTERVIEW SITUATIONS

I. Psychotic patients
   A. Short, concrete questions are better than long, abstract ones.
   B. Long silences, open-ended questions, and hypothetical questions may be disorganizing.
   C. Ask about the phenomenology of hallucinations if any are present (e.g., modality, intensity, clarity, context, response).
   D. Try to avoid signaling either belief or disbelief when asking about delusions.
   E. Delusions should not be directly challenged, but their fixity may be probed: "Do you ever wonder whether those things might not be true?"

II. Depressed patients
   A. The examiner may need to be more forceful and directive than usual; questions may need to be repeated.
   B. The presence of psychotic symptoms should be investigated.
   C. Suicidal thoughts and plans should be questioned. (This is true of all patients, not just those who are depressed.)
      1. Sample opening questions include, "Do you ever have thoughts of hurting yourself?" "Does it ever seem that life isn't worth living?"
      2. When a patient acknowledges suicidal thoughts, ask about intent, plans, means, and perceived consequences.

III. Agitated and potentially violent patients
   A. Most unpremeditated violence is preceded by a 30- to 60-minute prodrome of accelerating psychomotor agitation: pacing, fist pounding, loud and abusive language.
   B. Conduct the interview in a quiet, nonstimulating environment.
   C. Be certain that both patient and examiner have easy access to an exit.
   D. Avoid behavior that could be construed as menacing: standing over the patient, staring, touching.
   E. Do not bargain.
   F. Ask about weapons, but don't take them. Have them placed in a secure area.
   G. If the patient's agitation continues or worsens, terminate the interview if possible. If not, consider physical or chemical restraints.

IV. Patients from different cultures and backgrounds
   A. DSM-IV-TR has not been validated for use in all countries.
   B. Relative symptoms (e.g., social withdrawal) may be more difficult for a culturally naïve psychiatrist to assess than absolute symptoms (e.g., hallucinations).
   C. The vocabulary used to describe emotional distress varies from country to country.
   D. When interpreters are needed, they should be disinterested third parties, not family members or friends. Trained interpreters are better than untrained, and they should be instructed to translate verbatim, even if what the patient is saying is nonsensical.
   E. It is sometimes impossible to convey a formal thought disorder through translation.

V. Seductive patients
   A. Seductive behavior will have different meanings for different patients. For example, it may be a defense against feelings of inferiority, a habitual way of dealing with others, or an unconscious way of maintaining control in an anxiety-producing situation.
   B. Seductive behavior can include more than sexual flirtation; for example, it might be an offer of insider-trading information or a celebrity introduction.
   C. Gaining material or social benefit from a patient other than the agreed-upon fee is always unethical.
   D. The examiner must make it clear that seductive offerings will not be accepted, but in a way that preserves rapport and does not unnecessarily assault the patient's self-esteem.

VI. Patients who lie
   A. Patients may lie for primary gain (e.g., to obtain drugs or exemption from jury duty) or for secondary gain (e.g., for whatever psychological benefit is gained by assuming the sick role).
   B. The absence of biological markers may make it impossible to prove a patient is lying. However, suspicion may be aroused by subtle discrepancies, internal inconsistencies, or suspectedly atypical symptoms.
   C. The goal of a psychiatric evaluation should not be to avoid being taken in at all costs. The exaggerated suspiciousness of the examiner who is determined never to be deceived by a patient will disrupt rapport and make therapeutic work impossible.
   D. Not all patients' untruths are conscious lies. In describing an emotional reality, a patient may unwittingly deviate from historical reality. Patients with somatoform symptoms are giving an honest report of the symptoms as they are consciously experienced.

VII. Recording the results of the history and mental status examination

A. The differential diagnosis.
The purpose of the psychiatric examination is to establish a diagnosis. It may not be possible to make a definitive diagnosis, in which case all diagnoses that could possibly explain the patient's presenting signs and symptoms are listed in order of likelihood. This list is the differential diagnosis.

B. Major decision points.
Even in the absence of a single diagnosis, the examiner should be able to answer each of the following questions at the end of an evaluation:

1. Is the patient psychotic? Are psychotic symptoms present, such as hallucinations, delusions, serious formal thought disorders, or grossly disordered behavior?

TABLE 1-7
MULTIAXIAL EVALUATION REPORT FORM

The following form is offered as one possibility for reporting multiaxial evaluations. In some settings, this form may be used exactly as is; in other settings, the form may be adapted to satisfy special needs.

AXIS I: Clinical Disorders
    Other Conditions That May Be a Focus of Clinical Attention

Diagnostic code   DSM-IV name

___ ___ ___ . ___ ___   _____

___ ___ ___ . ___ ___   _____

___ ___ ___ . ___ ___   _____

AXIS II: Personality Disorders
    Mental Retardation

Diagnostic code   DSM-IV name

___ ___ ___ . ___ ___   _____

___ ___ ___ . ___ ___   _____

___ ___ ___ . ___ ___   _____

AXIS III: General Medical Conditions

ICD-9-CM code   ICD-9-CM name

___ ___ ___ . ___ ___   _____

___ ___ ___ . ___ ___   _____

AXIS IV: Psychosocial and Environmental Problems

Check:
- [ ] **Problems with primary support group** *Specify:* _____
- [ ] **Problems related to the social environment** *Specify:* _____
- [ ] **Educational problems** *Specify:* _____
- [ ] **Occupational problems** *Specify:* _____
- [ ] **Housing problems** *Specify:* _____
- [ ] **Economic problems** *Specify:* _____
- [ ] **Problems with access to health care services** *Specify:* _____
- [ ] **Problems related to interaction with the legal system/crime** *Specify:* _____
- [ ] **Other psychosocial and environmental problems** *Specify:* _____

AXIS V: Global Assessment of Functioning Scale   Score: _____

                                            Time frame: _____

2. Is the patient's condition likely to be the result of an underlying medical or drug-related problem?

3. Is the patient at risk for hurting himself or others?

C. Multiaxial diagnosis.   Five axes are listed in DSM-IV-TR. Assess and comment on each axis (Table 1–7).

Axis I: Clinical syndromes—list the mental disorder here (e.g., schizophrenia, bipolar I disorder). Other conditions that may be a focus of clinical attention (except borderline intellectual functioning) are also listed on Axis I. These are problems not sufficiently severe to warrant a psychiatric diagnosis (e.g., relational problems, bereavement).

Axis II: Personality disorders and mental retardation—mental retardation and personality disorders are listed here. Defense mechanisms and personality traits may also be listed here. Diagnoses on Axis I and Axis

TABLE 1–8
GLOBAL ASSESSMENT OF FUNCTIONING (GAF) SCALE

Consider psychological, social, and occupational functioning on a hypothetical continuum of mental health-illness. Do not include impairment in functioning due to physical (or environmental) limitations.

Code	Note: Use intermediate codes when appropriate (e.g., 45, 68, 72).
100	Superior functioning in a wide range of activities, life's problems never seem to get out of hand,
91	is sought out by others because of his or her many positive qualities. No symptoms.
90	Absent or minimal symptoms (e.g., mild anxiety before an exam), **good functioning in all areas,**
	interested and involved in a wide range of activities, socially effective, generally satisfied
	with life, no more than everyday problems or concerns (e.g., an occasional argument with
81	family members).
80	If symptoms are present, they are transient and expectable reactions to psychosocial stressors
	(e.g., difficulty concentrating after family argument); **no more than slight impairment in**
71	**social, occupational, or school functioning** (e.g., temporarily falling behind in schoolwork).
70	Some mild symptoms (e.g., depressed mood and mild insomnia) **OR some difficulty in social,**
	occupational, or school functioning (e.g., occasional truancy or theft within the household),
61	but generally functioning pretty well, has some meaningful interpersonal relationships.
60	Moderate symptoms (e.g., flat affect and circumstantial speech, occasional panic attacks)
	OR moderate difficulty in social, occupational, or school functioning (e.g., few friends,
51	conflicts with peers or coworkers).
50	Serious symptoms (e.g., suicidal ideation, severe obsessional rituals, frequent shoplifting) **OR**
	any serious impairment in social, occupational, or school functioning (e.g., no friends, unable
41	to keep a job).
40	Some impairment in reality testing or communication (e.g., speech is at times illogical, obscure,
	or irrelevant) **OR major impairment in several areas, such as work or school, family relations,**
	judgment, thinking, or mood (e.g., depressed man avoids friends, neglects family, and is
	unable to work; child frequently beats up younger children, is defiant at home, and is failing
31	at school).
30	Behavior is considerably influenced by delusions or hallucinations **OR serious impairment in**
	communication or judgment (e.g., sometimes incoherent, acts grossly inappropriately, suici-
	dal preoccupation) **OR inability to function in almost all areas** (e.g., stays in bed all day; no
21	job, home, or friends).
20	Some danger of hurting self or others (e.g., suicide attempts without clear expectation of
	death; frequently violent; manic excitement) **OR occasionally fails to maintain minimal**
	personal hygiene (e.g., smears feces) **OR gross impairment in communication** (e.g., largely
11	incoherent or mute).
10	Persistent danger of severely hurting self or others (e.g., recurrent violence) **OR persistent**
	inability to maintain minimal personal hygiene OR serious suicidal act with clear expectation
1	**of death.**
0	Inadequate information.

TABLE 1-9
GLOSSARY OF SPECIFIC DEFENSE MECHANISMS

acting out   The individual deals with emotional conflict or internal or external stressors by actions rather than reflections or feelings. This definition is broader than the original concept of the acting out of transference feelings or wishes during psychotherapy and is intended to include behavior arising both within and outside the transference relationship. Defensive acting out is not synonymous with "bad behavior" because it requires evidence that the behavior is related to emotional conflicts.

altrusim   The individual deals with emotional conflict or internal or external stressors by dedication to meeting the needs of others. Altruism differs from the self-sacrifice sometimes characteristic of reaction formation in that the individual receives gratification either vicariously or from the response of others.

anticipation   The individual deals with emotional conflict or internal or external stressors by experiencing emotional reactions in advance of, or anticipating consequences of, possible future events and considering realistic, alternative responses or solutions.

denial   The individual deals with emotional conflict or internal or external stressors by refusing to acknowledge some painful aspect of external reality or subjective experience that would be apparent to others. The term *psychotic denial* is used when gross impairment in reality testing is present.

displacement   The individual deals with emotional conflict or internal or external stressors by transferring a feeling about, or a response to, one object onto another (usually less threatening) substitute object.

dissociation   The individual deals with emotional conflict or internal or external stressors with a breakdown in the usually integrated functions of consciousness, memory, perception of self or the environment, or sensory/motor behavior.

humor   The individual deals with emotional conflict or external stressors by emphasizing the amusing or ironic aspects of the conflict or stressor.

idealization   The individual deals with emotional conflict or internal or external stressors by attributing exaggerated positive qualities to others.

intellectualization   The individual deals with emotional conflict or internal or external stressors by the excessive use of abstract thinking or the making of generalizations to control or minimize disturbing feelings.

isolation of affect   The individual deals with emotional conflict or internal or external stressors by the separation of ideas from the feelings originally associated with them. The individual loses touch with the feelings associated with a given idea (e.g., a traumatic event) while remaining aware of the cognitive elements of it (e.g., descriptive details).

omnipotence   The individual deals with emotional conflict or internal or external stressors by feeling or acting as if he or she possesses special powers or abilities and is superior to others.

projection   The individual deals with emotional conflict or internal or external stressors by falsely attributing to another his or her own unacceptable feelings, impulses, or thoughts.

projective identification   As in projection, the individual deals with emotional conflict or internal or external stressors by falsely attributing to another his or her own unacceptable feelings, impulses, or thoughts. However, the individual does not fully disavow what is projected, as in simple projection. Instead, the individual remains aware of his or her own affects or impulses but misattributes them as justifiable reactions to the other person. Not infrequently, the individual induces the very feelings in others that were first mistakenly believed to be there, making it difficult to clarify who did what to whom first.

rationalization   The individual deals with emotional conflict or internal or external stressors by concealing the true motivations for his or her own thoughts, actions, or feelings through the elaboration of reassuring or self-serving but incorrect explanations.

reaction formation   The individual deals with emotional conflict or internal or external stressors by substituting behavior, thoughts, or feelings that are diametrically opposed to his or her own unacceptable thoughts or feelings (this usually occurs in conjunction with their repression).

repression   The individual deals with emotional conflict or internal or external stressors expelling disturbing wishes, thoughts, or experiences from conscious awareness. The feeling component may remain conscious, detached from its associated ideas.

splitting   The individual deals with emotional conflict or internal or external stressors by compartmentalizing opposite affect states and failing to integrate the positive and negative qualities of the self or others into cohesive images. Because ambivalent affects cannot be experienced simultaneously, more balanced views and expectations of self or others are excluded from emotional awareness. Self and object images tend to alternate between polar opposites: exclusively loving, powerful, worthy, nurturant, and kind—or exclusively bad, hateful, angry, destructive, rejecting, or worthless.

sublimation   The individual deals with emotional conflict or internal or external stressors by channeling potentially maladaptive feelings or impulses into socially acceptable behavior (e.g., contact sports to channel angry impulses).

suppression   The individual deals with emotional conflict or internal or external stressors by intentionally avoiding thinking about disturbing problems, wishes, feelings or experiences.

undoing   The individual deals with emotional conflict or internal or external stressors by words or behavior designed to negate or to make amends symbolically for unacceptable thoughts, feelings, or actions.

From American Psychiatric Association. *Diagnostic and Statistical Manual of Mental Disorders*, text revision, 4th ed. Washington, DC: American Psychiatric Association, Copyright 2000, with permission.

II can coexist. The Axis I or Axis II condition that is responsible for bringing the patient to the psychiatrist or hospital is called the *principal* or *main diagnosis*.

Axis III: Physical disorders or conditions—if the patient has a physical disorder (e.g., cirrhosis), list that here.

Axis IV: Psychosocial and environmental problems—describe current stress in the patient's life (e.g., divorce, injury, death of a loved one).

Axis V: Global assessment of functioning (GAF)—rate the highest level of social, occupational, and psychological functioning of the patient according to the GAF scale (Table 1–8). Use the 12 months before the current evaluation as a reference point. Rate from 1 (lowest) to 100 (highest) or 0 (inadequate information).

A sample DSM-IV diagnosis could look like this:

Axis I	Schizophrenia, catatonic type
Axis II	Borderline personality disorder
Axis III	Hypertension
Axis IV	Psychosocial problem—death of mother
Axis V	Current GAF = 30 (behavior influenced by dementia)

A differential diagnosis and a multiaxial diagnosis are not the same thing. It is possible to combine them, however, by listing the multiple diagnostic possibilities of the differential on the appropriate axes.

D. The psychodynamic formulation.   For certain patients, particularly those being considered for a psychodynamic therapy, a psychodynamic formulation may be appropriate. It is based on psychoanalytic theory and provides a model to explain current symptomatology and interpersonal or functional limitations. It does not provide a DSM-IV-TR diagnosis. Commonly included in a psychodynamic formulation are the following:

1. Ego strengths.
   a. Principal defense mechanisms (Table 1–9).
   b. Regulation of drives.
   c. Interpersonal relationships.
   d. Reality testing.
2. Principal psychological conflicts.
3. Developmental history.

For a more detailed discussion of this topic, see Psychiatric Interview, History, and Mental Status Examination, Sec 7.1, p 652, in CTP/VII.

2

Psychiatric Clinical Signs and Symptoms

I. General introduction

Psychiatrists develop their ability to detect mental conditions for several reasons: to make accurate diagnoses, carry out effective treatments, offer reliable prognoses, analyze psychiatric issues as fully as possible, and communicate fruitfully with other clinicians. To accomplish these aims, they must become experts in the language of psychiatry; they must learn to recognize and define behavioral and emotional signs and symptoms and then become masters at rigorously observing and articulately describing the mental phenomena of psychiatry. Many psychiatric signs and symptoms are rooted in normal behavior and can be understood as various points on a spectrum ranging from normal to pathological.

A. Signs. Clinicians' observations and objective findings, such as a patient's constricted affect or psychomotor retardation.

B. Symptoms. The subjective experiences described by patients, such as a depressed mood or lack of energy.

C. Syndrome. A group of signs and symptoms that together make up a recognizable condition; a syndrome can be more equivocal than a specific disorder or disease.

II. Definitions of psychiatric signs and symptoms

Mental phenomena that relate to signs and symptoms are listed in alphabetical order and defined below.

abstract thinking Thinking characterized by the ability to grasp the essentials of a whole, break a whole into its parts, and discern common properties. Thinking symbolically.

abulia Reduced impulse to act and think (i.e., lack of will) associated with indifference to consequences of action. Occurs as a result of neurological deficit, depression, schizophrenia.

acalculia Loss of ability to perform calculations; not caused by anxiety or impairment of concentration. Occurs with neurological deficit, learning disorder.

acrophobia Dread of high places.

adiadochokinesia Inability to perform rapid alternating movements. Occurs with neurological deficit, cerebellar lesions.

affect The subjective and immediate experience of emotion attached to ideas or mental representations of objects. Affect has outward manifestations that may be classified as restricted, blunted, flattened, broad, labile, appropriate, or inappropriate. *See also* **mood**.

aggression   Forceful, goal-directed action that may be verbal or physical; the motor counterpart of the affect of rage, anger, or hostility. Seen in neurological deficit, temporal lobe disorder, impulse control disorders, mania, schizophrenia.

agitation   Severe anxiety associated with motor restlessness.

agoraphobia   Morbid fear of open places or leaving the familiar setting of the home. May be present with or without panic attacks.

akathisia   Subjective feeling of motor restlessness manifested by a compelling need to be in constant movement; may be seen as an extrapyramidal adverse effect of antipsychotic medication. May be mistaken for psychotic agitation.

akinesia   Lack of physical movement, as in the extreme immobility of catatonic schizophrenia; may also occur as an extrapyramidal effect of antipsychotic medication.

alexithymia   Inability to describe or be aware of one's emotions or moods, or to elaborate the fantasies associated with depression, substance abuse, and posttraumatic stress disorder.

ambivalence   Coexistence of two opposing impulses toward the same thing in the same person at the same time. Seen in schizophrenia, borderline states, obsessive-compulsive disorder.

amnesia   Partial or total inability to recall past experiences; may be organic (amnestic disorder) or emotional (dissociative amnesia) in origin.

anergia   Lack of energy.

anhedonia   Loss of interest in and withdrawal from all regular and pleasurable activities. Often associated with depression.

anomia   Inability to recall the names of objects.

anorexia   Loss of or decrease in appetite. In anorexia nervosa, appetite may be preserved, but patient refuses to eat.

anosognosia   Inability to recognize a physical deficit in oneself (e.g., patient denies limb paralysis).

anterograde amnesia   Loss of memory of events subsequent to the onset of amnesia; common after trauma. *Compare* **retrograde amnesia**.

anxiety   Feeling of apprehension caused by anticipation of danger, which may be internal or external.

apathy   Dulled emotional tone associated with detachment or indifference; observed in certain types of schizophrenia and depression.

aphasia   Any disturbance in the comprehension or expression of language caused by a brain lesion. For types of aphasia, see the specific term.

apraxia   Inability to perform a voluntary purposeful motor activity; cannot be explained by paralysis or other motor or sensory impairment. In constructional apraxia, a patient cannot draw two- or three-dimensional forms.

ataxia   Lack of coordination, either physical or mental. 1. In neurology, refers to loss of muscular coordination. 2. In psychiatry, the term **intrapsychic ataxia** refers to a lack of coordination between feelings and thoughts; seen in schizophrenia and severe obsessive-compulsive disorder.

attention   Concentration; the aspect of consciousness that relates to the amount of effort exerted in focusing on certain aspects of an experience, activity, or task. Usually impaired in anxiety and depressive disorders.

inappropriate affect   Emotional tone out of harmony with the idea, thought, or speech accompanying it. Seen in schizophrenia.

incoherence   Communication that is disconnected, disorganized, or incomprehensible. *See also* **word salad**.

incorporation   Primitive unconscious defense mechanism in which the psychic representation of another person or aspects of another person are assimilated into oneself through a figurative process of symbolic oral ingestion; represents a special form of introjection and is the earliest mechanism of identification.

insight   Conscious recognition of one's own condition. In psychiatry, it refers to the conscious awareness and understanding of one's own psychodynamics and symptoms of maladaptive behavior; highly important in effecting changes in the personality and behavior of a person.

irritability   Abnormal or excessive excitability, with easily triggered anger, annoyance, or impatience.

jamais vu   Paramnestic phenomenon characterized by a false feeling of unfamiliarity with a real situation that one has previously experienced.

judgment   Mental act of comparing or evaluating choices within the framework of a given set of values for the purpose of electing a course of action. If the course of action chosen is consonant with reality or with mature adult standards of behavior, judgment is said to be intact or normal; judgment is said to be impaired if the chosen course of action is frankly maladaptive, results from impulsive decisions based on the need for immediate gratification, or is otherwise not consistent with reality as measured by mature adult standards.

la belle indifférence   Inappropriate attitude of calm or lack of concern about one's disability. May be seen in patients with conversion disorder.

labile affect   Affective expression characterized by rapid and abrupt changes unrelated to external stimuli.

logorrhea   Copious, pressured, coherent speech; uncontrollable, excessive talking; observed in manic episodes of bipolar I disorder. Also called *tachylogia, verbomania, volubility.*

loosening of associations   Characteristic schizophrenic thinking or speech disturbance involving a disorder in the logical progression of thoughts, manifested as a failure to communicate verbally adequately; unrelated and unconnected ideas shift from one subject to another. *See also* **tangentiality**.

macropsia   False perception that objects are larger than they really are. *Compare* **micropsia**.

magical thinking   A form of dereistic thought; thinking similar to that of the preoperational phase in children (Jean Piaget), in which thoughts, words, or actions assume power (e.g., to cause or prevent events).

mania   Mood state characterized by elation, agitation, hyperactivity, hypersexuality, and accelerated thinking and speaking (flight of ideas). Seen in bipolar I disorder. *See also* **hypomania**.

mannerism   Ingrained, habitual involuntary movement.

memory   Process whereby what is experienced or learned is established as a record in the central nervous system (registration), where it persists with a variable degree of permanence (retention) and can be recollected or retrieved from storage at will (recall). For types of memory, see the specific term.

micropsia   False perception that objects are smaller than they really are. Sometimes called *Lilliputian hallucination.* *Compare* **macropsia.**

mood   Pervasive and sustained feeling tone that is experienced internally and that, in the extreme, can markedly influence virtually all aspects of a person's behavior and perception of the world. Distinguished from *affect,* the external expression of the internal feeling tone. For types of mood, see the specific term.

mood-congruent delusion   Delusion with content that is mood-appropriate (e.g., depressed patients who believe they are responsible for the destruction of the world).

mood-congruent hallucination   Hallucination with content that is consistent with either a depressed or manic mood (e.g., depressed patients who hear voices telling them that they are bad persons; manic patients who hear voices telling them that they have inflated worth, power, or knowledge).

mood-incongruent delusion   Delusion based on incorrect reference about external reality, with content that has no association to mood or is mood-inappropriate (e.g., depressed patients who believe that they are the new Messiah).

mood-incongruent hallucination   Hallucination not associated with real external stimuli, the content of which is not consistent with either depressed or manic mood (e.g., in depression, hallucinations not involving such themes as guilt, deserved punishment, or inadequacy; in mania, not involving such themes as inflated worth or power).

mutism   Organic or functional absence of the faculty of speech. *See also* **stupor.**

negativism   Verbal or nonverbal opposition or resistance to outside suggestions and advice; commonly seen in catatonic schizophrenia, in which the patient resists any effort to be moved or does the opposite of what is asked.

neologism   New word or phrase whose derivation cannot be understood; often seen in schizophrenia. The term has also been used to denote a word that has been incorrectly constructed but whose origins are nonetheless understandable (e.g., *head shoe* to mean *hat*), but such constructions are more properly referred to as *word approximations.*

nihilistic delusion   Depressive delusion that the world and everything related to it have ceased to exist.

obsession   Persistent and recurrent idea, thought, or impulse that cannot be eliminated from consciousness by logic or reasoning; obsessions are involuntary and ego-dystonic. *See also* **compulsion.**

olfactory hallucination   Hallucination primarily involving smell or odors; most common in medical disorders, especially those affecting the temporal lobe.

orientation   State of awareness of oneself and one's surroundings in terms of time, place, and person.

overvalued idea   False or unreasonable belief or idea that is sustained beyond the bounds of reason. It is less intense or of shorter duration than a delusion but is usually associated with mental illness.

panic   Acute, intense attack of anxiety associated with personality disorganization; the anxiety is overwhelming and accompanied by feelings of impending doom.

paranoid delusions   Include persecutory delusions and delusions of reference, control, and grandeur.

parapraxis   Faulty act, such as a slip of the tongue or the misplacement of an article. Freud ascribed parapraxes to unconscious motives.

perseveration   1. Pathological repetition of the same response to different stimuli, as in repetition of the same verbal response to different questions. 2. Persistent repetition of specific words or concepts in the process of speaking. Seen in cognitive disorders, schizophrenia, and other mental illness. *See also* **verbigeration**.

phobia   Persistent, pathological, unrealistic, intense fear of an object or situation; the phobic person may realize that the fear is irrational but nonetheless cannot dispel it. For types of phobias, see the specific term.

pressured speech   Increased amount of spontaneous speech; rapid, loud, accelerated speech, as occurs in mania, schizophrenia, and cognitive disorders.

psychomotor agitation   Physical and mental overactivity that is usually nonproductive and associated with a feeling of inner turmoil, as occurs in agitated depression.

restricted affect   Reduction in intensity of feeling tone that is less severe than in blunted affect but clearly present. *See also* **constricted affect**.

retrograde amnesia   Loss of memory of events preceding the onset of amnesia. *Compare* **anterograde amnesia**.

somatic delusion   Delusion pertaining to the functioning of one's body.

somatic hallucination   Hallucination involving the perception of a physical experience localized within the body.

stereotypy   Continuous mechanical repetition of speech or physical activities; observed in catatonic schizophrenia.

stupor   1. State of decreased reactivity to stimuli and less than full awareness of one's surroundings; as a disturbance of consciousness, it indicates a condition of partial coma or semicoma. 2. In psychiatry, used synonymously with *mutism* and does not necessarily imply a disturbance of consciousness; in catatonic stupor, patients are ordinarily aware of their surroundings.

suicidal ideation   Thoughts of taking one's own life.

tangentiality   Oblique, digressive, or even irrelevant manner of speech in which the central idea is not communicated.

thought broadcasting   Feeling that one's thoughts are being broadcast or projected into the environment. *See also* **thought withdrawal**.

thought disorder   Any disturbance of thinking that affects language, communication, or thought content; the hallmark feature of schizophrenia. Manifestations range from simple blocking and mild circumstantiality to profound loosening of associations, incoherence, and delusions; characterized by a failure to follow semantic and syntactic rules that is inconsistent with the person's education, intelligence, or cultural background.

thought insertion   Delusion that thoughts are being implanted in one's mind by other people or forces.

thought withdrawal   Delusion that one's thoughts are being removed from one's mind by other people or forces. *See also* **thought broadcasting**.

tic   Involuntary, spasmodic, stereotyped movement of small groups of muscles; seen predominantly in moments of stress or anxiety, rarely as a result of organic disease.

trance   Sleeplike state of reduced consciousness and activity.

vegetative signs   In depression, characteristic symptoms such as sleep disturbance (especially early morning awakening), decreased appetite, constipation, weight loss, and loss of sexual response.

verbigeration   Meaningless and stereotyped repetition of words or phrases, as seen in schizophrenia. Also called *cataphasia. See also* **perseveration.**

visual hallucination   Hallucination primarily involving the sense of sight.

waxy flexibility   Condition in which patients maintain the body position into which they are placed. Also called *catalepsy.*

word salad   Incoherent, essentially incomprehensible mixture of words and phrases, commonly seen in far-advanced cases of schizophrenia. *See also* **incoherence.**

For a more detailed discussion of this topic, see Signs and Symptoms in Psychiatry, Sec 7.3, p 677, in CTP/VII.

3

Diagnosis and Classification in Psychiatry

I. Introduction

Classification systems for psychiatric diagnoses have several purposes: (1) to distinguish one psychiatric diagnosis from another, so that clinicians can offer the most effective treatment; (2) to provide a common language among health care professionals, and (3) to explore the causes of any mental disorders that are still unknown. The two most important psychiatric classifications are found in the *Diagnostic and Statistical Manual of Mental Disorders* (DSM), used in the United States, and the *International Statistical Classification of Diseases and Related Health Problems* (ICD), used in Europe. The two systems differ in some respects, but they are mostly similar. The classification used in this book is based upon the text revision of the fourth edition of DSM (DSM-IV-TR), published in 2000 by the American Psychiatric Association.

II. DSM-IV-TR

DSM-IV-TR lists 17 major categories of mental disorders, comprising more than 400 discrete illnesses. The official DSM-IV-TR classification and code numbers (which are used in medical reports and insurance forms) are printed on the front and back pages of this handbook.

The DSM-IV-TR diagnostic system attempts to be reliable (i.e., different observers should obtain the same results) and valid (i.e., it should measure what it is supposed to measure; e.g., patients diagnosed with schizophrenia really are schizophrenic). DSM-IV-TR uses a descriptive approach, and the characteristic signs and symptoms of each disorder should be present before a diagnosis is made. The use of specific criteria increases the reliability of the diagnostic process among clinicians.

III. Definition of mental disorder

A mental disorder is an illness with psychological or behavioral manifestations associated with significant distress and impaired functioning caused by a biological, social, psychological, genetic, physical, or chemical disturbance. It is measured in terms of deviation from some normative concept. Each illness has characteristic signs and symptoms (see Chapter 2).

In addition to the DSM-IV-TR classifications, other terms that are used in psychiatry to describe mental illness are *psychotic, neurotic, functional, organic, primary,* and *secondary.*

Psychotic—loss of reality testing with delusions and hallucinations (e.g., schizophrenia).

Neurotic—no loss of reality testing; based on mainly intrapsychic conflicts or life events that cause anxiety; symptoms include obsession, phobia, and compulsion.

Functional—no known structural damage or clear-cut biological cause to account for impairment.

Organic—illness caused by a specific agent producing structural change in the brain; usually associated with cognitive impairment, delirium, or dementia (e.g., Pick's disease). The term *organic* is not used in DSM-IV-TR because it implies that some mental disorders do not have a biological component; however, it still remains in common use.

Primary—no known cause; also called *idiopathic* (similar to *functional*).

Secondary—known to be a symptomatic manifestation of a systemic or medical or cerebral disorder (e.g., delirium resulting from infectious brain disease).

IV. Classification of disorders in DSM-IV-TR

A. Disorders usually first diagnosed in infancy, childhood, or adolescence

1. **Mental retardation.** Below-average intellectual functioning; onset before age 10. Associated with impaired maturation and learning and social maladjustment; classified according to intelligence quotient (I.Q.) as **mild** (50–55 to 70), **moderate** (35–40 to 50–55), **severe** (20–25 to 35–40), or profound (below 20–25).

2. **Learning disorders.** Maturational deficits in development associated with difficulty in acquiring specific skills in **mathematics, writing,** and **reading.**

3. **Motor skills disorder.** Impairments in the development of motor coordination (**developmental coordination disorder**). Children with the disorder are often clumsy and uncoordinated.

4. **Communication disorders.** Developmental impairment resulting in difficulty in producing age-appropriate sentences (**expressive language disorder**), difficulty in using and understanding words (**mixed receptive-expressive language disorder**), difficulty in articulation (**phonologic disorder**), and disturbances in fluency, rate, and rhythm of speech (**stuttering**).

5. **Pervasive developmental disorders.** Characterized by autistic, atypical, and withdrawn behavior, gross immaturity, inadequate development, and failure to develop separate identity from mother; divided into **autistic disorder** (stereotyped behavior usually without speech), **Rett's disorder** (loss of speech and motor skills with decreased head growth), **childhood disintegrative disorder** (loss of acquired speech and motor skills before age 10), **Asperger's disorder** (stereotyped behavior with some ability to communicate), and a **not otherwise specified** (NOS) type.

6. **Attention-deficit and disruptive behavior disorders.** Characterized by inattention, overaggressiveness, delinquency, destructive-

ness, hostility, and feelings of rejection, negativism, or impulsiveness. Patients usually have inconsistent or punitive parental discipline. Divided into **attention-deficit/hyperactivity disorder** (poor attention span, impulsiveness), **conduct disorder** (delinquency), and **oppositional defiant disorder** (negativism).

7. **Feeding and eating disorders of infancy or early childhood.** Characterized by disturbed or bizarre feeding and eating habits that usually begin in childhood or adolescence and continue into adulthood. Divided into **pica** (eating nonnutritional substances) and **rumination disorder** (regurgitation or rechewing).

8. **Tic disorders.** Characterized by sudden, involuntary, recurrent, stereotyped movement or vocal sounds. Divided into **Tourette's disorder** (vocal tic and coprolalia), **chronic motor** or **vocal tic disorder**, and **transient tic disorder**.

9. **Elimination disorders.** Inability to maintain bowel control (**encopresis**) or bladder control (**enuresis**) because of physiological or psychological immaturity.

10. **Other disorders of infancy, childhood, or adolescence.** Selective mutism (voluntary refusal to speak), **reactive attachment disorder of infancy or early childhood** (severe impairment of ability to relate, beginning before age 5), **stereotypic movement disorder** (thumb sucking, head banging, nail biting, skin picking), and **separation anxiety disorder** (cannot separate from home because of anxiety).

B. **Delirium, dementia, and amnestic and other cognitive disorders.** Disorders characterized by change in brain structure and function that result in impaired learning, orientation, judgment, memory, and intellectual functions.

1. **Delirium.** Marked by short-term confusion and changes in cognition caused by a **general medical condition** (e.g., infection), **substances** (e.g., cocaine, opioids, phencyclidine), or **multiple etiologies** (e.g., head trauma and kidney disease). **Delirium NOS** may have other causes (e.g., sleep deprivation).

2. **Dementia.** Marked by severe impairment in memory, judgment, orientation, and cognition: **dementia of the Alzheimer's type**—usually occurs in persons over 65 and manifest by progressive intellectual disorientation and dementia, delusions, or depression; **vascular dementia**—caused by vessel thrombosis or hemorrhage; dementia caused by **other medical conditions**—HIV disease, head trauma; miscellaneous group—Pick's disease, Jakob-Creutzfelt disease (caused by slow-growing transmissible virus); also may be caused by toxin or medication (**substance-induced**)—gasoline fumes, atropine, or **multiple etiologies** and **NOS**.

3. **Amnestic disorder.** Marked by memory impairment and forgetfulness. Caused by **medical condition** (hypoxia), toxin, or **substance** (e.g., marijuana, diazepam [Valium]).

C. **Mental disorders caused by a general medical condition.** Signs and symptoms of psychiatric disorders that occur as a direct result of medical disease. Includes disorders associated with syphilis, encephalitis, abscess, cardiovascular disease or trauma, epilepsy, intracranial neoplasm, endocrine disorders, pellagra, avitaminosis, systemic infection (e.g., typhoid, malaria), and degenerative CNS diseases (e.g., multiple sclerosis). May produce **catatonic disorder** (e.g., immobility resulting from stroke) or **personality change** (e.g., resulting from brain tumor). Also may produce **delirium, dementia, amnestic disorder, psychotic disorder, mood disorder, anxiety disorder, sexual dysfunction,** and **sleep disorder.**

D. Substance-related disorders

1. **Substance use disorders.** **Dependence** on or **abuse** of any psychoactive drug (previously called *drug addiction*). Covers patients addicted to or dependent on such drugs as **alcohol, nicotine** (tobacco), and **caffeine.** Patients may be dependent on **opioids** (e.g., opium, opium alkaloids and their derivatives, and synthetic analgesics with morphine-like effects); **hallucinogens** [e.g., lysergic acid diethylamide (LSD)]; **phencyclidine; hypnotics, sedatives, or anxiolytics; cocaine; cannabis** (hashish, marijuana); **amphetamines;** and **inhalants.**

2. **Substance-induced disorders.** Psychoactive drugs and other substances may cause **intoxication** and **withdrawal** syndromes in addition to **delirium, persisting dementia, persisting amnestic disorder, psychotic disorder, mood disorder, anxiety disorder, sexual dysfunction,** and **sleep disorder.**

3. **Alcohol-related disorders.** Subclass of substance-related disorders that includes **alcohol intoxication** (simple drunkenness); **intoxication delirium** (from being drunk for several days); **alcohol withdrawal delirium** (also called *delirium tremens* [DTs]); **alcohol-induced psychotic disorder** (includes alcohol hallucinosis—differentiated from DTs by clear sensorium); **alcohol-induced persisting amnestic disorder** ([Korsakoff's syndrome]—often preceded by Wernicke's encephalopathy, a neurological condition of ataxia, ophthalmoplegia, and confusion, or the two may coexist [Wernicke-Korsakoff syndrome]); and **alcohol-induced persisting dementia** (differentiated from Korsakoff's syndrome by multiple cognitive deficits). **Mood disorder, anxiety disorder,** and **sleep disorder** induced by alcohol may also occur.

E. Schizophrenia and other psychotic disorders. Covers disorders manifested by disturbances of thinking and misinterpretation of reality, often with delusions and hallucinations.

1. **Schizophrenia.** Characterized by changes in affect (ambivalent, constricted, and inappropriate responsiveness; loss of empathy with others), behavior (withdrawn, aggressive, bizarre) and thinking (distortion of reality, sometimes with delusions and hallucinations). Schizophrenia includes five types: (1) **disorganized** (hebephrenic) **type**—disorganized thinking, giggling, shallow and inappropriate affect, silly and regressive behavior and mannerisms, frequent somatic complaints, and occasional transient and unorganized delusions and hallucinations; (2) **catatonic type**—the excited subtype is characterized by excessive and sometimes violent motor activity, and the withdrawn subtype is characterized by

generalized inhibition, stupor, mutism, negativism, waxy flexibility, and in some cases a vegetative state; (3) **paranoid type**—schizophrenia characterized by persecutory or grandiose delusions and sometimes by hallucinations or excessive religiosity, and the patient is often hostile and aggressive; (4) **undifferentiated type**—disorganized behavior with prominent delusions and hallucinations; and (5) **residual type**—signs of schizophrenia, after a psychotic schizophrenic episode, in patients who are no longer psychotic. (**Postpsychotic depressive disorder of schizophrenia** can occur during the residual phase.)

2. **Delusional (paranoid) disorder.** Psychotic disorder associated with persistent delusions (e.g., erotomanic, grandiose, jealous, persecutory, somatic, unspecified). Paranoia is a rare condition characterized by the gradual development of an elaborate delusional system with grandiose ideas; it has a chronic course; the rest of the personality remains intact.

3. **Brief psychotic disorder.** Psychotic disorder of less than 4 weeks' duration brought on by an external stressor.

4. **Schizophreniform disorder.** Similar to schizophrenia, with delusions, hallucinations, and incoherence, but lasts less than 6 months.

5. **Schizoaffective disorder.** Characterized by a mixture of schizophrenic symptoms and pronounced elation (bipolar type) or depression (depressive type).

6. **Shared psychotic disorder.** Same delusion occurs in two persons, one of whom is less intelligent than or more dependent on the other (also known as *shared delusional disorder, folie à deux*).

7. **Psychotic disorder resulting from a general medical condition.** Hallucinations or delusions that result from medical illness (e.g., temporal lobe epilepsy, avitaminosis, meningitis).

8. **Substance-induced psychotic disorder.** Symptoms of psychosis caused by psychoactive or other substances (e.g., hallucinogens, cocaine).

9. **Psychotic disorder NOS** (Also known as *atypical psychosis*). Psychotic features that are related to (1) a specific culture (koro—found in South and East Asia, fear of shrinking penis); (2) a certain time or event (postpartum psychosis—48 to 72 hours after childbirth); or (3) a unique set of symptoms (Capgras' syndrome—patients think they have a double).

F. **Mood disorders** (Previously called *affective disorders*). Characterized by a disorder of depression that dominates the patient's mental life and is responsible for diminished functioning. Mood disorders may be caused by a **medical condition** or by a **substance** (e.g., psychoactive drugs [cocaine] or medication [antineoplastic agents, reserpine]).

1. **Bipolar disorders.** Marked by severe mood swings between depression and elation and by remission and recurrence. **Bipolar I**—full manic or mixed episode, usually with major depressive episode; **bipolar II**—major depressive episode and hypomanic episode (less intense than mania) without manic or mixed episode; **cyclothymic disorder**—less severe type of bipolar disorder.

2. Depressive disorders. **Major depressive disorder**—severely depressed mood, mental and motor retardation, apprehension, uneasiness, perplexity, agitation, feelings of guilt, suicidal ideation, usually recurrent. **Dysthymic disorder**—less severe form of depression, usually caused by identifiable event or loss (also called *depressive neurosis*). **Postpartum depression** occurs within 1 month after childbirth. **Seasonal pattern depression** (also called *seasonal affective disorder* [SAD]) occurs most often during the winter months.

G. Anxiety disorders.   Characterized by massive and persistent anxiety (**generalized anxiety disorder**), often to the point of panic (**panic disorder**) and fears of going outside the home (**agoraphobia**); fear of specific situations or objects (**specific phobia**) or of performance and public speaking (**social phobia**); involuntary and persistent intrusions of thoughts, desires, urges, or actions (**obsessive-compulsive disorder**). Includes **posttraumatic stress disorder**—follows extraordinary life stress (war, catastrophe) and is characterized by anxiety, nightmares, agitation, and sometimes depression; **acute stress disorder**—similar to posttraumatic stress disorder but lasts for 4 weeks or less. May also be caused by a (1) **medical condition** (e.g., hyperthyroidism) or (2) **substance** (e.g., cocaine).

H. Somatoform disorders.   Marked by preoccupation with the body and fears of disease. Classified into **somatization disorder**—multiple somatic complaints without organic pathology; **conversion disorder** (previously called *hysteria, Briquet's syndrome*)—in which the special senses or voluntary nervous system is affected, with resultant blindness, deafness, anosmia, anesthesias, parethesias, paralysis, ataxia, akinesia, or dyskinesia; patients often show inappropriate lack of concern and may derive some benefits from their actions; **hypochondriasis** (hypochondriacal neurosis)—marked by preoccupation with the body and persistent fears of presumed disease; **pain disorder**—preoccupation with pain in which psychological factors play a part; **body dysmorphic disorder**—unrealistic concern that part of the body is deformed.

I. Factitious disorders.   Characterized by the intentional production or feigning of psychological symptoms, physical symptoms, or both to assume sick role (also called *Munchausen syndrome*).

J. Dissociative disorders.   Characterized by sudden, temporary change in consciousness or identity. **Dissociative** (psychogenic) **amnesia**—loss of memory without organic cause; **dissociative** (psychogenic) **fugue**—unexplained wandering from home; **dissociative identity disorder** (multiple personality disorder)—person has two or more separate identities; **depersonalization disorder**—feelings that things are unreal.

K. Sexual and gender identity disorders.   Divided into paraphilias, gender identity disorders, and sexual dysfunctions. In **paraphilias,** a person's sexual interests are primarily directed toward objects rather than other people, toward sexual acts not usually associated with coitus, or toward coitus performed under bizarre circumstances. Included are **exhibitionism, fetishism, frotteurism, pedophilia, sexual masochism, sexual sadism, transvestite fetishism** (cross-dressing), and **voyeurism.** Sexual dysfunctions include disorders of **desire** (**hypoactive sexual desire disorder, sex-**

ual aversion disorder), **arousal (female sexual arousal disorder, male erectile disorder** [i.e., impotence]), **orgasm (female orgasmic disorder** [i.e., anorgasmia]), **male orgasmic disorder** (i.e., delayed or retarded ejaculation, premature ejaculation]), and **sexual pain (dyspareunia, vaginismus**). Sexual dysfunction may caused by a **medical condition** (e.g., multiple sclerosis) or **substance abuse** (e.g., amphetamine). **Gender identity disorders** (including transsexualism) are characterized by persistent discomfort with one's biological sex and the desire to lose one's sex characteristics (e.g., castration).

L. Eating disorders. Characterized by marked disturbance in eating behavior. Includes **anorexia nervosa** (loss of body weight, refusal to eat) and **bulimia nervosa** (binge eating with or without vomiting).

M. Sleep disorders. Covers (1) **dyssomnias**, in which the person cannot fall asleep or stay asleep (**insomnia**) or sleeps too much (**hypersomnia**); (2) **parasomnias**, such as **nightmares, sleepwalking,** or **sleep terror disorder** (person wakes up in an immobilized state of terror); (3) **narcolepsy** (sleep attacks with loss of muscle tone [cataplexy]); (4) **breathing-related sleep disorders** (snoring, apnea); and (5) **circadian rhythm sleep disorder** (daytime sleepiness, jet lag). Sleep disorders can also be caused by **medical disease** (e.g., Parkinson's disease) and **substance abuse** (e.g., alcoholism).

N. Impulse-control disorders not elsewhere classified. Covers disorders in which persons cannot control impulses and act out. Includes **intermittent explosive disorder** (aggression), **kleptomania** (stealing), **pyromania** (setting fires), **trichotillomania** (pulling hair), and **pathological gambling**.

O. Adjustment disorder. Maladaptive reaction to a clearly defined life stress. Divided into subtypes depending on symptom—**with anxiety, depressed mood, mixed anxiety and depressed mood, disturbance of conduct,** and **mixed disturbance of emotions and conduct**.

P. Personality disorder. Disorders characterized by deeply ingrained, generally lifelong maladaptive patterns of behavior that are usually recognizable at adolescence or earlier.

1. **Paranoid personality disorder.** Characterized by unwarranted suspicion, hypersensitivity, jealousy, envy, rigidity, excessive self-importance, and a tendency to blame and ascribe evil motives to others.

2. **Schizoid personality disorder.** Characterized by shyness, oversensitivity, seclusiveness, avoidance of close or competitive relationships, eccentricity, no loss of capacity to recognize reality, daydreaming, and an ability to express hostility and aggression.

3. **Schizotypal personality disorder.** Similar to schizoid, but the person exhibits slight losses of reality testing, has odd beliefs, and is aloof and withdrawn.

4. **Obsessive-compulsive personality disorder.** Characterized by excessive concern with conformity and standards of conscience; patient may be rigid, overconscientious, overdutiful, overinhibited, and unable to relax (three *P*s—punctual, parsimonious, precise).

5. **Histrionic personality disorder.** Characterized by emotional instability, excitability, overreactivity, vanity, immaturity, dependency, and self-dramatization that is attention-seeking and seductive.

6. **Avoidant personality disorder.** Characterized by low levels of energy, easy fatigability, lack of enthusiasm, inability to enjoy life, and oversensitivity to stress.

7. **Antisocial personality disorder.** Covers persons in conflict with society. They are incapable of loyalty, selfish, callous, irresponsible, impulsive, and unable to feel guilt or learn from experience; they have a low level of frustration tolerance and a tendency to blame others.

8. **Narcissistic personality disorder.** Characterized by grandiose feelings, sense of entitlement, lack of empathy, envy, manipulativeness, and need for attention and admiration.

9. **Borderline personality disorder.** Characterized by instability, impulsiveness, chaotic sexuality, suicidal acts, self-mutilating behavior, identity problems, ambivalence, and feeling of emptiness and boredom.

10. **Dependent personality disorder.** Characterized by passive and submissive behavior; person is unsure of himself or herself and becomes entirely dependent on others.

Q. **Other conditions that may be a focus of clinical attention.** Include conditions in which no mental disorder is present, but the problem is the focus of diagnosis or treatment.

1. **Psychological factors affecting physical condition.** Disorders characterized by physical symptoms caused or affected by emotional factors; usually involve a single organ system with autonomic nervous system control or input. Examples are atopic dermatitis, backache, bronchial asthma, hypertension, migraine, ulcer, irritable colon, and colitis (also called *psychosomatic disorders*).

2. **Medication-induced movement disorders.** Disorders caused by medications, especially dopamine receptor antagonists (e.g., chlorpromazine [Thorazine]). Includes **parkinsonism, neuroleptic malignant syndrome** (muscle rigidity, hypothermia), **acute dystonia** (muscle spasm), **acute akathisia** (restlessness), **tardive dyskinesia** (choreiform movements), and **postural tremor**.

3. **Relational problems.** Impaired social interaction within a relational unit. Includes **parent–child problem, spouse** or **partner problem,** and **sibling problem**. May also result when one member is mentally or physically ill and the other is stressed as a result.

4. **Problems related to abuse or neglect.** Includes **physical abuse** and **sexual abuse** of children and adults.

R. **Additional conditions that may be a focus of clinical attention.** Conditions in which persons have problems not severe enough to warrant a psychiatric diagnosis but that interfere with functioning. Classified into **adult** and **child or adolescent antisocial behavior** (repeated criminal acts), **borderline intellectual functioning** (I.Q., 71 to 84), **malingering** (voluntary production of symptoms), **noncompliance with treatment, occupational** or **academic problem, phase of life problem** (parenthood, unemployment), **bereavement, age-related cognitive decline** (normal forgetfulness of old age), **identity problem** (career choice), **religious or spiritual problem,** and **acculturation problem** (immigration).

S. Other categories. In addition to the diagnostic categories listed above, other categories of illness are listed in DSM-IV-TR that require further study before they become an official part of DSM or that are controversial. These include the following:

1. **Postconcussional disorder.** Cognitive impairment, headache, sleep problems, irritability, dizziness, change in personality occurring after head injury.

2. **Mild neurocognitive disorder.** Disturbances in memory, comprehension, attention as a result of medical disease (e.g., electrolyte imbalance, hypothyroidism, early stages of multiple sclerosis).

3. **Caffeine withdrawal.** Fatigue, depression, headaches, anxiety after cessation of coffee intake.

4. **Postpsychotic depressive disorder of schizophrenia.** A depressive episode, which may be prolonged, arising in the aftermath of a schizophrenic illness.

5. **Simple deteriorative disorder (simple schizophrenia).** Characterized by oddities of conduct, inability to meet demands of society, blunting of affect, loss of volition, and social impoverishment. Delusions and hallucinations are evident.

6. **Minor depressive disorder, recurrent brief depressive disorder, and premenstrual dysphoric disorder. Minor depressive disorder** is associated with mild symptoms, such as worry and overconcern with minor autonomic symptoms (tremor and palpitations). **Recurrent brief depressive disorder** is characterized by recurrent episodes of depression, each of which lasts less than 2 weeks (typically 2 to 3 days) and each of which ends with complete recovery. **Premenstrual dysphoric disorder** occurs 1 week before menses (luteal phase) and is characterized by depressed mood, anxiety, irritability, lethargy, and sleep disturbances.

7. **Mixed anxiety-depressive disorder.** Characterized by symptoms of both anxiety and depression, neither of which predominates (sometimes called *neurasthenia*).

8. **Factitious disorder by proxy.** Also known as *Munchausen syndrome by proxy*; parents feign illness in their children.

9. **Dissociative trance disorder.** Marked by temporary loss of sense of personal identity and awareness of the surroundings; patient acts as if taken over by another personality, spirit or force.

10. **Binge-eating disorder.** Variant of bulimia nervosa, characterized by recurrent episodes of binge eating without self-induced vomiting and laxative abuse.

11. **Depressive personality disorder.** Marked by pessimism, anhedonia, chronic unhappiness, loneliness.

12. **Passive–aggressive personality disorder.** Marked by stubbornness, procrastination, intentional inefficiency multiplied by underlying aggression (also called *negativistic personality disorder*).

V. Severity of disorder

Depending on the clinical picture, the presence or absence of signs and symptoms, and their intensity, the severity of a disorder may be classified as follows:

A. Mild.   Few if any symptoms are present, and no more than minor impairment in social or occupational functioning.

B. Moderate.   Symptoms or functional impairment between *mild* and *severe* are present.

C. Severe.   Many symptoms or particularly severe symptoms that result in marked impairment in social or occupational functioning.

D. In partial remission.   The full criteria for the disorder were previously met, but currently only some of the symptoms or signs of the disorder remain.

E. In full remission.   No longer any symptoms or signs of the disorder.

F. Multiple diagnoses.   It is possible for a patient to have more than one diagnosis. The principal or main diagnosis is usually the one that was responsible for admission to a hospital or a visit to the psychiatrist. In some cases, it may not be possible to determine which diagnosis is the main one because each may have contributed equally to the need for treatment. In such cases, the term *dual diagnosis* is used (e.g., amphetamine dependence accompanied by schizophrenia).

For a more detailed discussion of this topic, see Classification of Mental Disorders, Ch 9, p 824, in CTP/VII.

4

Delirium, Dementia, Amnestic Disorders, and Other Cognitive Disorders, and Mental Disorders Due to a General Medical Condition

I. Overview

The cognitive disorders are characterized by significant impairment in functions such as memory, judgment, language, and attention. This impairment represents a change from baseline. Delirium is characterized by a disturbance of consciousness and the development of symptoms within a short period of time. Dementia is characterized by global cognitive impairments, including memory deficits, despite a normal level of alertness and arousal. Amnestic disorders are characterized by memory loss without other cognitive impairments. Mental disorders resulting from a general medical condition are defined as psychiatric symptoms that are directly caused by a medical or neurological disorder (e.g. depression resulting from a frontal lobe tumor). Cognitive disorders can also be caused by such problems as trauma, substance use disorder, toxins, or drugs. These disorders can coexist (e.g., acute delirium complicating long-standing dementia).

II. Clinical evaluation

A. **History.** Often requires collateral data from chart, staff, and family. Look for change from baseline functioning. Emphasize medical history, physical symptoms, medication used, and possible drugs of abuse. Include a complete review of systems in the history.

B. **Physical.** Emphasize neurological examination, but do not overlook other systems.

C. **Mental status.** Carefully evaluate cognition, but not to the point of missing other information, especially appearance and general behavior, mood, affect, and thought content and process. Look for nonspecific signs of brain dysfunction, such as the following:

1. Intellectual, memory, and cognitive impairment (paucity of thought, lack of intellectual flexibility, perseveration, poor judgment).
2. Alterations in level of consciousness (e.g., waking in the morning in a confused state).
3. Change in personality.
4. Disinhibition (inappropriateness or exacerbation of underlying personality traits).
5. Poverty of speech with decreased vocabulary and use of cliches.

6. Prominent visual hallucinations.
7. Mood initially may be depressed, anxious, and labile, but it may progress to apathy.
8. Affect may be shallow or flat.

D. Cognitive evaluation. Perform a screening assessment of cognition. Use the Mini-Mental State Examination (MMSE) to obtain a gross estimate of cognition. A score of 25 of a possible 30 points suggests impairment. A score of less than 20 indicates definite impairment (Table 4–1).

E. Consultation. Work closely with internists, neurologists, and other specialists. Be prepared to manage contributing illness.

F. Laboratory tests
1. Routine laboratory evaluation including complete blood cell count; measurement of electrolytes, red blood cell folate, and thyroid functions; drug screen; and serum liver chemistries. All are needed to detect treatable condition not readily apparent on screening tests such as MMSE.

TABLE 4–1
MINI-MENTAL STATE EXAMINATION

Orientation (score 1 point for correct response)
1. What is the year?
2. What is the season?
3. What is the date?
4. What is the day of the week?
5. What is the month?
6. Where are we? building or hospital?
7. Where are we? floor?
8. Where are we? town or city?
9. Where are we? county?
10. Where are we? state?

Registration (score 1 point for each object identified correctly, maximum of 3 points)
11. Name three objects at about one each second. Ask the patient to repeat them. If the patient misses an object, repeat them until all three are learned.

Attention and calculation (score 1 point for each correct answer up to maximum of 5 points)
12. Subtract 7s from 100 until 65 (or, as an alternative, spell "world" backwards).

Recall (score 1 point for each correct answer, maximum of 3)
13. Ask for names of three objects learned in question 11.

Language
14. Point to a pencil and a watch. Ask the patient to name each object. Score 1 point for each correct answer, maximum of 2 points.
15. Have the patient repeat "No *ifs, ands,* or *buts*." Score 1 point if correct.
16. Have the patient follow a three-stage command: "(1) Take the paper in your right hand. (2) Fold the paper in half. (3) Put the paper on the floor." Score 1 point for each command done correctly, maximum of 3 points.
17. Write the following in large letters: "CLOSE YOUR EYES." Ask the patient to read the command and perform the task. Score 1 point if correct.
18. Ask the patient to write a sentence of his or her own choice. Score 1 point if the sentence has a subject, an object, and a verb.
19. Draw the design printed below. Ask the patient to copy the design. Score 1 point if all sides and angles are preserved and if the intersecting sides form a quadrangle.

From Folstein MF, Folstein SE, McHugh PR. Mini-mental state. A practical method for grading the cognitive state of patients for the clinician. *J Psychiatr Res* 1975;12:189, with permission.

2. Psychometric assessment (psychological testing)—more sensitive to organicity, standardized, can utilize probabilities in interpretation, requires patient cooperation. Psychologist needs to be told where to focus assessment.

3. Skull roentgenogram, electroencephalogram (EEG), computed tomography (CT), magnetic resonance imaging (MRI), lumbar puncture, brain scan, and angiography, as indicated.

III. Delirium

A. **Definition.**   The hallmark symptom of delirium is an impairment of consciousness, usually accompanied by global impairments of cognitive functions; generally associated with emotional lability, hallucinations or illusions, and inappropriate, impulsive, irrational, or violent behavior. Generally considered to be an acute reversible disorder but can become irreversible.

B. **Epidemiology.**   Common among hospitalized patients—about 10% of all hospitalized patients, 20% of patients with burns, 30% of ICU patients, 30% of hospitalized AIDS patients. Very young and elderly patients are more susceptible to delirium. Patients with a history of delirium or brain damage are more likely to have an episode of delirium than the general population.

C. **Etiology.**   Delirium may be thought of as a common pathway for any brain insult. Major causes include systemic disease (e.g., cardiac failure), CNS disease (e.g., seizure disorders), and either intoxication with or withdrawal from prescribed pharmacological agents or drugs of abuse. Any drug a patient has taken (including over-the-counter medicines and herbal preparations) should be considered potential causes of delirium. Delirium is thought to involve dysfunction of the reticular formation and acetylcholine transmission. The dorsal tegmental pathway projecting from the reticular formation to the tectum and the thalamus has been implicated as the major pathway in delirium. Noradrenergic hyperactivity of the locus ceruleus has been associated with alcohol withdrawal delirium.

D. **Diagnosis, signs, and symptoms.**   Delirium is diagnosed according to etiology: delirium due to a medical condition (Table 4–2), substance intoxication delirium (Table 4–3) and substance withdrawal delirium, and delirium not otherwise specified (NOS). Key features include altered con-

TABLE 4–2
DSM-IV-TR DIAGNOSTIC CRITERIA FOR DELIRIUM DUE TO A GENERAL MEDICAL CONDITION

A. Disturbance of consciousness (i.e., reduced clarity of awareness of the environment) with reduced ability to focus, sustain, or shift attention.

B. A change in cognition (such as memory deficit, disorientation, language disturbance) or the development of a perceptual disturbance that is not better accounted for by a preexisting, established, or evolving dementia.

C. The disturbance develops over a short period of time (usually hours to days) and tends to fluctuate during the course of the day.

D. There is evidence from the history, physical examination, or laboratory findings that the disturbance is caused by the direct physiologic consequences of a general medical condition.

From American Psychiatric Association. *Diagnostic and Statistical Manual of Mental Disorders*, text revision, 4th ed. Washington, DC: American Psychiatric Association, Copyright 2000, with permission.

TABLE 4–3
DSM-IV-TR DIAGNOSTIC CRITERIA FOR SUBSTANCE INTOXICATION DELIRIUM

A. Disturbance of consciousness (i.e., reduced clarity of awareness of the environment) with reduced ability to focus, sustain, or shift attention.
B. A change in cognition (such as memory deficit, disorientation, language disturbance) or the development of a perceptual disturbance that is not better accounted for by a preexisting, established, or evolving dementia.
C. The disturbance develops over a short period of time (usually hours to days) and tends to fluctuate during the course of the day.
D. There is evidence from the history physical examination, or laboratory findings of either (1) or (2):
   (1) The symptoms in Criteria A and B developed during substance intoxication.
   (2) Medication use is etiologically related to the disturbance.

From American Psychiatric Association. *Diagnostic and Statistical Manual of Mental Disorders,* text revision, 4th ed. Washington, DC: American Psychiatric Association, Copyright 2000, with permission.

sciousness with hyperarousal, or hypoarousal with agitation or apathy; disorientation; memory impairment; illogical speech; perceptual disturbances, including auditory, visual, and tactile hallucinations; severe emotional lability; and reversed sleep–wake cycle or fragmented sleep. Associated neurological symptoms may include incoordination, dysphasia, tremor, asterixis, ataxia, and apraxia.

E. **Laboratory tests.**   Delirium is a medical emergency, and its cause must be identified as rapidly as possible. If the likely cause is not apparent, then a complete medical workup should be performed immediately. Even if an apparent cause is identified, multiple factors may be involved. The workup should include vital signs, complete blood cell count with differential, erythrocyte sedimentation rate, complete blood chemistries, liver and renal function tests, urinalysis, urine toxicology, ECG, chest roentgenography, CT of the head, and lumbar puncture (if indicated). The EEG often shows diffuse slowing throughout or focal areas of hyperactivity.

F. **Differential diagnosis**
   1. **Dementia.** See Table 4–4.
   2. **Schizophrenia and mania.** Usually do not have the rapidly fluctuating course of delirium, nor do they impair the level of consciousness or significantly impair cognition.
   3. **Dissociative disorders.** May show spotty amnesia but lack the global cognitive impairment and abnormal psychomotor and sleep patterns of delirium.

G. **Course and prognosis.**   Three-month mortality rate of 23–33% in patients who have an episode of delirium; 1-year mortality rate of 50%. The course is usually rapid. Symptoms usually recede 3 to 7 days after the causable factor is treated; symptom resolution may take 2 weeks. In some cases, the delirium may spontaneously clear.

H. **Treatment.**   Identify and treat the underlying cause. Correct metabolic abnormalities; ensure proper hydration, electrolyte balance, and nutrition; identify and where possible discontinue causative medication; optimize the sensory environment for the patient (e.g., decreased stimuli for a patient with delirium tremens and appropriate increased stimulation for a patient delirious from sensory deprivation). Low doses of a high-potency antipsychotic may be used for agitation, (e.g., 2 to 5 mg of haloperidol [Haldol] orally or intramuscularly every 4 hours). Benzodiazepines (e.g., 1 to 2 mg of lorazepam [Ativan] every 4 hours) can be used orally or intramuscularly every 4 hours as needed, and can also be used for agitation, especially in a patient who may be at risk for seizures (e.g., a patient suffering from alcohol or sedative-hypnotics withdrawal).

IV. Dementia

  A. **Definition.**   Dementia is a disorder characterized by multiple cognitive deficits, including memory loss. However, consciousness is not impaired in dementia, as it is in delirium. Affected functions include intelligence, language, problem solving, memory, learning, orientation, perception, attention, judgment, concentration, and social abilities. DSM-IV-TR requires that the defects represent a significant change from baseline and interfere with functioning.

  B. **Epidemiology.**   Primarily a syndrome of the elderly. About 5% of Americans over the age of 65 have severe dementia, and 15% have mild dementia. About 20% of Americans over the age of 80 have severe dementia. Increasing age is the most important risk factor. One fourth of demented patients have some treatable illness. In 15% of patients with dementia, the illness is reversible if timely treatment is initiated.

  C. **Etiology.**   See Table 4–5. Most common cause is Alzheimer's disease (50–60% of cases), followed by vascular disease (mixed forms are also common). Other common causes include head trauma, alcohol, movement disorders such as Huntington's and Parkinson's disease, and HIV infection.

  D. **Diagnosis, signs, and symptoms.**   The major defects in dementia involve orientation, memory, perception, intellectual functioning, and reasoning. Marked changes in personality, affect, and behavior can occur. Dementias are commonly accompanied by hallucinations (20–30% of pa-

TABLE 4–4
CLINICAL DIFFERENTIATION OF DELIRIUM AND DEMENTIA[a]

	Delirium	Dementia
History	Acute disease	Chronic disease
Onset	Rapid	Insidious (usually)
Duration	Days-weeks	Months-years
Course	Fluctuating	Chronically progressive
Level of consciousness	Fluctuating	Normal
Orientation	Impaired, at least periodically	Intact initially
Affect	Anxious, irritable	Labile but not usually anxious
Thinking	Often disordered	Decreased amount
Memory	Recent memory markedly impaired	Both recent and remote impaired
Perception	Hallucinations common (especially visual)	Hallucinations less common (except sundowning)
Psychomotor function	Retarded, agitated, or mixed	Normal
Sleep	Disrupted sleep–wake cycle	Less disruption of sleep–wake cycle
Attention and awareness	Prominently impaired	Less impaired
Reversibility	Often reversible	Majority not reversible

[a] Demented patients are more susceptible to delirium, and delirium superimposed on dementia is common.

TABLE 4–5
CAUSES OF DEMENTIA

Tumor	**Physiologic**
Primary cerebral[a]	Epilepsy[a]
Trauma	Normal-pressure hydrocephalus[a]
Hematomas[a]	**Metabolic**
Posttraumatic dementia[a]	Vitamin deficiencies[a]
Infection (chronic)	Chronic metabolic disturbances[a]
Metastatic[a]	Chronic anoxic states[a]
Syphilis	Chronic endocrinopathies[a]
Creutzfeldt-Jakob disease[b]	**Degenerative dementias**
AIDS dementia complex[c]	Alzheimer's disease[b]
Cardiac/vascular	Pick's disease (dementias of frontal lobe type)[b]
Single infarction[a]	Parkinson's disease[a]
Multiple infarctions[b]	Progressive supranuclear palsy[c]
Large infarction	Idiopathic cerebral ferrocalcinosis (Fahr's disease)[c]
Locunar infarction	Wilson's disease[c]
Binswanger's disease (subcortical	**Demyelinating disease**
arteriosclerotic encephalopathies)	Multiple sclerosis[c]
Hemodynamic type[a]	**Drugs and toxins**
Congenital/hereditary	Alcohol[a]
Huntington's disease[c]	Heavy metals[a]
Metachromatic leukodystrophy[c]	Carbon monoxide poisoning[a]
Primary psychiatric	Medications[a]
Pseudodementia[a]	Irradiation[a]

[a] Variable or mixed pattern.
[b] Predominantly cortical pattern.
[c] Predominantly subcortical pattern.
Table by Eric D. Caine, M.D., Hillel Grossman, M.D., and Jeffrey M. Lyness, M.D.

TABLE 4–6
DSM-IV-TR DIAGNOSTIC CRITERIA FOR DEMENTIA DUE TO OTHER GENERAL MEDICAL CONDITIONS

A. The development of multiple cognitive deficits manifested by both
    (1) memory impairment (impaired ability to learn new information or to recall previously learned information)
    (2) one (or more) of the following cognitive disturbances:
        (a) aphasia (language disturbance)
        (b) apraxia (impaired ability to carry out motor activities despite intact motor function)
        (c) agnosia (failure to recognize or identify objects despite intact sensory function)
        (d) disturbance in executive functioning (i.e., planning, organizing, sequencing, abstracting)
B. The cognitive deficits in Criteria A1 and A2 each cause significant impairment in social or occupational functioning and represent a significant decline from a previous level of functioning.
C. There is evidence from the history, physical examination, or laboratory findings that the disturbance is the direct physiological consequence of a general medical condition other than Alzheimer's disease or cerebrovascular disease (e.g., HIV infection, traumatic brain injury, Parkinson's disease, Huntington's disease, Pick's disease, Creutzfeldt-Jakob disease, normal-pressure hydrocephalus, hypothyroidism, brain tumor, or vitamin B_{12} deficiency).
D. The deficits do not occur exclusively during the course of delirium.

Code based on presence or absence of a clinically significant behavioral disturbance:
    Without behavioral disturbance: if the cognitive disturbance is not accompanied by any clinically significant behavioral disturbance.
    With behavioral disturbance: if the cognitive disturbance is accompanied by a clinically significant behavioral disturbance (e.g., wandering, agitation).

Coding note: Also code the general medical condition on Axis III (e.g., HIV infection, head injury, Parkinson's disease, Huntington's disease, Pick's disease, Creutzfeldt-Jakob disease).

From American Psychiatric Association. *Diagnostic and Statistical Manual of Mental Disorders*, text revision, 4th ed. Washington, DC: American Psychiatric Association, Copyright 2000, with permission.

tients) and delusions (30–40%). Symptoms of depression and anxiety are present in 40–50% of patients with dementia.

Dementia is diagnosed according to etiology: dementia of the Alzheimer's type (DAT), vascular dementia, dementia due to other general medical conditions (Table 4–6), substance-induced persisting dementia, dementia with multiple causes, and dementia NOS.

E. Laboratory tests. See Table 4–7. First identify a potentially reversible cause for the dementia, then identify other treatable medical conditions that may otherwise worsen the dementia (cognitive decline is often precipitated by other medical illness). The workup should include vital signs, complete blood cell count with differential sedimentation rate (ESR), complete blood chemistries, serum B_{12} and folate levels, liver and renal function tests, thyroid function tests, urinalysis, urine toxicology, ECG, chest roentgenography, CT or MRI of the head, and lumbar puncture. Single photon emission tomography (SPECT) can be used to detect patterns of brain metabolism in certain types of dementia.

TABLE 4-7
COMPREHENSIVE WORKUP OF DEMENTIA

Physical examination, including thorough neurologic examination
Vital signs
Mental status examination
Mini-Mental State Examination (MMSE)
Review of medications and drug levels
Blood and urine screens for alcohol, drugs, and heavy metals[a]
Physiological workup
Serum electrolytes/glucose/Ca^{++}, Mg^{++}
Liver, renal function tests
SMA-12 or equivalent serum chemistry profile
Urinalysis
Complete blood cell count with differential cell type count
Thyroid function tests (including TSH level)
RPR (serum screen)
FTA-ABS (if CNS disease suspected)
Serum B_{12}
Folate levels
Urine corticosteroids[a]
Erythrocyte sedimentation rate (Westergren)
Antinuclear antibody[a] (ANA), C_3C_4, Anti-DS DNA[a]
Arterial blood gases[a]
HIV screen[a,b]
Urine porphobilinogens[a]
Chest radiograph
Electrocardiogram
Neurological workup
CT or MRI of head[a]
SPECT[b]
Lumbar puncture[a]
EEG[a]
Neuropsychological testing[d]

[a] All indicated by history and physical examination.
[b] Requires special consent and counseling.
[c] May detect cerebral blood flow perfusion deficits.
[d] May be useful in differentiating dementia from other neuropsychiatric syndromes if it cannot be done clinically.
Adapted from Stoudemire A. Thompson TL. Recognizing and treating dementia. *Geriatrics* 1981;36:112, with permission.

F. Differential diagnosis

1. **Age-related cognitive decline (normal aging).** Associated with a decreased ability to learn new material and a slowing of thought processes as a consequence of normal aging. In addition, there is a syndrome of benign senescent forgetfulness, which does not show a progressively deteriorating course.

2. **Depression.** Depression in the elderly may present as symptoms of cognitive impairment, which has led to the term *pseudodementia*. The apparently demented patient is really depressed and responds well to antidepressant drugs or electroconvulsive therapy (ECT). Many demented patients also become depressed as they begin to comprehend their progressive cognitive impairment. In patients with both dementia and depression, a treatment trial with antidepressants or ECT is often warranted. Table 4–8 differentiates dementia from depression.

3. **Delirium.** Also characterized by global cognitive impairment. Demented patients often have a superimposed delirium. Dementia tends to be chronic and lacks the prominent features of rapid fluctuations, sudden onset, impaired attention, changing level of consciousness, psychomotor disturbance, acutely disturbed sleep–wake cycle, and prominent hallucinations or delusions that characterize delirium.

G. Course and prognosis.

Dementia may be progressive, remitting, or stable. Because about 15% of dementias are reversible (e.g., hypothyroidism, CNS syphilis, subdural hematoma, vitamin B_{12} deficiency, uremia, hypoxia), the course in these cases depends on how quickly the cause is reversed. If the cause is reversed too late, the patient may have residual deficits with a subsequently stable course if extensive brain damage has not occurred. For dementia with no identifiable cause (e.g., DAT), the course is likely to be one of slow deterioration. The patient may become lost in familiar places, lose the ability to handle money, later fail to recognize family members, and eventually become incontinent of stool and urine.

TABLE 4–8
DEMENTIA VERSUS DEPRESSION

Feature	Dementia	Pseudodementia
Age	Usually elderly	Nonspecific
Onset	Vague	Days to weeks
Course	Slow, worse at night	Rapid, even through day
History	Systemic illness or drugs	Mood disorder
Awareness	Unaware, unconcerned	Aware, distressed
Organic signs	Often present	Absent
Cognition[a]	Prominent impairment	Personality changes
Mental status examination	Consistent, spotty deficits	Variable deficits in different modalities
	Approximates, confabulates, perseverates	Apathetic, "I don't know"
	Emphasizes trivial accomplishments	Emphasizes failures
	Shallow or table mood	Depressed
Behavior	Appropriate to degree of cognitive impairment	Incongruent with degree of cognitive impairment
Cooperation	Cooperative but frustrated	Uncooperative with little effort
CT and EEG	Abnormal	Normal

[a] Benzodiazepines and barbiturates worsen cognitive impairments in the demented patient, whereas they help the depressed patient to relax.

H. Treatment. Treatment is generally supportive. Ensure proper treatment of any concurrent medical problems. Maintain proper nutrition, exercise, and activities. Provide an environment with frequent cues for orientation to day, date, place, and time. As functioning decreases, nursing home placement may be necessary. Often, cognitive impairment may become worse at night (sundowning). Some nursing homes have successfully developed a schedule of nighttime activities to help manage this problem.

1. **Psychological.** Supportive therapy, group therapy, and referral to organizations for families of demented patients can help them to cope and feel less frustrated and helpless.

2. **Pharmacological.** In general, barbiturates and benzodiazepines should be avoided because they can worsen cognition. For agitation, low doses of an antipsychotic are effective (e.g., 2 mg of haloperidol orally or intramuscularly or 0.25 to 1.0 mg of risperidone per day orally). Some clinicians suggest a short-acting benzodiazepine for sleep (e.g., 0.25 mg of triazolam [Halcion] orally), but this may cause further memory deficits the next day.

V. Dementia of the Alzheimer's type

A. Definition. A progressive dementia in which all known reversible causes have been ruled out. Two types—with late onset (onset after age 65) and with early onset (onset before or at age 65).

B. Diagnosis, signs, and symptoms. See Table 4–9.

C. Epidemiology. Most common cause of dementia. DAT accounts for 50–60% of all dementias. May affect as many as 5% of persons over age 65 and 15–20% of persons age 85 or older. Risk factors include female sex, history of head injury, and having a first-degree relative with the disorder. Incidence increases with age. Patients with DAT occupy more than 50% of nursing home beds.

D. Etiology. Genetic factors play a role; up to 40% of patients have a family history of DAT. Concordance rate for monozygotic twins is 43%, versus 8% for dizygotic twins. Several cases have documented autosomal dominant transmission. Down syndrome is associated with DAT. The gene for amyloid precursor protein on chromosome 21 may be involved. The neurotransmitters most often implicated are acetylcholine and norepinephrine. Both are believed to be hypoactive. Degeneration of cholinergic neurons in the nucleus basalis of Meynert in addition to decreased brain concentrations of acetylcholine and its key synthetic enzyme choline acetyltransferase have been noted. Further evidence for a cholinergic hypothesis includes the beneficial effects of cholinesterase inhibitors and the further impairment of cognition associated with anticholinergics. Some evidence has been found of a decrease in norepinephrine-containing neurons in the locus ceruleus. Decreased levels of corticotropin and somatostatin may also be involved. Other proposed causes include abnormal regulation of cell membrane phospholipid metabolism and aluminum toxicity.

TABLE 4-9
DSM-IV-TR DIAGNOSTIC CRITERIA FOR DEMENTIA OF THE ALZHEIMER'S TYPE

A. The development of multiple cognitive deficits manifested by both
    (1) memory impairment (impaired ability to learn new information or to recall previously learned information)
    (2) one (or more) of the following cognitive disturbances:
        (a) aphasia (language disturbance)
        (b) apraxia (impaired ability to carry out motor activities despite intact motor function)
        (c) agnosia (failure to recognize or identify objects despite intact sensory function)
        (d) disturbance in executive functioning (i.e., planning, organizing, sequencing, abstracting)
B. The cognitive deficits in Criteria A1 and A2 each cause significant impairment in social or occupational functioning and represent a significant decline from a previous level of functioning.
C. The course is characterized by gradual onset and continuing cognitive decline.
D. The cognitive deficits in Criteria A1 and A2 are not due to any of the following:
    (1) other central nervous system conditions that cause progressive deficits in memory and cognition (e.g., cerebrovascular disease, Parkinson's disease, Huntington's disease, subdural hematoma, normal-pressure hydrocephalus, brain tumor)
    (2) systemic conditions that are known to cause dementia (e.g., hypothyroidism, vitamin B_{12} or folic acid deficiency, niacin deficiency, hypercalcemia, neurosyphilis, HIV infection)
    (3) substance-induced conditions
E. The deficits do not occur exclusively during the course of a delirium.
F. The disturbance is not better accounted for by another Axis I disorder (e.g., major depressive disorder, schizophrenia).

Code based on presence or absence of a clinically significant behavioral disturbance:
    Without behavioral disturbance: if the cognitive disturbance is not accompanied by any clinically significant behavioral disturbance.
    With behavioral disturbance: if the cognitive disturbance is accompanied by a clinically significant behavioral disturbance (e.g., wandering, agitation).

Specify subtype:
    With early onset: if onset is at age 65 years or below
    With late onset: if onset is after age 65 years

Coding note: Also code Alzheimer's disease on Axis III. Indicate other prominent clinical features related to the Alzheimer's disease on Axis I (e.g., mood disorder due to Alzheimer's disease, with depressive features, and personality change due to Alzheimer's disease, aggressive type).

From American Psychiatric Association. *Diagnostic and Statistical Manual of Mental Disorders*, text revision, 4th ed. Washington, DC: American Psychiatric Association; Copyright 2000, with permission.

    E. Neuropathology.   The characteristic neuropathological changes, first described by Alois Alzheimer, are neurofibrillary tangles, senile plaques, and granulovacuolar degenerations. These changes can also appear with normal aging, but they are always present in the brains of DAT patients. Pathological findings are predominantly parietal–temporal. They are most prominent in the amygdala, hippocampus, cortex, and basal forebrain. A definitive diagnosis of Alzheimer's disease can be made only by histopathology. The aluminum toxicity etiological theory is based on the fact that these pathological structures in the brain contain high amounts of aluminum. The clinical diagnosis of DAT should be considered only either possible or probable in Alzheimer's disease.

    Other abnormalities that have been found in DAT patients include diffuse cortical atrophy on CT or MRI, enlarged ventricles, and decreased brain acetylcholine metabolism. The finding of low levels of acetylcholine explains why these patients are highly susceptible to the effects of anticholinergic medication and has led to development of choline-replacement strategies for treatment.

VIII. Creutzfeldt-Jakob disease

This rapidly progressive degenerative dementing disease is caused by a prion infection. A prion is a replicative protein that causes a variety of spongiform diseases. Prions can be transmitted by the use of contaminated dura mater or corneal grafts, or by ingesting meat from cattle infected with bovine spongiform encephalopathy. The onset usually is in a patient's 40s or 50s. The very first signs of this disease may be vague somatic complaints or unspecified feelings of anxiety. Other signs include ataxia, extrapyramidal signs, choreoathetosis, and dysarthria. Myoclonic jerks are often present. Usually fatal within 6 to 12 months of diagnosis. CT shows atrophy in cortex and cerebellum. A characteristic EEG in later stages usually consists of a bilateral synchronous spike-and-wave pattern that later gives way to synchronous triphasic sharp-wave complexes; spike activity may correspond to myoclonic jerks. There is no known treatment.

IX. Huntington's disease

A. Definition.   A genetic autosomal dominant disease with complete penetrance (chromosome 4) characterized by choreoathetoid movement and dementia. The chance for the development of the disease in a person who has one parent with Huntington's disease is 50%.

B. Diagnosis.   Onset usually is in a patient's 30s to 40s (the patient frequently already has children). Choreiform movements usually present first and become progressively more severe. Dementia presents later, often with psychotic features. Dementia may first be described by the patient's family as a personality change. Look for a family history.

C. Associated psychiatric symptoms and complications

1. Personality changes (25%).

2. Schizophreniform (25%).

3. Mood (50%).

4. Presentation with sudden-onset dementia (25%).

5. Development of dementia in 90% of patients.

D. Epidemiology.   Incidence is two to six cases a year per 100,000 persons. More than 1,000 cases have been traced to two brothers who immigrated to Long Island from England. Incidence is equal in men and women.

E. Pathophysiology.   Atrophy of brain with extensive involvement of the basal ganglia and the caudate nucleus in particular.

F. Differential diagnosis.   When choreiform movements are first noted, they are often misinterpreted as inconsequential habit spasms or tics. Up to 75% of patients with Huntington's disease are initially misdiagnosed with a primary psychiatric disorder. Features distinguishing it from DAT are the high incidence of depression and psychosis and the classic choreoathetoid movement disorder.

G. Course and prognosis.   The course is progressive and usually leads to death 15 to 20 years after diagnosis. Suicide is common.

H. Treatment. Institutionalization may be needed as chorea progresses. Symptoms of insomnia, anxiety, and depression can be relieved with benzodiazepines and antidepressants. Psychotic symptoms can be treated with high-potency antipsychotics or serotonin-dopamine antagonists. Genetic counseling is the most important intervention.

X. Parkinson's disease

A. Definition. An idiopathic movement disorder with onset usually late in life, characterized by bradykinesia, resting tremor, pill-rolling tremor, masklike face, cogwheel rigidity, and shuffling gait. Intellectual impairment is common, and 40–80% of patients become demented. Depression is extremely common.

B. Epidemiology. Annual prevalence in the Western Hemisphere is 200 cases per 100,000 persons.

C. Etiology. Unknown for most patients. Characteristic findings are decreased cells in the substantia nigra, decreased dopamine, and degeneration of dopaminergic tracts. Parkinsonism can be caused by repeated head trauma and a contaminant of an illicitly made synthetic heroin, N-methyl-4-phenyl-1,2,3,6-tetrahydropyridine (MPTP).

D. Treatment. Levodopa (Larodopa) is a dopamine precursor and is often prepared with carbidopa (Sinemet), a dopa decarboxylase inhibitor, to increase brain dopamine levels. Amantadine (Symadine) has also been used synergistically with levodopa. Some surgeons have tried implanting adrenal medulla tissue into the brain to produce dopamine, with equivocal results. Depression is treatable with antidepressants or ECT.

XI. Other dementias

See Table 4–5. Other dementias include those associated with Wilson's disease, supranuclear palsy, normal-pressure hydrocephalus (dementia, ataxia, incontinence), brain tumors, Lewy body disease, and Binswanger's disease.

Systemic causes of dementia include thyroid disease, pituitary diseases (Addison's disease and Cushing's disease), liver failure, dialysis, nicotinic acid deficiency (pellagra causes the three Ds: dementia, dermatitis, diarrhea), vitamin B_{12} deficiency, folate deficiency, infections, heavy-metal intoxication, and chronic alcohol abuse.

XII. Amnestic disorder

A. Definition. Impaired recent, short-term memory and long-term memory attributed to a specific organic cause (i.e., drug or medical disease). Patient is normal in other areas of cognition.

B. Diagnosis, signs, and symptoms. Amnestic disorders are diagnosed according to their etiology: amnestic disorder resulting from a general medical condition (Table 4–11), substance-induced persisting amnestic disorder, and amnestic disorder NOS.

C. Etiology. See Table 4–12. Most common form is caused by thiamine deficiency associated with alcohol dependence. May also result from head trauma, surgery, hypoxia, infarction, and herpes simplex encephalitis. Typically, any process that damages certain diencephalic and medial temporal structures (e.g., mamillary bodies, fornix, hippocampus) can cause the disorder.

D. Differential diagnosis. Amnesia also is a part of delirium and dementia, but these disorders involve impairments in many other areas of cognition. Factitious disorders may simulate amnesia, but the amnestic deficits will be inconsistent. Patients with dissociative disorders are more likely to have lost their orientation to self and may have more selective memory deficits than do patients with amnestic disorders. Dissociative disorders are also often associated with emotionally stressful life events involving money, the legal system, or troubled relationships.

E. Treatment. Identify the cause and reverse it if possible; otherwise, institute supportive medical procedures (e.g., fluids, blood pressure maintenance).

XIII. Transient global amnesia

A. Abrupt episodes of profound amnesia in all modalities.

B. Patient is fully alert, distant memory is intact.

C. Usually occurs in late middle age or old age.

D. Usually lasts several hours.

TABLE 4–11
DSM-IV-TR DIAGNOSTIC CRITERIA FOR AMNESTIC DISORDER DUE TO A GENERAL MEDICAL CONDITION

A. The development of memory impairment as manifested by impairment in the ability to learn new information or the inability to recall previously learned information.
B. The memory disturbance causes significant impairment in social or occupational functioning and represents a significant decline from a previous level of functioning.
C. The memory disturbance does not occur exclusively during the course of a delirium or a dementia.
D. There is evidence from the history, physical examination, or laboratory findings that the disturbance is the direct physiologic consequence of a general medical condition (including physical trauma).

Specify if:
   Transient: if memory impairment lasts for 1 month or less.
   Chronic: if memory impairment lasts for more than 1 month.

Coding note: Include the name of the general medical condition on Axis I, e.g., amnestic disorder due to head trauma: also code the general medical condition on Axis III.

From American Psychiatric Association. *Diagnostic and Statistical Manual of Mental Disorders.* Text revision, 4th ed. Washington, DC: American Psychiatric Association, Copyright 2000, with permission.

TABLE 4–12
MAJOR CAUSES OF AMNESTIC DISORDERS

Systemic medical conditions	Hypoxia (including nonfatal hanging attempts
Thiamine deficiency (Korsokoff's syndrome)	and carbon monoxide poisoning)
Hypoglycemia	Transient global amnesia
Primary brain conditions	Electroconvulsive therapy
Seizures	Multiple sclerosis
Head trauma (closed and penetrating)	**Substances**
Cerebral tumors (especially thalamic and	Alcohol
temporal lobe)	Neurotoxins
Cerebrovascular diseases (especially thalamic	Benzodiazepines (and other sedative-hypnotics)
and temporal lobe)	Many over-the-counter preparations
Surgical procedures on the brain	
Encephalitis due to herpes simplex	

E. Patient is bewildered and confused after an episode and may repeatedly ask others about what happened.

F. Usually associated with cerebrovascular disease, but also with episodic medical conditions (e.g., seizures).

XIV. Mental disorders resulting from a general medical condition

The disorders are characterized by a medical condition (e.g., cerebrovascular disease, head trauma) that directly causes psychiatric symptoms (e.g., catatonia, depression, anxiety). (The medical condition is coded on Axis III.) Causes include endocrinopathies, deficiency states, connective tissue diseases, CNS disorders, and toxic effects of medication. Some disorders caused by a general medical condition include amnestic, psychotic, mood, anxiety, and sleep disorders; personality change; and sexual dysfunction. Similar to functional diagnoses except that prominent symptoms are caused by a specific organic factor; patient is normal in other areas of cognition.

XV. Other disorders that cause psychiatric syndromes

A. **Degenerative disorders.** Disorders of the basal ganglia that are commonly associated with movement disorders and depression, dementia, and psychosis:
   1. Parkinson's disease—see prior discussion.
   2. Huntington's disease—see prior discussion.
   3. Wilson's disease—autosomal recessive disease that results in destruction of lenticular nuclei.
   4. Fahr's disease—rare hereditary disorder involving calcification and destruction of the basal ganglia.

B. **Epilepsy**
   1. Ictal and postictal confusional syndromes.
   2. Prevalence of psychosis in epilepsy is 7%.
   3. Epilepsy is three to seven times more common in psychotic patients.
   4. Lifetime prevalence of psychosis in epileptics is 10%.
   5. Seizures versus pseudoseizures (Table 4–13).
   6. Temporal lobe epilepsy (TLE).
      a. TLE is the most likely type to produce psychiatric symptoms.
      b. Often involves schizophrenia-like psychosis.

TABLE 4–13
CLINICAL FEATURES DISTINGUISHING SEIZURES AND PSEUDOSEIZURES[a]

Feature	Seizure	Pseudoseizure
Aura	Common stereotyped	Rare
Timing	Nocturnal common	Only when awake
Incontinence	Common	Rare
Cyanosis	Common	Rare
Postictal confusion	Yes	No
Body movement	Tonic or clonic	Nonstereotyped and asynchronous
Self-injury	Common	Rare
EEG	May be abnormal	Normal
Affected by suggestion	No	Yes
Secondary gain	No	Yes

[a] Some patients with organic seizure disorders may also have pseudoseizures.

    c. Often difficult to distinguish from schizophrenia with aggressiveness.

    d. Varied and complex auras that may masquerade as functional illness (e.g., hallucinations, depersonalization, derealization).

    e. Automatisms, autonomic effects, and visceral sensations (e.g., epigastric aura, stomach churning, salivation, flushing, tachycardia, dizziness).

    f. Altered perceptual experiences (e.g., distortions, hallucinations, depersonalization, feeling remote, feeling something has a peculiar significance [*déjà vu, jamais vu*]).

    g. Hallucinations of taste and smell are common and may be accompanied by lip smacking or pursing, chewing, or tasting and swallowing movements.

    h. Subjective disorders of thinking and memory.

    i. Strong affective experiences, most commonly fear and anxiety.

C. Brain tumors

1. Neurological signs, headache, nausea, vomiting, seizures, visual loss, papilledema, virtually any psychiatric symptoms are possible.

2. Symptoms often are caused by raised intracranial pressure or mass effects rather than by direct effects of tumor.

3. Suicidal ideation is present in 10% of patients, usually during headache paroxysms.

4. Although rarely seen in a psychiatric practice, most patients with brain tumors have psychiatric symptoms.

    a. Slow tumors produce personality change.

    b. Rapid tumors produce cognitive change.

5. Frontal lobe tumors—depression, inappropriate affect, disinhibition, dementia, impaired coordination, psychotic symptoms. Often misdiagnosed as primary degenerative dementia; neurological signs often are absent. May have bowel or bladder incontinence.

6. Temporal lobe tumors—anxiety, depression, hallucinations (especially gustatory and olfactory), TLE symptoms, schizophrenia-like psychosis. May have impaired memory and speech.

7. Parietal lobe tumors—fewer psychiatric symptoms (anosognosia, apraxia, aphasia); may be mistaken for hysteria.

8. Colloid cysts—not a tumor. Located in third ventricle and can place pressure on diencephalon. Can produce depression, psychosis, mood lability, and personality change. Classically produces position-dependent intermittent headaches.

D. Head trauma

1. Wide range of acute and chronic clinical pictures.

2. Duration of disorientation is an approximate guide to prognosis.

3. Brain imaging shows classic *contrecoup* lesion, edema acutely.

4. Acute—amnesia (posttraumatic amnesia often resolves abruptly), agitation, withdrawn behavior, psychosis (acute posttraumatic psychosis), delirium.

5. Chronic—amnesia, psychosis, mood disorder, personality change, and (rarely) dementia.

6. Factors affecting course—premorbid personality, epilepsy (very strongly affects work ability), environment, litigation, emotional repercussion of injury, response to intellectual losses, and amount and location of brain damage.

7. Generally, the patient's coping mechanisms may affect the eventual course much more than the actual amount of brain damage.

E. Demyelinating disorders

1. Multiple sclerosis

a. More common in Northern Hemisphere.

b. Psychiatric changes are common (75%).

c. Depression is seen early in course.

d. Later, with frontal lobe involvement, disinhibition and manic-like symptoms occur, including euphoria.

e. Intellectual deterioration is common (60%), ranging from mild memory loss to dementia.

f. Psychosis is reported, but rates are unclear.

g. Hysteria is common, especially late in disease.

h. Symptoms are exacerbated by physical or emotional trauma.

i. MRI is needed for workup.

2. Amyotrophic lateral sclerosis

a. Rare progressive noninherited disease causing asymmetric muscle atrophy.

b. Atrophy of all muscle except cardiac and ocular.

c. Deterioration of anterior horn cells.

d. Rapidly progressive, usually fatal within 4 years.

e. Concomitant dementia rare. Patients with pseudobulbar palsy may show emotional lability.

F. Infectious diseases

1. Herpes encephalitis (herpes simplex virus).
Most common type of local encephalitis; usually affects the frontal and temporal lobes. Neuropsychiatric disorder caused by CNS infection with herpes simplex virus. Symptoms often involve anosmia, olfactory and gustatory hallucinations, personality changes, and bizarre and psychotic behavior; onset usually is sudden or rapid. (Microcephaly, mental retardation, intracranial calcification, and ocular abnormalities may result from infection during birth.)

a. **Laboratory tests.** EEG abnormalities in the acute stage include slowing (diffuse or focal) and high-voltage sharp waves in the temporal regions. CT, MRI, and SPECT often reveal structural changes or reduced blood flow in the temporal lobes and orbitofrontal regions.

b. **Treatment.** Arabinosyladenine reduces mortality and morbidity if initiated early.

2. Rabies encephalitis

a. Incubation period of 10 days to 1 year.

b. Symptoms include restlessness, overactivity, and agitation.

  c. Hydrophobia—an intense fear of drinking water in up to 50% of patients. Fear is caused by severe laryngeal and diaphragmatic spasms that occur when they drink water.

  d. Disease is fatal within days to weeks of development.

3. Neurosyphilis (general paresis)

  a. Appears 10 to 15 years after primary *Treponema* infection.

  b. Rare since penicillin, but now more commonly seen in association with AIDS.

  c. Frontal lobes usually affected.

4. Chronic meningitis

  a. Seen in association with AIDS.

  b. Usual causes are *Mycobacterium tuberculosis, Cryptococcus,* and *Coccidia.*

  c. Usual symptoms include memory impairment, confusion, fever, and headache.

5. Subacute sclerosing panencephalitis

  a. Disease of early childhood with male-to-female ratio of 3:1.

  b. Onset follows measles infection or vaccine.

  c. Initial symptoms may be behavioral change, temper tantrums, sleepiness, hallucinations.

  d. Progresses to myoclonus, ataxia, seizures, and intellectual deterioration.

  e. Outcome is coma, then death within 1 to 2 years.

G. Immune disorders

 1. AIDS. The major immune disorder in contemporary society. See Chapter 5.

 2. Systemic lupus erythematosus (SLE)

  a. One of the autoimmune diseases with direct CNS involvement (others include polyarteritis nodosa and temporal arteritis).

  b. Mental symptoms are common (approximately 50%) and may occur early.

  c. No characteristic form or pattern.

  d. Delirium is the most common mental syndrome.

  e. Psychotic depression is more common than schizophrenia-like features.

  f. May progress to dementia.

  g. Seizures are common (50%), including grand mal and temporal lobe types.

  h. A variety of movement disorders.

  i. Treatment with corticosteroids may induce further psychiatric complications, including psychosis and mania.

H. Endocrine disorders

 1. Thyroid disorders

  a. Hyperthyroidism

   (1) Can cause confusion, anxiety and agitated depression, mania, hallucinations, delusions, and cognitive impairments.

   (2) Common symptoms: weariness, fatigue, weight loss with increased appetite, tremulousness, palpitations.

b. Hypothyroidism

    (1) Myxedema can cause paranoia, depression, hypomania, hallu-
cinations, slowed thinking, and delirium (myxedema madness).

    (2) Physical symptoms include weight gain; thin, dry hair; cold in-
tolerance; deep voice; impaired hearing.

    (3) Ten percent of patients have residual neuropsychiatric impair-
ments after hormone replacement.

    (4) Subtle, subclinical hypothyroidism may resemble refractory
mood disorders.

2. Parathyroid disorders. Hypoparathyroidism causes hypercalcemia.

    a. Can result in delirium and personality change.

    b. Muscle weakness, reduced reflexes may also be seen.

    c. Symptoms of hypocalcemia include cataract formation, seizures,
extrapyramidal symptoms, and increased intracranial pressure.

3. Adrenal disorders

    a. Addison's disease—adrenal insufficiency.

        (1) Most common causes are adrenocortical atrophy or tubercular
or fungal infection.

        (2) Patients may have apathy, irritability, fatigue, and depression.

        (3) Rarely have confusion or psychosis.

        (4) Treatment with cortisone or the equivalent is usually effective.

    b. Cushing's syndrome

        (1) Excessive cortisol produced by an adrenocortical tumor or hy-
perplasia.

        (2) Causes secondary mood disorder of agitated depression and of-
ten suicide.

        (3) Patient may have memory deficits, decreased concentration,
psychosis.

        (4) Physical findings include truncal obesity, moon facies, buffalo
hump, purple striae, hirsutism, and excessive bruising.

I. Metabolic disorders

    1. Common cause of organic brain dysfunction.

    2. Consider in the presence of recent and rapid change in behavior, think-
ing, and consciousness.

    3. Metabolic encephalopathies can progress from delirium to stupor,
coma, and death.

    4. Hepatic encephalopathy can cause changes in memory, personality,
and intellectual skills. Changes in consciousness range from drowsiness to apathy to coma. Common features include asterixis, hyperventilation, and EEG abnormalities.

    5. Uremia—alterations in memory, orientation, and consciousness. As-
sociated symptoms are restlessness, crawling sensations, muscle
twitching, persistent hiccups.

    6. Hypoglycemic encephalopathy—caused by excessive endogenous or
exogenous insulin. Symptoms may include nausea, sweating, tachy-

cardia, hunger, restlessness, apprehension and hallucinations. A persistent residual dementia sometimes develops.

7. Acute intermittent porphyria—autosomal dominant disorder of heme biosynthesis resulting in accumulation of porphyrins. Onset is between the ages of 20 and 50; more women than men are affected. Symptom triad is abdominal pain, motor polyneuropathy, and psychosis. Other psychiatric symptoms include anxiety, lability, and depression. Barbiturates can precipitate and aggravate the disorder and are contraindicated.

J. Nutritional disorders

1. Niacin (nicotinic acid) deficiency

a. Associated with pellagra, a nutritional deficiency disease associated with vegetarian diets, alcohol abuse, poverty.

b. Three *d*s: dementia, dermatitis, diarrhea.

c. Other symptoms: irritability, insomnia, depression, peripheral neuropathies.

d. Good response to treatment with nicotinic acid, but patient may have permanent dementia.

2. Thiamine (vitamin B_1) deficiency

a. Beriberi—secondary to familial poverty; causes neurological and cardiovascular symptoms.

b. Wernicke-Korsakoff syndrome—caused by chronic alcohol abuse or dependence.

c. Symptoms include apathy, irritability, anxiety, depression, and severe memory impairment if deficiency is prolonged.

3. Vitamin B_{12} deficiency

a. Caused by failure of gastric mucosa to secrete intrinsic factor.

b. Chronic macrocytic megaloblastic anemia (pernicious anemia).

c. Neurological changes in 30% of patients.

d. Apathy, depression, irritability common.

e. Encephalopathy with associated delirium, dementia, and psychotic symptoms (megaloblastic madness).

f. Parenteral vitamin therapy early in course can arrest neurologic symptoms.

K. Toxins

1. Lead.
Abdominal colic, lead neuropathy, lead encephalopathy. May present suddenly as delirium, seizures, elevated blood pressure, impaired memory and concentration, headache, tremor, deafness, transient aphasia, and hemianopsia. Depression, weakness, vertigo, hyperesthesia for visual and auditory stimuli. Treatment with calcium lactate, milk, chelating agents.

2. Mercury.
Mad hatter's syndrome (thermometers, photoengravers, ore workers, fingerprinters, chemical workers, repairers of electric meters, felt hat industry)—gastritis, bleeding gums, excessive salivation, coarse tremor with jerky movements. Patients are irritable and quarrelsome, lose temper easily, and have cognitive impairments.

3. **Manganese** (ore workers, dry batteries, bleaching, welding). Headache; asthenia; torpor; hypersomnia; erectile dysfunction; uncontrollable laughter and crying; impulses to run, dance, sing, or talk; may commit senseless crimes. Parkinsonism develops later.

4. **Arsenic** (fur and glass industries, insecticides). Long-term exposure—dermatitis, conjunctivitis, lacrimation, anorexia, headache, vertigo, apathy, drowsiness, intellectual impairment, peripheral neuritis. May eventually present as Korsakoff's psychosis.

5. **Thallium** (from pesticides). Tingling, abdominal pain, vomiting, headache, tachycardia, gastritis, offensive breath, alopecia, ataxia, paresthesias, peripheral neuropathy, retrobulbar neuritis, tremor, chorea, athetosis, myoclonic jerking, impaired consciousness, depression, seizures, delirium.

For a more detailed discussion of this topic, see Delirium, Dementia, and Amnestic and Other Cognitive Disorders, Ch 10, p 854, in CTP/VII.

V. Neurobiological aspects of HIV infection

A. Introduction. An extensive array of disease processes can affect the brain of HIV-infected patients, even in the absence of other signs or symptoms of AIDS. Primary neurobiological complications are those attributed directly to the virus itself. Secondary complications are those that arise from HIV-associated illnesses and treatments. Mental disorders associated with HIV infection include dementia, acute psychosis, mood disorder, and personality change resulting from a general medical condition. Diseases that occasionally cause dementia in patients with AIDS include cerebral toxoplasmosis, cryptococcal meningitis, and primary brain lymphoma. The neurobiological complications of HIV-1 infection are listed in Table 5–6.

B. Neurocognitive disorders. In HIV infection of brain macrophage microglia, neurotoxins are produced that ultimately cause neuronal injury. Cardinal features include impaired cognition, motor slowing, incoordination, and mood disturbances. Table 5–7 summarizes HIV-1 cognitive disorders.

1. **Asymptomatic neurocognitive impairment.** Subclinical neuropsychological impairments that do not affect functioning.

2. **Mild neurocognitive disorder.** Asymptomatic and mild neurocognitive disorders occur in 50% of AIDS patients. Prevalence increases with disease progression. These conditions appear to be stable or slowly progressive. Typical features includes difficulty concentrating, subjective slowing, mental fatigability, subjective memory loss, slowing of

---

TABLE 5–6
NEUROBIOLOGICAL COMPLICATIONS OF HIV-1 INFECTION

I. Primary neurobiological complications
  A. HIV-1 neurocognitive disorders
    1. Asymptomatic neurocognitive impairment
    2. HIV-1 mild neurocognitive disorder
    3. HIV-1–associated dementia
  B. Other HIV-1 neurobiological complications
    1. HIV-1 meningitis
    2. HIV-1 vacuolar myelopathy
    3. HIV-1 neuropathies
      a. Acute demyelinating (Guillain-Barré) syndrome
      b. Relapsing or progressive demyelinating disease (e.g., mononeuritis multiplex)
      c. Predominantly sensory polyneuropathy
    4. HIV-1 myopathy
II. Secondary neurobiological complications (generally causing delirium)
  A. Infections
    1. *Toxoplasma* encephalitis/abscess
    2. *Cryptococcus* meningitis
    3. Cytomegalovirus (CMV) encephalitis
    4. Progressive multifocal leukoencephalopathy
    5. Other infections of the CNS
  B. Neoplasia
    1. Primary or secondary CNS lymphoma
    2. Kaposi's sarcoma of the CNS
    3. Other neoplasia
  C. Cerebrovascular disease related to HIV infection
  D. Other delirium
    1. Adverse effects of drugs
    2. Hypoxemia, hypercapnia (e.g., with *Pneumocytis carinii* pneumonia)
    3. Other metabolic and nutritional disorders

Table by Igor Grant, M.D., F.R.C.P.(C), and J. Hampton Atkinson, Jr., M.D.

TABLE 5-7
HIV-1–ASSOCIATED COGNITIVE DISORDERS

As Defined by Grant and Atkinson	As Proposed by American Academy of Neurology (AAN) Working Group
HIV-1–associated neurocognitive disorders	HIV-1–associated cognitive/motor complex
A. HIV-1–associated dementia	A. Probable[b] HIV-1–associated dementia complex
1. *Marked acquired impairment in cognitive functioning,* involving at least two ability domains (e.g., memory, attention); typically the impairment is in multiple domains, especially in learning of new information, slowed information processing, and defective attention or concentration. The cognitive impairment can be ascertained by history, mental status examination, or neuropsychological testing.	1. *Acquired abnormality in at least two of the following cognitive abilities* (present for at least 1 month): attention/concentration; speed of information processing; abstraction/reasoning; visuospatial skills; memory/learning; speech/language. *Cognitive dysfunction causes impairment in work or activities of daily living.*
2. The cognitive impairment produces *marked interference with day-to-day functioning* (work, home life, social activities).	2. At least one of the following: a. Acquired abnormality in motor functioning. b. Decline in motivation or emotional control or change in social behavior.
3. The marked cognitive impairment has been present for at least 1 month.	3. Absence of clouding of consciousness during a period long enough to establish presence of No. 1.
4. The pattern of cognitive impairment *does not meet criteria for delirium* (e.g., clouding of consciousness is not a prominent feature); or, if delirium is present, criteria for dementia need to have been met on a prior examination when delirium was not present.	4. Absence of another cause of the above cognitive, motor, or behavioral symptoms or signs (e.g., active CNS opportunistic infection or malignancy, psychiatric disorders, substance abuse).
5. There is *no evidence of another, preexisting cause* that could explain the dementia (e.g., other CNS infection, CNS neoplasm, cerebrovascular disease, preexisting neurological disease, or severe substance abuse compatible with CNS disorder).	
B. HIV-1–associated mild neurocognitive disorder (MND)	B. Probable[b] HIV-1–associated minor cognitive/motor disorder
1. Acquired impairment in cognitive functioning, involving at least two ability domains, documented by performance of at least 1.0 standard deviation below the mean for age- or education-appropriate norms on standardized neuropsychological tests. The neuro-psychological assessment must survey at least the following abilities: verbal/language; attention/speeded processing; abstraction/executive; memory (learning, recall); complex perceptual-motor performance; motor skills.	1. Acquired cognitive/motor/behavior abnormalities (must have both *a* and *b*) a. At least two of the following symptoms present for at least 1 month verified by a reliable history: (1) Impaired attention or concentration. (2) Mental slowing. (3) Impaired memory. (4) Slowed movements. (5) Incoordination. b. Acquired cognitive/motor abnormality verified by clinical neurological examination or neuropsychological testing.
2. The cognitive impairment produces at least mild interference in daily functioning (at least one of the following): a. Self-report of reduced mental acuity, inefficiency in work, homemaking, or social functioning. b. Observation by knowledgeable others that the individual has undergone at least mild decline in mental acuity with resultant inefficiency in work, homemaking, or social functioning.	2. Cognitive/motor/behavioral abnormality causes mild impairment of work or activities of daily living (objectively verifiable or by report of key informant).
3. The cognitive impairment has been present for at least 1 month.	3. Absence of another cause of the above cognitive/motor/behavioral abnormality (e.g., active CNS opportunistic infection or malignancy, psychiatric disorders, substance abuse).

TABLE 5–7—*continued*

As Defined by Grant and Atkinson	As Proposed by American Academy of Neurology (AAN) Working Group
4. Does not meet criteria for delirium or dementia.	
5. There is no evidence of another preexisting cause for the MND.[a]	

[a] If the individual with suspected MND also satisfies criteria for a major depressive episode or substance dependence, the diagnosis of MND should be deferred to a subsequent examination conducted at a time when the major depression has remitted or at least 1 month has elapsed following termination of dependent substance use.

[b] The designation *probable* is used when criteria are met, there is no other likely cause, and data are complete. The designation *possible* is used if another potential cause is present whose contribution is unclear, when a dual diagnosis is possible, or if the evaluation is not complete.

Table by Igor Grant, M.D., F.R.C.P.(C), and J. Hampton Atkinson, Jr., M.D.

simple motor performance, and difficulties with problem solving and abstract reasoning. Neuropsychological findings are consistent with subcortical deficits. The rate of CD4+ decline may be related to the severity of cognitive impairment. The CSF viral load may correlate with severity. The results of electroencephalogram (EEG) and brain imaging studies are usually normal.

3. **Dementia.** More profound abnormalities include severe forgetfulness, poor concentration, marked mental slowing, and problems with naming and word finding. Major deficits are present on neuropsychological tests, even if the Mini-Mental State Examination results are mildly abnormal. Dementia can progress to severe apathy, confusion, and total disability. Neurologic findings include frontal lobe release signs, hyperreflexia, incoordination, and motor weakness. Brain imaging may reveal cerebral atrophy and white matter lucencies on computed tomography (CT) and abnormal areas of high signal on magnetic resonance imaging (MRI), in addition to metabolic abnormalities on positron emission tomography (PET) and single-photon emission computed tomography (SPECT). EEG reveals slowing. The CSF examination reveals high levels of β_2-microglobulin and increased levels of neopterin and quinolinic acid. The size of the CSF viral load is related to the severity of dementia. Neuropathological examination reveals multinucleated giant cells, microglial nodules, perivascular infiltrate, and demyelination. The development of dementia is a poor prognostic sign, with 50–75% of patients dying within 6 months. The incidence of dementia has declined substantially with the use of antiviral therapy.

C. **Psychiatric syndromes**

1. **Delirium.** Can result from the same variety of causes that lead to dementia in HIV-infected patients. Delirium is probably underdiagnosed.

2. **Anxiety disorders.** Patients with HIV infection may have any of the anxiety disorders, but generalized anxiety disorder, posttraumatic stress disorder, and obsessive-compulsive disorder are particularly common.

3. **Adjustment disorder.** Adjustment disorder with anxiety or depressed mood reportedly occurs in 5–20% of HIV-infected patients.

4. **Depressive disorders.** The range of HIV-infected patients reported to meet the diagnostic criteria for depressive disorders is 4–40%.

5. **Substance abuse.** Patients may be tempted to use drugs regularly in an attempt to deal with depression or anxiety.

6. **Suicide.** Suicidal ideation and suicide attempts may be increased in patients with HIV infection and AIDS. The risk factors for suicide are having friends who died of AIDS-related causes, recent notification of HIV seropositivity relapse, difficult social issues relating to homosexuality, inadequate social and financial support, and dementia or delirium and substance abuse.

7. **Worried well.** Persons in high-risk groups who, although they are seronegative and disease-free, are anxious or have an obsession about contracting the virus. Symptoms can include generalized anxiety, panic attacks, obsessive-compulsive disorder, and hypochondriasis. Repeated negative serum test results can reassure some patients. For those who cannot be reassured, psychotherapy or pharmacotherapy may be indicated.

VI. Treatment

A. **Prevention.**   All persons at any risk for HIV infection should be informed about safe sex practices and the need to avoid sharing hypodermic needles. Preventive strategies are complicated by the complex societal values surrounding sexual acts, sexual orientation, birth control, and substance abuse.

1. **Safe sex.** A common question that physicians should be prepared to answer is, "What is safe and unsafe sex?" Patients should be advised about the guidelines listed in Table 5–8, which should be followed.

TABLE 5–8
AIDS SAFE SEX GUIDELINES

Remember: Any activity that allows for exchange of body fluids of one person and the mouth, anus, vagina, bloodstream, cuts, or sores of another person is considered *unsafe* at this time.

Safe sex practices
Massage, hugging, body-to-body rubbing
Dry social kissing
Masturbation
Acting out sexual fantasies (that do not include any unsafe sex practices)
Using vibrators or other instruments (provided they are not shared)

Low-risk sex practices (these activities are not considered completely safe)
French (wet) kissing (without mouth sores)
Mutual masturbation
Vaginal and anal intercourse with a condom
Oral sex, male (fellatio) with a condom
Oral sex, female (cunnilingus), with barrier
External contact with semen or urine provided there are no breaks in the skin

Unsafe sex practices
Vaginal or anal intercourse without a condom
Semen, urine, or feces in the mouth or vagina
Unprotected oral sex (fellatio or cunnilingus)
Blood contact of any kind
Sharing sex instruments or needles

From Moffatt B, Spiegel J, Parrish S, Helquist M. *AIDS: A Self-Care Manual.* Santa Monica, CA: IBS Press, 1987;125, with permission.

TABLE 5–9
ANTIRETROVIRAL AGENTS

Generic Name	Trade Name	Usual Abbreviation
Nucleoside reverse transcriptase inhibitors		
Zidovudine	Retrovir	AZT or ZDV
Didanosine	Videx	ddl
Zalcitabine	Hivid	ddC
Stavudine	Zerit	d4T
Lamivudine	Epivir	3TC
Abacavir	Ziagen	
Nonnucleoside reverse transcriptase inhibitors		
Nevirapine	Viramune	
Delavirdine	Rescriptor	
Efavirenz	Sustiva	
Protease inhibitors		
Saquinavir	Invirase, Fortovase	
Ritonavir	Norvir	
Indinavir	Crixivan	
Nelfinavir	Viracept	
Amprenavir	Agenerase	

Adapted from Igor Grant, M.D., F.R.C.P.(C), and J. Hampton Atkinson, Jr., M.D.

   2. Postexposure prophylaxis. Prompt administration of antiretroviral therapy following exposure to HIV can reduce the likelihood of infection developing by 80%. Combination treatment with zidovudine (Retrovir) and lamivudine (Epivir) for 4 weeks is usually recommended.
 B. Pharmacotherapy
   1. Antiretroviral therapy (Table 5–9). The goal of antiretroviral therapy is full viral suppression, as the viral load governs the rate of CD4-cell decline. Combination therapy with agents that act at different points in viral transcription has become standard. The two classes of agents used are the reverse transcriptase inhibitors of the nucleoside and nonnucleoside types and the protease inhibitors. Treatment is recommended when plasma HIV RNA levels are more than 5,000 to 10,000 copies per mL, regardless of the CD4-cell count. Triple therapy is recommended to cover all possible resistant HIV genotypes. Strict adherence to complex treatment regimens is required for efficacy and to prevent emergence of resistance. Drug combinations are used based on mechanism of action and drug–drug interactions. Indications for changing treatment include upswing in viral load toxicity, nonadherence, and medication intolerance. These agents are used in combination with drugs that prevent or treat the HIV-associated complications caused by various opportunistic infections. Antiviral therapy and aggressive prophylaxis and treatment of opportunistic infections have greatly increased the longevity and quality of life of HIV-infected patients.
   2. Antiretroviral therapy of neurocognitive disorders. High-dosage zidovudine monotherapy can be used to treat HIV-associated neurocognitive impairment in part because of its good blood–brain barrier penetration. Stavudine (Zerit) and nevirapine (Viramune) show reasonable CSF concentrations. Despite their inability to penetrate the blood-brain barrier, protease inhibitors in combination with earlier-gen-

eration agents such as zidovudine appear to prevent or reverse the progression of HIV-related neurocognitive disorders. A significant percentage of patients show improvement on neuropsychological testing and improvement in pattern and severity of white matter signal abnormalities on MRI within 2 to 3 months of beginning therapy.

3. **Drug therapy of HIV-associated psychiatric syndromes.** Psychiatric syndromes associated with HIV should be treated as they would be in non–HIV-infected persons. In patients with more advanced HIV-related disease, lower drug doses should be used (initial doses of one half to one fourth of the usual starting doses) because of their heightened sensitivity to side effects. Agitation associated with delirium and dementia or psychosis can be treated with low doses of high-potency antipsychotics (e.g., 0.5 mg of haloperidol [Haldol] initially) or serotonin-dopamine antagonists (e.g., 0.25 mg of risperidone [Risperdal] initially, 2.5 mg of olanzapine [Zyprexa] initially). One must be aware of the increased risk for anticholinergic delirium, seizures, and extrapyramidal side effects in this population. Patients with neurocognitive syndromes may benefit from psychostimulants (e.g., 2.5 mg of methylphenidate twice a day with slow increases up to 20 mg/d). Depression may also be treated with stimulants if a rapid response is required or typical antidepressants are not effective. For depression, selective serotonin reuptake inhibitors (SSRIs) are typically used, or tricyclics with the lowest possible anticholinergic burden, such as desipramine (Norpramin, Pertofrane). Injections of up to 400 mg of testosterone (DEPO-Testosterone) biweekly for 8 weeks may be effective for major depression and fatigue–anergia syndromes. Electroconvulsive therapy has also been effective. Anxiety states are generally treated with benzodiazepines of short or medium half-life or buspirone (BuSpar). Manic states can be treated with lithium or anticonvulsant mood stabilizers. It appears that the anticonvulsants are better tolerated than lithium in this population. Mania secondary to zidovudine has been successfully treated with lithium to allow continuation of zidovudine. Medical, environmental, and social support are needed in addition to pharmacotherapy.

4. **Interactions of psychotropic drugs and antiretroviral drugs.** Protease inhibitors are metabolized primarily by cytochrome isoenzyme P450 3A (CYP 3A) and secondarily by the 2D6 system. These pathways are shared by many psychotropic drugs. It is good practice to anticipate drug interactions and monitor patients for treatment-related emergent adverse events and, when possible, check plasma drug concentrations. All protease inhibitors increase psychotropic drug concentrations if the major route of metabolism of the psychotropic is the CYP 3A system. If 2D6 is the primary route of metabolism, as it is for SSRIs and tricyclics, then ritonavir (Norvir) will specifically inhibit their metabolism. Protease inhibitors may inhibit the metabolism of antidepressants, antipsychotics, and benzodiazepines. Alprazolam (Xanax), midazolam (Versed), triazolam (Halcion), and zolpidem (Ambiem) concentrations may be increased, and dosage reductions may be needed to prevent

oversedation. Protease inhibitors have been reported to increase levels of bupropion (Wellbutrin), nefazodone (Serzone), and fluoxetine (Prozac) to toxic levels and to increase desipramine levels by 100% to 150%. Zidovudine in particular may increase the blood concentration of antipsychotics. Levels of methadone (Dolophine, Methadose) and meperidine (Demerol) may also be elevated. Carbamazepine (Tegretol) and phenobarbital (Solfoton) may reduce serum concentrations of protease inhibitors. Nefazodone and fluoxetine have been reported to re-

TABLE 5-10
NEUROPSYCHIATRIC SIDE EFFECTS OF THERAPEUTIC DRUGS FOR HIV

Agent	Effects
Antiinfective	
Acyclovir	Depressed mood, agitation, auditory and visual hallucinations, depersonalization, tearfulness, confusion, hyperesthesia, hyperacusis, insomnia, thought insertion, headache
Amphotericin-β	Delirium
Cephalosporins	Confusion, disorientation, paranoia
Cycloserine	Anxiety, confusion, depression, disorientation, hallucinations, paranoia, loss of appetite, fatigue
Dapsone	Agitation, hallucinations, insomnia
Didanosine	Mania
Ethambutol	Headache, dizziness, confusion, visual disturbances
Ethionamide	Depression, drowsiness, hallucinations, neuritis
5-Flucytosine	Delirium, headache, persisting neurocognitive impairment
Indinavir	Insomnia
Isoniazid	Depression, agitation, hallucinations, paranoia
Ketoconazole	Dizziness, headache, photosensitivity
Lamivudine	Possible depressed mood
Metronidazole	Depression, agitation, delirium, seizures
Nelfinavir	Anxiety, possible depressed mood, insomnia
Pentamidine	Delirium, hallucinations
Rifampin	Headache, fatigue, loss of appetite
Ritonavir	Agitation, anxiety, confusion, hallucinations, possible depressed mood
Saquinavir	Anxiety, irritability, hallucinations
Sulfonamides	Headache, neuritis, insomnia, loss of appetite, photosensitivity
Thiabendazole	Hallucinations
Trimethoprim-sulfamethoxazole	Delirium, mutism, depression, loss of appetite, insomnia, apathy, headache, neuritis
Zalcitabine	Agitation, anxiety, mania, hallucinations
Zidovudine	Depressed mood, agitation, headache, myalgia, insomnia, mania
Antineoplastic	Delirium
Methotrexate	Mania
Procarbazine	Depression, loss of appetite, headache, neuritis
Vinblastine	Ataxia, headache, hallucinations, neuritis
Vincristine	Depression, weakness, anergic-apathetic states
Interferon alfa	
Other	Visual hallucinations
Amantadine	Excitement, hyperactivity, hallucinations, depression
Barbiturates	Delirium, drowsiness, amnesia, excitement
Benzodiazepines	Confusion, depression, hallucinations, mania, paranoia
Corticosteroids	Delirium
Meperidine	Depression, mania
Metoclopramide	Delirium, agitation
Morphine	Confusion, delirium, euphoria
Phenytoin	Drowsiness, mania, delirium, insomnia
Tricyclic antidepressants	

Table by Igor Grant, M.D., F.R.C.P.(C), and J. Hampton Atkinson, Jr., M.D.

duce the metabolism of protease inhibitors, with an increase in protease inhibitor adverse effects. Table 5–10 lists the side effects of HIV drug therapy.

C. Psychotherapy.   The role of both individual and group psychotherapy is important in helping patients deal with issues of self-blame, self-esteem, and possible death. Many patients infected with HIV feel they are being punished for a deviant lifestyle. Difficult health care decisions (e.g., regarding antiretroviral drugs, terminal care, and life support systems) should be explored. In addition, all infectious persons must be educated concerning safe sex practices. Involving the patient's spouse or lover is often warranted. The treatment of gay and bisexual persons with AIDS involves helping them approach their families and deal with possible issues of rejection, guilt, and anger. Practical themes involve employment, medical benefits, life insurance, career plans, dating and sex, and relationships with family and friends.

The advent of protease inhibitors and hope for a cure have brought about new therapeutic tasks, such as dealing with unrealistic expectations, fears of treatment failure, and anger over not responding to regimens that have benefited others. The possibility of avoiding death from AIDS—the so-called second-life agenda—has created new challenges for both patients and caregivers.

For more detailed discussion of this topic, see Neuropsychiatric Aspects of HIV Infection and AIDS, Sec 2.8, p 308, in CTP/VII.

friends or relatives have told the patient to cut down on drinking. Always look for subtle signs of alcohol abuse, and always inquire about the use of other substances. Physical findings may include palmar erythema, Dupuytren's contractures, and telangiectasia. Does the patient seem to be accident-prone (head injury, rib fracture, motor vehicle accidents)? Is he or she often in fights? Often absent from work? Are there social or family problems? Laboratory assessment can be helpful. Patients may have macrocytic anemia secondary to nutritional deficiencies. Serum liver enzymes and γ-glutamyltransferase (GGT) may be elevated. An elevation of liver enzymes can also be used as a marker of a return to drinking in a previously abstinent patient (Table 6–6).

G. **Treatment.** The goal is the prolonged maintenance of total sobriety. Relapses are common. Initial treatment requires detoxification, on an inpatient basis if necessary, and treatment of any withdrawal symptoms. Coexisting mental disorders should be treated when the patient is sober.

1. **Insight.** Critically necessary but often difficult to achieve. The patient must acknowledge that he or she has a drinking problem. Severe denial may have to be overcome before the patient will cooperate in seeking treatment. Often, this requires the collaboration of family, friends, employers, and others. The patient may need to be confronted with the potential loss of career, family, and health if he or she continues to drink. Individual psychotherapy has been used, but group therapy may

TABLE 6–4
CLINICAL COURSE OF ALCOHOL DEPENDENCE

Age at first drink[a]	13–15 years
Age at first intoxication[a]	15–17 years
Age at first problem[a]	16–22 years
Age at onset of dependence	25–40 years
Age at death	60 years
Fluctuating course of abstention, temporary control, alcohol problems	
Spontaneous remission in 20%	

[a] Same as general population.
Table from Marc A. Schuckitt, M.D.

TABLE 6–5
DSM-IV-TR DIAGNOSTIC CRITERIA FOR ALCOHOL OR SUBSTANCE ABUSE

A. A maladaptive pattern of substance use leading to clinically significant impairment or distress, as manifested by one (or more) of the following, occurring within a 12-month period:
   (1) recurrent substance use resulting in a failure to fulfill major role obligations at work, school, or home (e.g., repeated absences or poor work performance related to substance use; substance-related absences, suspensions, or expulsions from school; neglect of children or household)
   (2) recurrent substance use in situations in which it is physically hazardous (e.g., driving an automobile or operating a machine when impaired by substance use)
   (3) recurrent substance-related legal problems (e.g., arrests for substance-related disorderly conduct)
   (4) continued substance use despite having persistent or recurrent social or interpersonal problems caused or exacerbated by the effects of the substance (e.g., arguments with spouse about consequences of intoxication, physical fights)
B. The symptoms have never met the criteria for substance dependence for this class of substance.

TABLE 6-6
STATE MARKERS OF HEAVY DRINKING USEFUL IN SCREENING FOR ALCOHOLISM

Test	Relevant Range of Results
γ-Glutamyltransferase (GGT)	>30 U/L
Carbohydrate-deficient transferrin (CDT)	>20 mg/L
Mean corpuscular volume (MCV)	>91 μm^3
Uric acid	>6.4 mg/dL for men
	>5.0 mg/dL for women
Aspartate aminotransferase (AST)	>45 IU/L
Alanine aminotransferase (ALT)	>45 IU/L
Triglycerides	>160 mg/dL

Adapted from Marc A. Schuckitt, M.D.

be more effective. Group therapy may also be more acceptable to many patients who perceive alcohol dependence as a social problem rather than a personal psychiatric problem.

2. **Alcoholics Anonymous (AA) and Al-Anon.** Supportive organizations, such as AA (for patients) and Al-Anon (for families of patients), can be effective in maintaining sobriety and helping the family to cope. AA emphasizes the inability of the member to cope alone with addiction to alcohol and encourages dependence on the group for support; AA also utilizes many techniques of group therapy.

3. **Psychosocial interventions.** Often necessary and very effective. Family therapy should focus on describing the effects of alcohol use on other family members. Patients must be forced to relinquish the perception of their right to be able to drink and recognize the detrimental effects on the family.

4. **Psychopharmacotherapy**

   a. **Disulfiram (Antabuse).** A daily dosage of 25 to 500 mg of disulfiram may be used if the patient desires enforced sobriety. The usual dosage is 250 mg/day. Patients taking disulfiram have an extremely unpleasant reaction when they ingest even small amounts of alcohol. The reaction, caused by an accumulation of acetaldehyde resulting from the inhibition of aldehyde dehydrogenase, includes flushing, headache, throbbing in the head and neck, dyspnea, hyperventilation, tachycardia, hypotension, sweating, anxiety, weakness, and confusion. Life-threatening complications, although uncommon, can occur. Patients with preexisting heart disease, cerebral thrombosis, diabetes, and several other conditions cannot take disulfiram because of the risk for a fatal reaction. Disulfiram is useful only temporarily to help establish a long-term pattern of sobriety and to change long-standing alcohol-related coping mechanisms.

   b. **Naltrexone (ReVia).** This agent decreases the craving for alcohol, probably by blocking the release of endogenous opioids, thereby aiding the patient to achieve the goal of abstinence by preventing relapse and decreasing alcohol consumption. A dosage of 50 mg once daily is recommended for most patients.

       c. Other agents. Acamprosate (Campral) in dosages of 2,000 mg/day as part of a comprehensive treatment program appears to increase rates of abstinence. It may affect the γ-aminobutyric acid (GABA) or NMDA systems. It is not yet available in the United States. Buspirone may also be of use in the treatment of alcoholism.

    5. After recovery. Most experts recommend that a recovered alcohol-dependent patient maintain lifelong sobriety and discourage attempts by recovered patients to learn to drink normally. (A dogma of AA is, "It's the first drink that gets you drunk.")

  H. Medical complications. Alcohol is toxic to numerous organ systems. Complications of chronic alcohol abuse and dependence (or associated nutritional deficiencies) are listed in Table 6–7. Alcohol use during pregnancy is toxic to the developing fetus and can cause congenital defects in addition to fetal alcohol syndrome.

III. Alcohol intoxication

  A. Definition. Alcohol intoxication, also called simple drunkenness, is the recent ingestion of a sufficient amount of alcohol to produce acute maladaptive behavioral changes.

  B. Diagnosis, signs, and symptoms. Whereas mild intoxication may produce a relaxed, talkative, euphoric, or disinhibited person, severe intoxication often leads to more maladaptive changes, such as aggressiveness, irritability, labile mood, impaired judgment, and impaired social or work functioning, among others.

    Persons exhibit at least one of the following: slurred speech, incoordination, unsteady gait, nystagmus, memory impairment, stupor, and flushed face. Severe intoxication can lead to withdrawn behavior, psychomotor retardation, blackouts, and eventually obtundation, coma, and death. Common complications of alcohol intoxication include motor vehicle accidents, head injury, rib fracture, criminal acts, homicide, and suicide. Blood alcohol concentrations and corresponding effects are presented in Table 6–8.

    1. Evaluation. A thorough medical evaluation should be conducted; consider a possible subdural hematoma or a concurrent infection. Always evaluate for possible intoxication with other substances. Alcohol is frequently used in combination with other CNS depressants, such as benzodiazepines and barbiturates. The CNS depressant effects of such combinations can be synergistic and potentially fatal.

      An appropriate examination of the patient's mental status and the diagnosis of concurrent mental disorders usually require reevaluation after the patient is no longer intoxicated because almost any psychiatric symptom may acutely be caused by alcohol intoxication. Blood alcohol levels are seldom important in the clinical evaluation (except to determine legal intoxication) because tolerance varies.

    2. Alcohol idiosyncratic intoxication. Maladaptive behavior (often aggressive or assaultive) after the ingestion of a small amount of alcohol that would not cause intoxication in most people (i.e., pathological intoxication). Uncommon and controversial. The behavior

TABLE 6–7
NEUROLOGICAL AND MEDICAL COMPLICATIONS OF ALCOHOL USE

Alcohol intoxication
  Acute intoxication
  Pathological intoxication (atypical, complicated, unusual)
  Blackouts
Alcohol withdrawal syndromes
  Tremulousness (shakes or jitters)
  Alcoholic hallucinosis (horrors)
  Withdrawal seizures (rum fits)
  Delirium tremens (shakes)
Nutritional diseases of the nervous system secondary to alcohol abuse
  Wernicke-Korsakoff syndrome
  Cerebellar degeneration
  Peripheral neuropathy
  Optic neuropathy (tobacco–alcohol amblyopia)
  Pellagra
Alcoholic diseases of uncertain pathogenesis
  Central pontine myelinolysis
  Marchiafava-Bignami disease
  Fetal alcohol syndrome
  Myopathy
  Alcoholic dementia (?)
  Alcoholic cerebral atrophy
Systemic diseases due to alcohol with secondary neurological complications
  Liver disease
    Hepatic encephalopathy
    Acquired (nonwilsonian) chronic hepatocerebral degeneration
  Gastrointestinal diseases
    Malabsorption syndromes
    Postgastrectomy syndromes
    Possible pancreatic encephalopathy
  Cardiovascular diseases
    Cardiomyopathy with potential cardiogenic emboli and cerebrovascular disease
    Arrhythmias and abnormal blood pressure leading to cerebrovascular disease
  Hematologic disorders
    Anemia, leukopenia, thrombocytopenia (could possibly lead to hemorrhagic cerebrovascular
      disease)
  Infectious disease, especially meningitis (especially pneumococcal and meningococcal)
  Hypothermia and hyperthermia
  Hypotension and hypertension
  Respiratory depression and associated hypoxia
  Toxic encephalopathies (alcohol and other substances)
  Electrolyte imbalances leading to acute confusional states and rarely focal neurological signs and
    symptoms
    Hypoglycemia
    Hyperglycemia
    Hyponatremia
    Hypercalcemia
    Hypomagnesemia
    Hypophosphatemia
Increased incidence of trauma
  Epidural, subdural, and intracerebral hematoma
  Spinal cord injury
  Posttraumatic seizure disorders
  Compressive neuropathies and brachial plexus injuries (Saturday night palsies)
  Posttraumatic symptomatic hydrocephalus (normal-pressure hydrocephalus)
  Muscle crush injuries and compartmental syndromes

Reprinted from Rubino FA. Neurologic complications of alcoholism. *Psychiatr Clin North Am* 1992;15:361, with permission.

TABLE 6–8
IMPAIRMENT LIKELY TO BE SEEN AT DIFFERENT BLOOD ALCOHOL CONCENTRATIONS

Level	Likely Impairment
20–30 mg/dL	Slowed motor performance and decreased thinking ability
30–80 mg/dL	Increases in motor and cognitive problems
80–200 mg/dL	Increases in incoordination and judgment errors
	Mood lability
	Deterioration in cognition
200–300 mg/dL	Nystagmus, marked slurring of speech, and alcoholic blackouts
>300 mg/dL	Impaired vital signs and possible death

Table from Marc A. Schuckitt, M.D.

must be atypical for the person when he or she is not drinking. Brain-damaged persons may also be more susceptible to alcohol idiosyncratic intoxication.

C. **Treatment**
   1. Usually only supportive.
   2. May give nutrients (especially thiamine, vitamin B_{12}, folate).
   3. Observation for complications (e.g., combativeness, coma, head injury, falling) may be required.

D. **Blackouts.** Periods of intoxication during which the patient exhibits complete anterograde amnesia and appears awake and alert. They occasionally can last for days, during which the intoxicated person performs complex tasks, such as long-distance travel, with no subsequent recollection. Brain-damaged persons may be more susceptible to blackouts.

IV. **Alcohol-induced psychotic disorder, with hallucinations (previously known as alcohol hallucinosis)**

   Vivid, persistent hallucinations (often visual and auditory), without delirium, following (usually within 2 days) a decrease in alcohol consumption in an alcohol-dependent person. May persist and progress to a more chronic form that is clinically similar to schizophrenia. Rare. The male-to-female ratio is 4:1. The condition usually requires at least 10 years of alcohol dependence. If the patient is agitated, possible treatments include benzodiazepines (e.g., 1 to 2 mg of lorazepam [Ativan] orally or intramuscularly, 5 to 10 mg of diazepam [Valium]) or low doses of a high-potency antipsychotic (e.g., 2 to 5 mg of haloperidol [Haldol] orally or intramuscularly as needed every 4 to 6 hours).

V. **Alcohol withdrawal**

   Begins within several hours after cessation of, or reduction in, prolonged (at least days) heavy alcohol consumption. At least two of the following must be present: autonomic hyperactivity, hand tremor, insomnia, nausea or vomiting, transient illusions or hallucinations, anxiety, grand mal seizures, and psychomotor agitation. May occur with perceptual disturbances (e.g., hallucinations) and intact reality testing.

VI. Alcohol withdrawal delirium (delirium tremens (DTs))

Usually occurs only after recent cessation of or reduction in severe, heavy alcohol use in medically compromised patients with a long history of dependence. Less common than uncomplicated alcohol withdrawal. Occurs in 1–3% of alcohol-dependent patients.

A. Diagnosis, signs, and symptoms
1. Delirium.
2. Marked autonomic hyperactivity—tachycardia, sweating, fever, anxiety, or insomnia.
3. Associated features—vivid hallucinations that may be visual, tactile, or olfactory; delusions; agitation; tremor; fever; and seizures or so-called rum fits (if seizures develop, they always occur before delirium).
4. Typical features—paranoid delusions, visual hallucinations of insects or small animals, and tactile hallucinations.

B. Medical workup
1. Complete history and physical.
2. Laboratory tests—complete blood cell count with differential; measurement of electrolytes, including calcium and magnesium; blood chemistry panel; liver function tests; measurement of bilirubin, blood urea nitrogen, creatinine, fasting glucose, prothrombin time, albumin, total protein, hepatitis type B surface antigen, vitamin B, folate, serum amylase; stool guaiac; urinalysis and urine drug screen; electrocardiogram (ECG); chest roentgenography. Other possible tests: electroencephalogram (EEG), lumbar puncture, computed tomography of the head, and gastrointestinal series.

C. Treatment
1. Take vital signs every 6 hours.
2. Observe the patient constantly.
3. Decrease stimulation.
4. Correct electrolyte imbalances and treat coexisting medical problems (e.g., infection, head trauma).
5. If the patient is dehydrated, hydrate.
6. Chlordiazepoxide (Librium): 25 to 100 mg orally every 6 hours (other sedative-hypnotics can be substituted, but this is the convention). Use as needed for agitation, tremor, or increased vital signs (temperature, pulse, blood pressure) (Table 6–9).
7. Thiamine: 100 mg orally one to three times a day.
8. Folic acid: 1 mg orally daily.
9. One multivitamin daily.
10. Magnesium sulfate: 1 g intramuscularly every 6 hours for 2 days (in patients who have had post-withdrawal seizures).
11. After the patient is stabilized, taper chlordiazepoxide by 20% every 5 to 7 days.
12. Provide medication for adequate sleep.
13. Treat malnutrition if present.

TABLE 6–9
DRUG THERAPY FOR ALCOHOL INTOXICATION AND WITHDRAWAL

Clinical Problem	Drug	Route	Dosage[a]	Comment
Tremulousness and mild to moderate agitation	Chlordiazepoxide	Oral	25–100 mg every 4–6 h	Initial dose can be repeated every 2 h until patient is calm; subsequent doses must be individualized and titrated.
	Diazepam	Oral	5–20 mg every 4–6 h	
Hallucinosis	Lorazepam	Oral	2–10 mg every 4–6 h	
Extreme agitation	Chlordiazepoxide	Intravenous	0.5 mg/kg at 12.5 mg/min	Give until patient is calm; subsequent doses must be individualized and titrated.
Withdrawal seizures	Diazepam	Intravenous	0.15 mg/kg at 2.5 mg/min	
Delirium tremens	Lorazepam	Intravenous	0.1 mg/kg at 2.0 mg/min	

[a] Scheduled doses should be held for somnolence.
Adapted from Koch-Weser J, Sellers EM, Kalant J. Alcohol intoxication and withdrawal. *N Engl J Med* 1976;294:757, with permission.

14. This regimen allows for a very flexible dosage of chlordiazepoxide. If prescribing a sedative on a standing regimen, be sure that the medication will be held if the patient is asleep or not easily aroused. The necessary total dose of benzodiazepine varies greatly among patients owing to inherent individual differences, differing levels of alcohol intake, and concomitant use of other substances. Because many of these patients have impaired liver function, it also may be difficult to estimate the elimination half-life of the sedative accurately.

15. Generally antipsychotics should be used cautiously because they can precipitate seizures. If the patient is agitated, psychotic, and shows signs of benzodiazepine toxicity (ataxia, slurred speech) despite being agitated, then consider using a high-potency antipsychotic such as haloperidol or fluphenazine (Prolixin, Permitil), which is less likely to precipitate seizures than are low-potency antipsychotics.

VII. Alcohol-induced persisting amnestic disorder

Disturbance in short-term memory resulting from prolonged heavy use of alcohol; rare in persons under the age of 35. The classic names for the disorder are *Wernicke's encephalopathy* (an acute set of neurological symptoms) and *Korsakoff's syndrome* (a chronic condition).

A. Wernicke's encephalopathy (also known as *alcoholic encephalopathy*). An acute syndrome caused by thiamine deficiency. Characterized by nystagmus, abducens and conjugate gaze palsies, ataxia, and global confusion. Other symptoms may include confabulation, lethargy, indifference, mild delirium, anxious insomnia, and fear of the dark. Thiamine deficiency usually is secondary to chronic alcohol dependence. Treat with 100 to 300 mg of thiamine per day until ophthalmoplegia resolves. The patient may also require magnesium (a cofactor for thiamine metabolism). With treatment, most symptoms resolve except ataxia, nystagmus, and sometimes peripheral neuropathy. The syndrome may clear in a few days or weeks or progress to Korsakoff's syndrome.

B. Korsakoff's syndrome   (also known as *Korsakoff's psychosis*). A chronic condition, usually related to alcohol dependence, wherein alcohol represents a large portion of the caloric intake for years. Caused by thiamine deficiency. Rare. Characterized by retrograde and anterograde amnesia. The patient also often exhibits confabulation, disorientation, and polyneuritis. In addition to thiamine replacement, clonidine (Catapres) and propranolol (Inderal) may be of some limited use. Often coexists with alcohol-related dementia. Twenty-five percent of patients recover fully, and 50% recover partially with long-term oral administration of 50 to 100 mg of thiamine per day.

VIII. Substance-induced persisting dementia

This diagnosis should be made when other causes of dementia have been excluded and a history of chronic heavy alcohol abuse is evident. The symptoms persist past intoxication or withdrawal states. The dementia is usually mild. Management is similar to that for dementia of other causes.

For a more detailed discussion of this topic, see Alcohol-Related Disorders, Ch 11, p 924, in CTP/VII.

7
Other Substance-Related Disorders

I. Introduction

Substance-related disorders are a widespread public health problem, causing disability in multiple areas of functioning. Thirty-seven percent of the population have used an illicit substance at one time. More than 15% of the U.S. population over the age of 18 have serious substance use problems. Approximately two thirds to three fourths of patients with substance use disorders have comorbid psychiatric diagnoses. Substance-induced syndromes can mimic the full range of psychiatric illnesses, including major mood, psychotic, and anxiety disorders. These phenomena hold rich possibilities for psychiatric research (as in the phencyclidine model of schizophrenia, with resultant investigation of N-methyl-D-aspartate [NMDA] receptor activity). In clinical practice, substance use disorders must always be considered when psychiatric disorders are being diagnosed and treated. Conversely, patients who present with primary substance use disorders must be evaluated for psychiatric comorbidity (dual diagnosis) that may be contributing to the substance abuse or dependence.

A. Epidemiology. See Table 7–1.

B. Evaluation. Substance-abusing patients are often difficult to detect and evaluate. Not easily categorized, they almost always underestimate the amount of substance used, are prone to use denial, are often manipulative, and often fear the consequences of acknowledging the problem. Because these patients may be unreliable, it is necessary to obtain information from other sources, such as family members.

When dealing with these patients, clinicians must present clear, firm, and consistent limits, which will be tested frequently. Such patients usually require a confrontational approach. Although clinicians may feel angered by being manipulated, they should not act on these feelings.

Psychiatric conditions are difficult to evaluate properly in the presence of ongoing substance abuse, which itself causes symptoms. Substance abuse is frequently associated with personality disorders (e.g., antisocial, borderline, and narcissistic). Depressed, anxious, or psychotic patients may self-medicate with either prescribed or nonprescribed substances. Substance-induced disorders should always be considered in the evaluation of depression, anxiety, or psychosis. Underlying substance use is often present when psychiatric disorders do not respond to usual treatments.

1. Toxicology. Urine or blood tests are useful in confirming suspected substance use. The two types of tests are screening and confirmatory. Screening tests are sensitive but not specific (many false-positives).

TABLE 7-1
USE OF ILLICIT DRUGS, ALCOHOL, AND TOBACCO IN THE U.S. POPULATION BY AGE GROUPS

Drug	Lifetime Use (%)				Past-Year Use (%)				Past-Month Use (%)			
	12 to 17	18 to 25	26 to 34	>35	12 to 17	18 to 25	26 to 34	>35	12 to 17	18 to 25	26 to 34	>35
Any illicit drug[a]	23.7	48.0	53.1	29.0	16.7	26.8	14.6	5.3	9.0	15.6	8.4	2.9
Marijuana and hashish	16.8	44.0	50.5	27.0	13.0	23.8	11.3	3.8	7.1	13.2	6.3	2.0
Cocaine	1.9	10.2	20.9	8.9	1.4	4.7	3.5	0.9	0.6	2.0	1.5	0.4
Crack	0.7	3.0	4.4	1.6	0.4	1.3	1.1	0.4	0.2	0.6	0.5	0.2
Inhalants	5.9	10.8	8.3	3.6	4.0	3.0	1.1	0.3	1.7	1.0	0.3	0.1
Hallucinogens	5.6	16.3	15.4	7.3	4.3	6.9	1.1	0.2	2.0	2.3	0.2	0.1
PCP	1.2	2.3	4.2	3.4	0.7	0.5	0.0	0.1	0.2	0.1	—[b]	0.0
LSD	4.3	13.9	11.7	5.8	2.8	4.6	0.5	—[b]	0.8	0.9	0.1	—[b]
Heroin	0.5	1.3	1.3	1.2	0.3	0.9	0.2	0.0	0.2	0.4	0.1	0.0
Nonmedical use of any psychotherapeutic[c]	6.8	12.7	13.4	8.3	4.7	6.7	4.2	1.8	1.9	2.9	1.9	0.9
Stimulants	2.2	4.3	6.5	4.7	1.5	2.0	1.3	0.4	0.5	0.6	0.4	0.3
Sedatives	1.1	1.3	2.9	2.5	0.4	0.7	0.5	0.2	0.2	0.3	0.2	0.0
Tranquilizers	1.7	5.0	5.8	3.1	1.0	2.6	1.6	0.7	0.2	0.9	0.5	0.4
Analgesics	5.5	8.9	7.5	4.2	3.7	4.9	2.5	1.1	1.5	2.0	1.1	0.5
Any illicit drug other than marijuana[d]	13.0	26.6	30.2	15.1	9.3	12.7	7.2	2.7	4.6	6.3	3.6	1.4
Alcohol	38.8	83.8	90.3	87.8	32.7	75.3	77.2	64.9	18.8	60.0	61.6	51.7
"Binge" alcohol use[e]	—[f]	—	—	—	—	—	—	—	7.2	32.0	22.8	11.3
Heavy alcohol use[e]	—	—	—	—	—	—	—	—	2.9	12.9	7.1	3.8
Cigarettes	36.3	68.5	73.8	77.8	24.2	44.7	39.2	29.1	18.3	38.3	35.0	27.0
Smokeless tobacco	10.0	23.4	24.4	14.8	4.6	9.7	7.2	2.9	1.9	6.1	4.9	2.3

[a] Use at least once of marijuana or hashish, cocaine (including crack), inhalants, hallucinogens (including PCP and LSD), heroin, or any prescription-type psychotherapeutic used nonmedically.
[b] Low precision; no estimate reported.
[c] Does not include over-the-counter-drugs.
[d] Use at least once of any of these listed drugs, regardless of marijuana use; marijuana users who also have used any of the other listed drugs are included.
[e] Drinking five or more drinks on the same occasion on at least 1 day in the past 30 days. "Occasion" means at the same time or within a couple hours of each other. Heavy alcohol use is defined as drinking five or more drinks on the same occasion on each of five or more days in the past 30 days; all heavy alcohol users are also "binge" alcohol users.
[f] Not available.
From National Household Survey on Drug Abuse. Substance Abuse and Mental Health Services Administration (SAMHSA) Office of Applied Studies. Department of Health and Human Services, preliminary data, June 1997.

Confirm positive screening results with a specific confirmatory test for an identified drug. Although most drugs are well detected in urine, some are best detected in blood (e.g., barbiturates and alcohol). Absolute blood concentrations can sometimes be useful (e.g., a high concentration in the absence of clinical signs of intoxication would imply tolerance). Urine toxicology is usually positive for up to 2 days after the ingestion of most drugs (see Table 26–5 in Chapter 26).

2. Physical examination

a. Carefully consider whether concomitant medical conditions are substance-related. Look specifically for the following:

    (1) **Subcutaneous or intravenous abusers**—AIDS, scars from intravenous or subcutaneous injections, abscesses, infections from contaminated injections, bacterial endocarditis, drug-induced or infectious hepatitis, thrombophlebitis, tetanus.

    (2) **Snorters of cocaine, heroin, or other drugs**—deviated or perforated nasal septum, nasal bleeding, rhinitis.

    (3) **Cocaine freebasers; smokers of crack, marijuana, or other drugs; inhalant abusers**—bronchitis, asthma, chronic respiratory conditions.

b. Determine the pattern of abuse. Is it continuous or episodic? When, where, and with whom is the substance taken? Is the abuse recreational or confined to certain social contexts? Find out how much of the patient's life is associated with obtaining, taking, withdrawing from, and recovering from substances. How much do the substances affect the patient's social and work functioning? How does he or she get and pay for the substances? Always specifically describe the substance and route of administration rather than the category (i.e., use "intravenous heroin withdrawal" rather than "opioid withdrawal"). If describing polysubstance abuse, list all substances. Substance abusers typically abuse multiple substances.

C. Diagnoses. See Table 7–2.

D. Treatment. See Table 7–3. In general, the management of intoxication involves observation for possible overdose, evaluation for polysubstance intoxication and concomitant medical conditions, and supportive treatment, such as protecting the patient from injury. The management of abuse or dependence involves abstinence and long-term treatment.

1. Period of abstinence. Anything that improves abstinence should be used.

2. Long-term treatment lasting at least 6 months. Relapse is common. A variety of methods may help, including individual therapy, group therapy, self-help groups (e.g., Alcoholics Anonymous, Narcotics Anonymous), therapeutic communities, family groups (e.g., Al-Anon), chemical maintenance (e.g., methadone [Dolophine], disulfiram [Antabuse], naltrexone [ReVia], and a variety of philosophical approaches, including addictive, medical, and moral [or inspirational] models).

TABLE 7-2
DSM-IV-TR DIAGNOSES ASSOCIATED WITH CLASS OF SUBSTANCES

	Dependence	Abuse	Intoxication	Withdrawal	Intoxication Delirium	Withdrawal Delirium	Dementia	Amnestic Disorder	Psychotic Disorders	Mood Disorders	Anxiety Disorders	Sexual Dysfunctions	Sleep Disorders
Alcohol	X	X	X	X	I	W	P	P	I/W	I/W	I/W	I	I/W
Amphetamines	X	X	X	X	I	—	—	—	I	I/W	I	I	I/W
Caffeine	—	—	X	—	—	—	—	—	—	—	I	—	I
Cannabis	X	X	X	—	I	—	—	—	I	—	I	—	—
Cocaine	X	X	X	X	I	—	—	—	I/W	I/W	I/W	I	I/W
Hallucinogens	X	X	X	—	I	—	—	—	I[a]	I	I	—	—
Inhalants	X	X	X	—	I	—	P	—	I	I	I	—	—
Nicotine	X	—	—	X	—	—	—	—	—	—	—	—	—
Opioids	X	X	X	X	I	—	—	—	I	I	—	I	I/W
Phencyclidine	X	X	X	—	I	—	—	—	I	I	I	—	—
Sedatives, hypnotics, or anxiolytics	X	X	X	X	I	W	P	P	I/W	I/W	W	I	I/W
Polysubstance	X	—	—	—	—	—	—	—	—	—	—	—	—
Other	X	X	X	X	I	W	P	P	I/W	I/W	I/W	I	I/W

[a] Also hallucinogen persisting perception disorder (flashbacks).

X, I, W, I/W, or P indicates that the category is recognized in DSM-IV-TR. In addition, I indicates that the specifier "with onset during intoxication" may be noted for the category (except for intoxication delirium); W indicates that the specifier "with onset during withdrawal" may be noted for the category (except for withdrawal delirium); and I/W indicates that either "with onset during intoxication" or "with onset during withdrawal" may be noted for the category. P indicates that the disorder is "persisting."

From American Psychiatric Association. *Diagnostic and Statistical Manual of Mental Disorders*, text revision, 4th ed. Washington, DC: American Psychiatric Association, Copyright 2000, with permission.

E. Definitions
  1. **Intoxication.** Maladaptive behavior associated with recent drug ingestion. The effects of intoxication of any drug can vary widely among persons and depend on such factors as dose, circumstances, and underlying personality (Table 7–4).
  2. **Withdrawal.** Psychoactive substance-specific syndrome following cessation of heavy use (implies tolerance and indicates dependence (Table 7–5).
  3. **Tolerance.** More of a substance is needed to become intoxicated, or the same amount of a drug produces a decreased effect with continued or heavy use (tachyphylaxis).
  4. **Abuse.** A maladaptive pattern of substance use resulting in repeated problems and adverse consequences (e.g., use in hazardous situations; legal, social, and occupational problems).
  5. **Dependence.** Psychological or physical need to continue taking the substance. Dependence on a drug may be physical, psychological, or both. **Psychological dependence,** also referred to as *habituation,* is characterized by a continuous or intermittent craving for the substance. **Physiologic dependence** is characterized by **tolerance,** a need to take the substance to prevent the occurrence of a withdrawal or abstinence syndrome. **Note:** The presence of withdrawal symptoms on abstinence usually implies dependence. Other than for short-term treatment of withdrawal symptoms, the distinction between abuse and dependence is of limited clinical significance.
  6. **Addiction.** A nonscientific term that implies psychological dependence, drug-seeking behavior, physical dependence and tolerance, and associated deterioration of physical and mental health. It still appears despite its official removal from the medical nosology.
  7. **Discontinuation syndrome.** A new term, used to refer to transient withdrawal signs and symptoms after the use of a prescribed medication is stopped.

II. Opioids

The lifetime rate of heroin use in the United States is about 2%. Opioid use has been on the rise because of an increase in heroine purity and a decrease in price. Opioids include opium derivatives and synthetic drugs: opium, morphine, heroin, methadone, codeine, oxycodone, hydromorphone (Dilaudid), levorphanol (Levo-Dromoran), pentazocine (Talwin), meperidine (Demerol), and propoxyphene (Darvon). Table 7–5 lists the duration of action of opioids. Opioids affect opioid receptors. μ-Opioid receptors mediate analgesia, respiratory depression, constipation, and dependence; κ-opioid receptors mediate analgesia, diuresis, and sedation; and δ-opioid receptors may produce analgesia. Opioids also affect dopaminergic and nonadrenergic systems. Dopaminergic reward pathways mediate addiction. Heroin is more lipid-soluble than morphine and more potent. It crosses the blood–brain barrier more rapidly, has a faster onset of action, and is more addictive.
  A. Route of administration. Depends on the drug. Opium is smoked. Heroin is typically injected (intravenously or subcutaneously) or inhaled

TABLE 7–3
PSYCHOACTIVE DRUG-RELATED CONDITIONS AND TREATMENTS

Drug	Behavioral Effects	Physical Effects	Laboratory Findings	Treatment
Opioids: opium, morphine, heroin, meperidine, methadone, pentazocine	Euphoria, drowsiness, anorexia, decreased sex drive, hypoactivity, change in personality	Miosis, pruritus, nausea, bradycardia, constipation, needle tracks in arms, legs, groin	Detected in blood up to 24 h after last dose	For gradual withdrawal: methadone 5–10 mg every 6 h for 24 h, then decrease dose for 10 d. For overdose: naloxone 0.4 mg IM every 20 min for 3 doses, keep airway open; give O_2
Amphetamine and other sympathomimetics (including cocaine) and amphetamine-like substances	Alertness, loquaciousness, euphoria, hyperactivity, irritability, aggressiveness, agitation, paranoid trends, impotence, visual and tactile hallucinations	Mydriasis, tremor, halitosis, dry mouth, tachycardia, hypertension, weight loss, arrhythmics, fever, convulsions, perforated nasal septum (with snorting)	Detected in blood and urine	For agitation: diazepam IM or PO 5–10 mg every 3 h; for tachyarrhythmias: propranolol (Inderal) 10–20 mg PO every 4 h, vitamin C 0.5 g QID PO may increase urinary excretion by acidifying urine
Hallucinogens: LSD, psilocybin (mushrooms), mescaline (peyote), DET, DMT, DOM or STP, MDA	Duration of 8–12 h with flashback after abstinence, visual hallucinations, paranoid ideation, false sense of achievement and strength, suicidal or homicidal tendencies, depersonalization, derealization	Mydriasis, ataxia, hyperemic conjunctiva, tachycardia, hypertension	None	Emotional support (talking down); for mild agitation: diazepam 10 mg IM or PO every 2 h for 4 doses; for severe agitation: haloperidol 1–5 mg IM and repeat every 6 h pm. May have to continue haloperidol 1–2 mg/d PO for weeks to prevent flashback syndrome. Phenothiazines may be used only with LSD. **Caution:** phenothiazines can produce *fatal* results is used with other hallucinogens (e.g., DET, DMT), especially if they are adulterated with strychnine or belladonna alkaloids
PCP and phencyclidine-like substances (including ketamine, TCP)	Duration of 8–12 h (about 2 h for ketamine), hallucinations, paranoid ideation, labile mood, loose associations (may mimic schizophrenia), catatonia, violent behavior, convulsions	Nystagmus, mydriosis, ataxia, tachycardia, hypertension	Detected in urine up to 5 days after ingestion	Phenothiazines contraindicated for first week after ingestion; for violent delusions: haloperidol 1–4 mg IM or PO every 2–4 h until patient is calm

CNS depressants: barbiturates, methaqualone (illegal), meprobamate, benzodiazepines, glutethimide	Drowsiness, confusion, inattentiveness	Diaphoresis, ataxia, hypotension, seizures, delirium, miosis	Detected in blood	For barbiturates: substitute 30 mg of liquid phenobarbital for every 100 mg barbiturates abused and give in divided doses every 6 h and then decrease by 20% every other day; may also substitute diazepam for barbiturate abused. Give 10 mg every 2–4 h for 24 h and then reduce dose. For benzodiazepines: gradual reduction of diazepam every other day over 10-day period
Volatile hydrocarbons and petroleum derivatives; glue, benzene, gasoline, varnish thinner, lighter fluid, aerosols	Euphoria, clouded sensorium, slurred speech, ataxia, hallucinations in 50% of cases psychoses, permanent brain damage if used daily over 6 mo	Odor on breath, tachycardia with possible ventricular fibrillation, possible damage of brain, liver, kidneys, myocardium	Relevant to determine tissue damage (aspartate aminotransferase)	For agitation: haloperidol 1–5 mg every 6 h until calm; avoid epinephrine because of myocardial sensitization
Other inhalants: nitrous oxide	Euphoria, drowsiness, ataxia, confusion	Analgesia, respiratory depression, hypotension	None	Hypoxia is treated with O_2 inhalation
Alcohol	Poor judgment, loquaciousness, mood change, aggression, impaired attention, amnesia	Nystagmus, flushed face, ataxia, slurred speech	Blood level between 100 and 200 mg/dL	For delirium: diazepam 5–10 mg IM or PO every 3 h. IM vitamin B complex, hydration. For hallucinosis: haloperidol 1–4 mg every 6 h IM or PO
Belladonna alkaloids (found in OTC medications and morning glory seeds): stramonium, homatropine, atropine, scopolamine, hyoscyamine	Hot skin, erythema, weakness, thirst, blurred vision, confusion, excitement, delirium, stupor, coma (anticholinergic delirium)	Dry mouth and throat, mydriasis, twitching, dysphagia, light sensitivity, pyrexia, hypertension followed by shock, urinary retention	None	Antidote is physostigmine 2 mg IV every 20 min; IV should be controlled at no more than 1 mg/min; watch for copious salivary secretion because of anticholinesterase activity. Propranolol for tachyarrhythmias

Adapted from New York State Medical Society.

(snorted) nasally, and it may be combined with stimulants for intravenous injection (speedball). Heroin snorting and smoking are increasingly popular owing to increased drug purity and concerns about HIV risk. Pharmaceutically available opioids are typically taken orally, but some are also injectable. Heroin is exclusively a drug of abuse and is most commonly used by patients of lower socioeconomic status, who often engage in criminal activities to pay for drugs.

TABLE 7–4
SIGNS AND SYMPTOMS OF SUBSTANCE INTOXICATION AND WITHDRAWAL

Substance	Intoxication	Withdrawal
Opioid	Drowsiness Slurred speech Impaired attention or memory Analgesia Anorexia Decreased sex drive Hypoactivity	Craving for drug Nausea, vomiting Muscle aches Lacrimation, rhinorrhea Pupillary dilation Piloerection Sweating Diarrhea Fever Insomnia Yawning
Amphetamine or cocaine	Perspiration, chills Tachycardia Pupillary dilation Elevated blood pressure Nausea, vomiting Tremor Arrhythmia Fever Convulsions Anorexia, weight loss Dry mouth Impotence Hallucinations Hyperactivity Irritability Aggressiveness Paranoid ideation	Dysphoria Fatigue Sleep disorder Agitation Craving
Sedative, hypnotic, or anxiolytic	Slurred speech Incoordination Unsteady gait Impaired attention or memory	Nausea, vomiting Malaise, weakness Autonomic hyperactivity Anxiety, irritability Increased sensitivity to light and sound Coarse tremor Marked insomnia Seizures

TABLE 7–5
DURATION OF ACTION OF OPIOIDS

Drug	Duration of Action (h)
Heroin	3–4
Levomethadyl acetate	48–96
Meperidine	2–4
Morphine, hydromorphone	4–5
Methadone	12–24
Propoxyphene	12
Pentazocine	2–3

B. **Dose.**   Often difficult to determine by history for two reasons. First, the abuser has no way of knowing the concentration of the heroin he or she has bought and may underestimate the amount taken (which can lead to accidental overdose if the person suddenly obtains one bag containing 15% heroin when the typical amount is 5%). Second, the abuser may overstate the dosage in an attempt to get more methadone.

C. **Intoxication**
   1. **Objective signs and symptoms.** CNS depression, decreased gastrointestinal motility, respiratory depression, analgesia, nausea and vomiting, slurred speech, hypotension, bradycardia, pupillary constriction, seizures (in overdose). Tolerant patients still have pupillary constriction and constipation.
   2. **Subjective signs and symptoms.** Euphoria (heroin intoxication, described as a total-body orgasm), at times anxious dysphoria, tranquility, decreased attention and memory, drowsiness, and psychomotor retardation.

D. **Overdose.**   Can be a medical emergency and is usually accidental. Can result from incorrect estimation of dose or erratic pattern of use in which person has lost previous tolerance to drug. Often results from combined use with other CNS depressants (e.g., alcohol or sedative-hypnotics). Clinical signs include pinpoint pupils, respiratory depression, CNS depression.
   1. **Treatment**
      a. ICU admission and support of vital functions (e.g., intravenous fluids).
      b. Immediately administer 0.8 mg of naloxone (Narcan) (0.01 mg/kg for neonates), an opioid antagonist, intravenously and wait 15 minutes.
      c. If no response, give 1.6 mg intravenously and wait 15 minutes.
      d. If still no response, give 3.2 mg intravenously and suspect another diagnosis.
      e. If successful, continue at 0.4 mg/h intravenously.
   2. Always consider possible polysubstance overdose. A patient successfully treated with naloxone may wake up briefly only to succumb to subsequent overdose symptoms from another, slower-acting drug (e.g., sedative-hypnotic) taken simultaneously. Remember that naloxone will precipitate rapid withdrawal symptoms. It has a short half-life and must be administered continuously until the opioid has been cleared (up to 3 days for methadone). Babies born to opioid-abusing mothers may experience intoxication, overdose, or withdrawal.

E. **Tolerance, dependence, and withdrawal.**   Develop rapidly with long-term opioid use, which changes the number and sensitivity of opioid receptors and increases the sensitivity of dopaminergic, cholinergic, and serotonergic receptors. Produce profound effects on noradrenergic systems. Occur after cessation of long-term use or after abrupt cessation, as with administration of an opioid antagonist. Symptoms are primarily related to rebound hyperactivity of noradrenergic neurons of the locus ceruleus. Withdrawal is seldom a medical emergency. Clinical signs are flu-like and include drug craving, anxiety, lacrimation, rhinorrhea, yawning, sweating, insomnia, hot and cold flashes, muscle aches, abdominal cramping, dilated pupils, piloerection, tremor, restlessness, nausea and vomiting, diarrhea, and increased vital signs. Intensity depends on previous dose and on rate of decrease. Less intense with drugs that have long half-lives, such as methadone; more intense with drugs that have short half-lives, such as meperidine. Patients have severe craving for opioid drugs and will demand and manipulate for opioids. Beware of malingerers and look for piloerection, dilated pupils, tachycardia, hypertension. If objective signs are absent, do not give opioids for withdrawal. The goal of detoxification is to minimize withdrawal symptoms (to prevent the patient from abandoning treatment) while steadily decreasing the opioid dose. Untreated opioid withdrawal results in no serious medical sequelae in otherwise healthy people.

1. **Detoxification.** If objective withdrawal signs are present, give 10 mg of methadone. If withdrawal persists after 4 to 6 hours, give an additional 5 to 10 mg, which may be repeated every 4 to 6 hours. Total dose in 24 hours equals the dose for the second day (seldom > 40 mg). Give twice a day or every day and decrease dosage by 5 mg/day for heroin withdrawal; methadone withdrawal may require slower detoxification. Pentazocine-dependent patients should be detoxified on pentazocine because of its mixed opioid receptor agonist and antagonist properties. Many nonopioid drugs have been tried for opioid detoxification, but the only promising one is clonidine (Catapres), which is a centrally acting agent that effectively relieves the nausea, vomiting, and diarrhea associated with opioid withdrawal (it is not effective for most other symptoms). Give 0.1 to 0.2 mg every 3 hours as needed, not to exceed 0.8 mg/d. Titrate dose according to symptoms. When dosage is stabilized, taper over 2 weeks. Hypotension is a side effect. Clonidine is short-acting and not a narcotic.

   The general approach in withdrawal is one of support, detoxification, and progression to methadone maintenance or abstinence. Patients dependent on multiple drugs (e.g., an opioid and a sedative-hypnotic) should be maintained on a stable dosage of one drug while being detoxified from the other. Naltrexone (a long-acting oral opioid antagonist) can be used with clonidine to expedite detoxification. It is orally effective, and when given three times a week (100 mg on weekdays and 150 mg on weekends), it blocks the effects of heroin. After detoxification, oral naltrexone has been effective in helping to maintain abstinence for up to 2 months.

   Ultrarapid detoxification is the procedure of precipitating withdrawal with opioid antagonists under general anesthesia. Further research is needed to determine whether the use of this expensive and intensive method, which adds anesthetic risk to the detoxification process, is of any benefit.

2. **Opioid substitutes.** The main long-term treatment for opiate dependence, methadone maintenance, is a slow, extended detoxification. Most patients can be maintained on daily doses of 60 mg or less. Al-

though often criticized, methadone maintenance programs do decrease rates of heroin use. A sufficient methadone dosage is necessary; the use of plasma methadone concentrations may help to determine the appropriate dosage.

Levomethadyl (ORLAAM, also known as LAAM) is a longer-acting opioid than methadone. It can be given in doses of 30 to 80 mg three times per week for maintenance treatment. Treatment with LAAM is increasing. Buprenorphine is a partial μ-opioid receptor agonist that may be of use for both detoxification and maintenance treatment.

3. **Therapeutic communities.** Residential programs that emphasize abstinence and group therapy in a structured environment (e.g., Phoenix House).

4. **Other interventions.** Education about HIV transmission, free needle-exchange programs, individual and group psychotherapies, self-help groups (e.g., Narcotics Anonymous), and outpatient drug-free programs are also of benefit.

III. Sedatives, hypnotics, and anxiolytics

Drugs of this class are used to treat insomnia and anxiety. They all have agonist effects on the γ-aminobutyric acid type A (GABA$_A$) receptor complex. Sedatives, hypnotics, and anxiolytics are the most commonly prescribed psychoactive drugs. The prevalence of benzodiazepine use is outlined in Table 7–6. Sedative-hypnotics are taken orally. Usually, dependence develops only after at least several months of daily use, but persons vary widely in this respect. Many middle-aged patients begin taking benzodiazepines for insomnia or anxiety, become dependent, and then seek multiple physicians to prescribe them. Sedative-hypnotics are used illicitly for their euphoric effects, to augment the effects of other CNS depressant drugs (e.g., opioids and alcohol), and to temper the excitatory and anxiety-producing effects of stimulants (e.g., cocaine).

The major complication of sedative, hypnotic, or anxiolytic intoxication is overdose with associated CNS and respiratory depression. Although mild intoxication is not in itself dangerous (unless the patient is driving or operating machinery), the possibility of a covert overdose must always be considered.

TABLE 7–6
PREVALENCE OF BENZODIAZEPINE USE

- Retail sales of benzodiazepines reached their highest level in 1973–1975 at 87 million a year but have declined gradually since then.
- The United States has the highest volume of sales in the world, but per capita sales are at the median of the nine countries with the largest sales.
- Sales of drugs with short elimination half-lives (e.g., alprazolam) have increased in comparison with drugs with long half-lives (e.g., diazepam).
- A survey of the United States population showed that self-reported medical use of a tranquilizer declined from 10.9% to 8.3% from 1970 to 1990; hypnotic use declined from 3.5% to 2.6% during the same period.
- Persons who abuse alcohol and drugs use and abuse benzodiazepines at higher rates than do anxiety disorder patients without substance abuse histories.

Adapted from Domenic A. Ciraulo, M.D., and Ofra Sarid-Segal, M.D.

The lethality of benzodiazepine overdose has been reduced by the use of the specific benzodiazepine antagonist flumazenil (Romazicon) in emergency department settings.

Sedative, hypnotic, or anxiolytic intoxication is similar to alcohol intoxication, but idiosyncratic aggressive reactions are uncommon. These drugs are often taken with other CNS depressants (e.g., alcohol), which can produce additive effects. Withdrawal is dangerous and can lead to delirium or seizures.

A. Drugs. See Chapter 25 for a complete list of drugs in this category.

1. **Benzodiazepines.** Diazepam (Valium), chlordiazepoxide (Librium), flurazepam (Dalmane), lorazepam (Ativan), alprazolam (Xanax), triazolam (Halcion), oxazepam (Serax), temazepam (Restoril), and others.

2. **Barbiturates.** Secobarbital (Seconal), pentobarbital (Nembutal), and others.

3. **Similarly acting drugs.** Meprobamate (Miltown), methaqualone (Quaalude), glutethimide (Doriden), ethchlorvynol (Placidyl), chloral hydrate.

B. Intoxication. See Table 7–4. Intoxication also can cause disinhibition and amnesia.

C. Withdrawal. See Table 7–4. Can range from a minor to a potentially life-threatening condition requiring hospitalization. Individual differences in tolerance are large. All sedatives, hypnotics, and anxiolytics are cross-tolerant with each other and with alcohol. Drugs with a short half-life (e.g., alprazolam) may induce a more rapid onset of withdrawal and a more severe withdrawal than drugs with a long half-life (e.g., diazepam). The degree of tolerance can be measured with the pentobarbital challenge test (Table 7–7), which identifies the dose of pentobarbital needed to prevent withdrawal. True withdrawal, a return of original anxiety symptoms (recurrence) or worsening of original anxiety symptoms (rebound), can be precipitated by drug discontinuation. Guidelines for treatment of benzodiazepine withdrawal are presented in Table 7–8. Dose equivalents are presented in Table 7–9.

IV. Amphetamines and amphetamine-like substances (stimulants)

Amphetamine-like substances exert their major effect by releasing catecholamines, primarily dopamine, from presynaptic stores, particularly in the

TABLE 7–7
PENTOBARBITAL[a] CHALLENGE TEST

1. Give 200 mg of pentobarbital orally.
2. Observe patient for intoxication after 1 h (e.g., sleepiness, slurred speech, or nystagmus).
3. If patient is not intoxicated, give another 100 mg of pentobarbital every 2 h (maximum 500 mg over 6 hs).
4. Total dose given to produce mild intoxication is equivalent to daily abuse level of barbiturates.
5. Substitute 30 mg of phenobarbital (longer half-life) for each 100 mg of pentobarbital.
6. Decrease dose by about 10% a day.
7. Adjust rate if signs of intoxication or withdrawal are present.

[a] Other drugs can also be used.

"reward pathway" of dopaminergic neurons projecting from the ventral tegmentum to the cortex. Legitimate indications include attention-deficit disorders, narcolepsy, and depression. In the United States, 4.5% of adults have reported nonmedical use of amphetamines. Methylphenidate (Ritalin) appears less addictive than other amphetamines, possibly because it has a different mechanism of action (inhibits dopamine reuptake). Effects are euphoric and anorectic. Amphetamines are usually taken orally but also can be injected,

---

TABLE 7–8
GUIDELINES FOR TREATMENT OF BENZODIAZEPINE WITHDRAWAL

1. Evaluate and treat concomitant medical and psychiatric conditions.
2. Obtain drug history and urine and blood samples for drug and ethanol assay.
3. Determine required dose of benzodiazepine or barbiturate for stabilization, guided by history, clinical presentation, drug-ethanol assay, and (in some cases) challenge dose.
4. Detoxification from supratherapeutic dosages:
   a. Hospitalize if there are medical or psychiatric indications, poor social supports, or polysubstance dependence or the patient is unreliable.
   b. Some clinicians recommend switching to longer-acting benzodiazepine for withdrawal (e.g., diazepam, clonazepam); others recommend stabilizing on the drug that the patient was taking or on phenobarbital.
   c. After stabilization, reduce dosage by 30% on the second or third day and evaluate the response, keeping in mind that symptoms occur sooner after decreases in benzodiazepines with short elimination half-lives (e.g., lorazepam) than after decreases in those with longer elimination half-lives (e.g., diazepam).
   d. Reduce dosage further by 10% to 25% every few days if tolerated.
   e. Use adjunctive medications if necessary; carbamazepine, β-adrenergic receptor antagonists, valproate, clonidine, and sedative antidepressants have been used, but their efficacy in the treatment of the benzodiazepine abstinence syndrome has not been established.
5. Detoxification from therapeutic dosages:
   a. Initiate 10% to 25% dose reduction and evaluate response.
   b. Dose, duration of therapy, and severity of anxiety influence the rate of taper and need for adjunctive medications.
   c. Most patients taking therapeutic doses have uncomplicated discontinuation.
6. Psychological interventions may assist patients in detoxification from benzodiazepines and in the long-term management of anxiety.

Adapted from Domenic A. Ciraulo M.D., and Ofra Sarid-Segal, M.D.

TABLE 7–9
APPROXIMATE THERAPEUTIC EQUIVALENT DOSES OF BENZODIAZEPINES

Generic Name	Trade Name	Dose (mg)
Alprazolam	Xanax	1
Chlordiazepoxide	Librium	25
Clonazepam	Klonopin	0.5–1
Clorazepate	Tranxene	15
Diazepam	Valium	10
Estazolam	ProSom	1
Flurazepam	Dalmane	30
Lorazepam	Ativan	2
Oxazepam	Serax	30
Prazepam	Paxipam	80
Temazepam	Restoril	20
Triazolam	Halcion	0.25
Quazepam	Doral	15
Zolpidem[a]	Ambiem	10

[a] An imidazopyridine benzodiazepine agonist.
Adapted from Domenic A. Ciraulo, M.D., and Ofra Sarid-Segal, M.D.

nasally inhaled, or smoked. The clinical syndromes associated with amphetamines are similar to those associated with cocaine, although the oral route of amphetamine administration produces a less rapid euphoria and consequently is less addictive. Intravenous amphetamine abuse is highly addictive. Amphetamines are commonly abused by students, long-distance truck drivers, and other persons who desire prolonged wakefulness and attentiveness. Amphetamines can induce a paranoid psychosis similar to paranoid schizophrenia. Intoxication usually resolves in 24 to 48 hours. Amphetamine abuse can cause severe hypertension, cerebrovascular disease, and myocardial infarction and ischemia. Neurological symptoms range from twitching to tetany to seizures, coma, and death as doses escalate. Tremor, ataxia, bruxism, shortness of breath, headache, fever, and flushing are common but less severe physical effects.

A. **Drugs**
   1. **Major amphetamines.** Amphetamine, dextroamphetamine (Dexedrine), methamphetamine (Desoxyn, "speed"), methylphenidate, pemoline (Cylert).
   2. **Related substances.** Ephedrine, phenylpropanolamine (PPA), khat, methcathinone ("crank").
   3. **Substituted (designer) amphetamines** (also classified as hallucinogens). Have neurochemical effects on both serotonergic and dopaminergic systems; have both amphetamine-like and hallucinogen-like behavioral effects (e.g., 3,4-methylenedioxymethamphetamine [MDMA, "ecstasy"], N-ethyl-3,4-methylenedioxyamphetamine [MDEA], 5-methoxy-3,4-methylenedioxyamphetamine [MMDA]). MDMA use is associated with increased self-confidence and sensory sensitivity; peaceful feelings with insight, empathy, and a sense of personal closeness with other people. Effects are activating and energizing with a hallucinogenic character but less disorientation and perceptual disturbance than are seen with classic hallucinogens. MDMA is associated with hyperthermia, particularly when used in close quarters in combination with increased physical activity, as is common at "raves." Heavy or long-term use may be associated with serotoninergic nerve damage.
   4. **"Ice."** Pure form of methamphetamine (inhaled, smoked, injected). Particularly powerful. Psychological effects can last for hours. Synthetic, manufactured domestically.

B. **Intoxication and withdrawal.** See Table 7–4.
C. **Treatment.** Symptomatic. See Table 7–3.

V. Cocaine

One of the most addictive of the commonly abused substances, referred to as *coke, blow, cane, freebase.* The effects of cocaine are pharmacologically similar to those of other stimulants, but its widespread use warrants a separate discussion.

Before it was well-known that cocaine is highly addictive, it was widely used as a stimulant and euphoriant. Cocaine is usually inhaled but can be smoked or injected. Crack is smoked, has a rapid onset of action, and is highly addictive.

The onset of action of smoked cocaine is comparable with that of intravenously injected cocaine, and the drug is equally addictive in this circumstance. The euphoria is intense, and a risk for dependence develops after only one dose. Like amphetamines, cocaine can be taken in binges lasting up to several days. This phenomenon is partly the result of greater euphoric effects derived from subsequent doses (sensitization). During binges, the abuser takes the cocaine repeatedly until exhausted or out of drug. There follows a crash of lethargy, hunger, and prolonged sleep, followed by another binge. With repeated use, tolerance develops to the euphoriant, anorectic, hyperthermic, and cardiovascular effects.

Intravenous cocaine use is associated with risks for the same conditions as other forms of intravenous drug abuse, including AIDS, septicemia, and venous thrombus. Long-term snorting can lead to a rebound rhinitis, which is often self-treated with nasal decongestants; it also causes nosebleeds and eventually may lead to a perforated nasal septum. Other physical sequelae include cerebral infarctions, seizures, myocardial infarctions, cardiac arrhythmias, and cardiomyopathies.

A. Cocaine intoxication.   See Table 7–4. Can cause restlessness, agitation, anxiety, talkativeness, pressured speech, paranoid ideation, aggressiveness, increased sexual interest, heightened sense of awareness, grandiosity, hyperactivity, and other manic symptoms. Physical signs include tachycardia, hypertension, pupillary dilation, chills, anorexia, insomnia, and stereotyped movements. Cocaine use has also been associated with sudden death from cardiac complications and delirium. Delusional disorders are typically paranoid. Delirium may involve tactile or olfactory hallucinations. Delusions and hallucinations may occur in up to 50% of all persons who use cocaine. Delirium may lead to seizures and death.

B. Withdrawal.   The most prominent sign of cocaine withdrawal is the craving for cocaine. The tendency to develop dependence is related to the route of administration (lower with snorting, higher with intravenous injection or smoking freebase cocaine). Withdrawal symptoms include fatigue, lethargy, guilt, anxiety, and feelings of helplessness, hopelessness, and worthlessness. Long-term use can lead to depression, which may require antidepressant treatment. Observe for possible suicidal ideation. Withdrawal symptoms usually peak in several days, but the syndrome (especially depressive symptoms) may last for weeks.

C. Treatment.   Treatment is largely symptomatic. Agitation can be treated with restraints, benzodiazepines, or, if severe (delirium or psychosis), low doses of high-potency antipsychotics (only as a last resort because the medications lower the seizure threshold). Somatic symptoms (e.g., tachycardia, hypertension) can be treated with β-adrenergic receptor antagonists (beta blockers). Evaluate for possible medical complications.

VI. Cannabis (marijuana)

About one third of Americans have tried marijuana. Marijuana and hashish contain Δ-9-tetrahydrocannabinol (THC), which is the main active euphoriant (many other active cannabinoids are probably responsible for the other varied effects). Sometimes, purified THC also is abused. Cannabinoids usually are smoked but also can be eaten (onset of effect is delayed, but one can eat very large doses).

A. **Cannabis intoxication.**   When cannabis is smoked, euphoric effects appear within minutes, peak in 30 minutes, and last 2 to 4 hours. Motor and cognitive effects can last 5 to 12 hours. Symptoms include euphoria or dysphoria, anxiety, suspiciousness, inappropriate laughter, time distortion, social withdrawal, impaired judgment, and the following objective signs: conjunctival injection, increased appetite, dry mouth, and tachycardia. It also causes a dose-dependent hypothermia and mild sedation. Often used with alcohol, cocaine, and other drugs. Can cause depersonalization and, rarely, hallucinations. More commonly causes mild persecutory delusions, which seldom require medication. In very high doses, can cause mild delirium with panic symptoms or a prolonged cannabis psychosis (may last up to 6 weeks). Long-term use can lead to anxiety or depression and an apathetic amotivational syndrome. Chronic respiratory disease and lung cancer are long-term risks secondary to inhalation of carcinogenic hydrocarbons. Results of urinary testing for THC are positive for up to 4 weeks after intoxication.

B. **Cannabis dependence.**   Dependence and withdrawal are controversial diagnoses; there are certainly many psychologically dependent abusers, but forced abstinence, even in heavy users, does not consistently cause a characteristic withdrawal syndrome.

C. **Therapeutic uses.**   Cannabis and its primary active components (Δ-9-THC) have been used successfully to treat nausea secondary to cancer chemotherapy, to stimulate appetite in patients with AIDS, and in the treatment of glaucoma.

D. **Treatment.**   Treatment of intoxication usually is not required. Anxiolytics for anxiety, antipsychotics for hallucinations or delusions.

VII. Hallucinogens

Hallucinogen use has increased in the last decade. The use of lysergic acid diethylamide (LSD) is most likely to occur between the ages of 18 and 25.

A. **Drugs**
   1. LSD.
   2. Psilocybin (from some mushrooms).
   3. Mescaline (peyote cactus).
   4. Harmine and harmaline.
   5. Ibogaine.
   6. Substituted amphetamines (e.g., MDMA, MDEA, 2,5-dimethoxy-4-methylamphetamine [DOM, STP], dimethyltryptamine [DMT], MMDA, trimethoxyamphetamine [TMA]), which are also commonly classified with amphetamines.

B. **General considerations.**   Hallucinogens usually are eaten, sucked out of paper (buccally ingested), or smoked. This category includes many different drugs with different effects. Hallucinogens act as sympathomimetics and cause hypertension, tachycardia, hyperthermia, and dilated pupils. Psychological effects range from mild perceptual changes to frank hallucinations; most users experience only mild effects. Usually used sporadically because of tolerance, which develops rapidly and remits within several days of abstinence. Physical dependence or withdrawal does not occur, but psychological dependence can develop. Hallucinogens often are contaminated with anticholinergic drugs. Hallucinogen potency is associated with binding affinity at the serotonin-5-HT$_2$ receptor, where these drugs act as partial agonists.

C. **Hallucinogen intoxication (hallucinosis)**
   1. **Diagnosis, signs, and symptoms.** In a state of full wakefulness and alertness, maladaptive behavioral changes (anxiety, depression, ideas of reference, paranoid ideation); changes in perception (hallucinations, illusions, depersonalization); pupillary dilation, tachycardia or palpitations, sweating, blurring of vision, tremors, and incoordination. Panic reactions ("bad trips") can occur even in experienced users. The user typically becomes convinced that the disturbed perceptions are real. In the typical bad trip, the user feels as if he or she is going mad, has damaged his or her brain, and will never recover.
   2. **Treatment.** Involves reassurance and keeping the patient in contact with trusted, supportive people (friends, nurses). Diazepam (20 mg orally) can rapidly curtail hallucinogen intoxication and is considered superior to "talking down" the patient, which may take hours. If the patient is psychotic and agitated, high-potency antipsychotics, such as haloperidol (Haldol), fluphenazine (Prolixin), or thiothixene (Navane), may be used (avoid low-potency antipsychotics because of anticholinergic effects). A controlled environment is necessary to prevent possible dangerous actions resulting from grossly impaired judgment. Physical restraints may be required. Prolonged psychosis resembling schizophreniform disorder occasionally develops in vulnerable patients. Delusional syndromes and mood (usually depressive) disorders may also develop.

D. **Posthallucinogen perception disorder.** A distressing repeated experience of impaired perception after cessation of hallucinogen use (i.e., a **flashback**). The patient may require low doses of a benzodiazepine (for an acute episode) or antipsychotic drug (if persistent).

VIII. **Phencyclidine (PCP) and similarly acting drugs**

   PCP is a dissociative anesthetic with hallucinogenic effects. Similarly acting drugs include ketamine (Ketalar), also referred to as *special K*. PCP commonly causes paranoia and unpredictable violence, which often brings abusers to medical attention. The primary pharmacodynamic effect is antagonism of the NMDA subtype of glutamate receptors.

A. **PCP intoxication**
   1. **Diagnosis, signs, and symptoms.** Belligerence, assaultiveness, agitation, impulsiveness, unpredictability, and the following signs: nystagmus, increased blood pressure or heart rate, numbness or diminished response to pain, ataxia, dysarthria, muscle rigidity, seizures, and hyperacusis.

Typically, PCP is smoked with marijuana (a laced joint) or tobacco, but it can be eaten, injected, or inhaled nasally. PCP should be considered in patients who describe unusual experiences with marijuana or LSD. PCP may remain detectable in blood and urine for more than 1 week.

Effects are dose-related. At low doses, PCP acts as a CNS depressant, producing nystagmus, blurred vision, numbness, and incoordination. At moderate doses, PCP produces hypertension, dysarthria, ataxia, increased muscle tone (especially in the face and neck), hyperactive reflexes, and sweating. At higher doses, PCP produces agitation, fever, abnormal movements, rhabdomyolysis, myoglobinuria, and renal failure. Overdose can cause seizures, severe hypertension, diaphoresis, hypersalivation, respiratory depression, stupor (with eyes open), coma, and death. Violent actions are common with intoxication. Because of the analgesic effects of PCP, patients may have no regard for their own bodies and may severely injure themselves while agitated and combative. Psychosis, sometimes persistent (may resemble schizophreniform disorder), may develop. This is especially likely in patients with underlying schizophrenia. Other possible complications include delirium, mood disorder, and delusional disorder.

2. **Treatment.** Isolate the patient in a nonstimulating environment. Do not try to talk down the intoxicated patient, as you might with a patient with anxiety disorder; wait for the PCP to clear first. Urine acidification may increase drug clearance (ascorbic acid or ammonium chloride), but it may be ineffective and increase the risk for renal failure. Screen for other drugs. If the patient is acutely agitated, use benzodiazepines. If agitated and psychotic, a high-potency antipsychotic may be used. Avoid antipsychotics with potent intensive anticholinergic properties, as high-dose PCP has anticholinergic actions. If physical restraint is required, immobilize the patient completely to prevent self-injury. Recovery is usually rapid. Protect the patient and staff. Always evaluate for concomitant medical conditions.

IX. Inhalants

A wide variety of glues, solvents, and cleaners are volatile and can be inhaled for psychotropic effects. Most are aromatic hydrocarbons; they include gasoline, kerosene, plastic and rubber cements, airplane and household glues, paints, lacquers, enamels, paint thinners, aerosols, polishes, fingernail polish remover, nitrous oxide, amyl nitrate, butyl nitrate, and cleaning fluids.

Inhalants typically are abused by adolescents in lower socioeconomic groups. Some persons use "poppers" (amyl nitrate, butyl nitrate) during sex to intensify orgasm through vasodilation, which produces light-headedness, giddiness, and euphoria.

Symptoms of mild intoxication are similar to intoxication with alcohol or sedative-hypnotics. Psychological effects include mild euphoria, belligerence, assaultiveness, impaired judgment, and impulsiveness. Physical effects in-

TABLE 7–10
TYPICAL CAFFEINE CONTENT OF FOODS AND MEDICATIONS

Substance	Caffeine Content
Brewed coffee	100 mg/6 oz
Instant coffee	70 mg/6 oz
Decaffeinated coffee	4 mg/6 oz
Leaf or bag tea	40 mg/6 oz
Instant tea	25 mg/6 oz
Caffeinated soda	45 mg/12 oz
Cocoa beverage	5 mg/6 oz
Chocolate milk	4 mg/6 oz
Dark chocolate	20 mg/1 oz
Milk chocolate	6 mg/1 oz
Caffeine-containing cold remedies	25–50 mg/tablet
Caffeine-containing analgesics	25–65 mg/tablet
Stimulants	100–350 mg/tablet
Weight-loss aids	75–200 mg/tablet

Adapted from DSM-IV-TR and Barone JJ, Roberts HR. Caffeine consumption. *Food Chem Toxicol* 1996;34:119, with permission.

clude ataxia, confusion, disorientation, slurred speech, dizziness, depressed reflexes, and nystagmus. These can progress to delirium and seizures. Possible toxic effects include brain damage, liver damage, bone marrow depression, peripheral neuropathies, and immunosuppression. Although not recognized by DSM-IV-TR, rarely a withdrawal syndrome can develop. It is characterized by irritability, sleep disturbances, jitters, sweats, nausea, vomiting, tachycardia, and sometimes hallucinations and delusions. Short-term treatment is supportive medical care (e.g., fluids and monitoring of blood pressure).

X. Caffeine

Caffeine is present in coffee, tea, chocolate, cola and other carbonated beverages, cocoa, cold medications, and over-the-counter stimulants. (See Table 7–10 for the typical caffeine content of foods and medications.) Intoxication is characterized by restlessness, nervousness, excitement, insomnia, flushed face, diuresis, gastrointestinal disturbance, muscle twitching, rambling flow of thought and speech, tachycardia or cardiac arrhythmia, periods of inexhaustibility, and psychomotor agitation. High doses can increase symptoms of psychiatric disorders (e.g., anxiety, psychosis). Tolerance develops. Withdrawal is usually characterized by headache and lasts 4 to 5 days.

XI. Nicotine

Nicotine is taken through tobacco smoking and chewing. Nicotine dependence is the most prevalent and deadly substance use disorder. About 25% of Americans smoke, 25% are former smokers, and 50% have never smoked cigarettes. Nicotine activates nicotine acetylcholine receptors in addition to the dopamine reward system and increases multiple stimulatory neurohormones.

A. Nicotine dependence. Develops rapidly and is strongly affected by environmental conditioning. Often coexists with dependence on other substances (e.g., alcohol, marijuana). Treatments for dependence include hypnosis, aversive therapy, acupuncture, nicotine nasal sprays and gums, transdermal nicotine (nicotine patches), clonidine, and a variety of other nonnicotine psychopharmacologic agents. Bupropion (Zyban) at doses of 300 mg/d may increase the quit rate in smokers with and without depression. The combined use of systemic nicotine administration and behavioral counseling has resulted in sustained abstinence rates of 60%. (See Table 7–11 for the treatment of nicotine dependence.) High relapse rates. Psychiatrists should be aware of the effects of abstinence from smoking on blood concentrations of psychotropic drugs (Table 7–12). Smoking is more habit-forming than chewing. Smoking is associated with chronic obstructive pulmonary disease, cancers, coronary heart disease, and peripheral vascular disease. Tobacco chewing is associated with peripheral vascular disease.

   B. Nicotine withdrawal.   Characterized by nicotine craving, irritability, frustration, anger, anxiety, difficulty concentrating, restlessness, bradycardia, and increased appetite. The withdrawal syndrome may last for up to several weeks and is often superimposed on withdrawal from other substances.

XII. Anabolic steroids

   Anabolic steroids are Drug Enforcement Agency Schedule III controlled substances that are illegally used to enhance physical performance and appearance and to increase muscle bulk. Examples of commonly used anabolic

TABLE 7–11
SCIENTIFICALLY PROVEN TREATMENTS FOR SMOKING

Psychosocial therapy
  Behavior therapy
Pharmacological therapies
  Nicotine gum
  Nicotine patch
  Nicotine gum + patch
  Nicotine nasal spray
  Nicotine inhaler
  Bupropion
  Bupropion + nicotine patch
  Clonidine[a]
  Nortriptyline[a]

[a] Not an FDA-approved use.
Adapted from John R. Hughes, M.D.

TABLE 7–12
EFFECT OF ABSTINENCE FROM SMOKING ON BLOOD CONCENTRATIONS OF PSYCHIATRIC MEDICINES

Abstinence increases blood concentrations			
Clomipramine	Desmethyldiazepam	Haloperidol	Nortriptyline
Clozapine	Doxepin	Imipramine	Propranolol
Desipramine	Fluvoxamine	Oxazepam	
Abstinence does not increase blood concentrations			
Amitriptyline	Ethanol	Midazolam	
Chlordiazepoxide	Lorazepam	Triazolam	
Effects of abstinence unclear			
Alprazolam	Chlorpromazine	Diazepam	

Adapted from John R. Hughes, M.D.

TABLE 7–13
EXAMPLES OF COMMONLY USED ANABOLIC STEROIDS[a]

Compounds usually administered orally
Fluoxymesterone (Halotestin, Android-F, Ultandren)
Methandienone (formerly called *methandrostenolone*) (Dianabol)
Methyltestosterone (Android, Testred, Virilon)
Mibolerone (Cheque Drops)[b]
Oxandrolone (Anavar)
Oxymetholone (Anadrol, Hemogenin)
Mesterolone (Mestoranum, Proviron)
Stanozolol (Winstrol)
Compounds usually administered intramuscularly
Nandrolone decanoate (Deca-Durabolin)
Nandrolone phenpropionate (Durabolin)
Methenolone enanthate (Primobolan depot)
Boldenone undecylenate (Equipoise)[b]
Stanozolol (Winstrol-V)[b]
Testosterone esters blends (Sustanon, Sten)
Testosterone cypionate
Testosterone enanthate (Delatestryl)
Testosterone propionate (Testoviron, Androlan)
Testosterone undecanoate (Andriol, Restandol)
Trenbolone acetate (Finajet, Finaplix)[b]
Trenbolone hexahydrobencylcarbonate (Parabolan)

[a] Many of the brand names listed are foreign but are included because of the widespread illicit use of foreign steroid preparations in the United States.
[b] Veterinary compound.
Adapted from Harrison G. Pope, Jr., M.D., and Kirk J. Brower, M.D.

steroids are listed in Table 7–13. An estimated 1 million Americans have used illegal steroids at least once. Use has been increasing among male adolescents and young adults. People drawn to these drugs are usually involved in athletics. Reinforcement occurs when the drugs produce desired results, such as enhanced performance and appearance. Anabolic steroid users typically use a variety of ergogenic (performance-enhancing) drugs to gain muscle, lose fat, or lose water for body-building competitions. These drugs include thyroid hormones and stimulants. Dehydroepiandrosterone (DHEA) and androstenedione are adrenal androgens marketed as food supplements and sold over the counter. Steroids initially produce euphoria and hyperactivity, which can give way to hostility, irritability, anxiety, somatization, depression, manic symptoms, and violent outbursts ("roid rage"). Steroids are addictive. Abstinence can produce depression, anxiety, and worry about physical appearance. Physical complications of abuse include acne, premature balding, gynecomastia, testicular atrophy, yellowing of the skin and eyes, clitoral enlargement, menstrual abnormalities, and hirsutism.

Gamma hydroxybutyrate (GHB, "liquid ecstasy") has been used by body builders as a steroid alternative. It is a naturally occurring transmitter in the brain that is related to sleep regulation. Abuse can produce intoxication in addition to nausea, vomiting, seizures, brain damage, coma, and death.

Treatment includes psychotherapy to cope with body image distortions and the profound physical side effects of prolonged steroid use. As with other substances of abuse, abstinence is the goal. Frequent urine testing is indicated.

For more detailed discussion of this topic, see Substance-Related Disorders, Ch 11, p 924, in CTP/VII.

8

Schizophrenia

I. Definition

Schizophrenia is a psychotic disorder of unknown etiology and divergent presentations. It is characterized by positive and negative (deficit) symptoms (Table 8–1). Although not a cognitive disorder, schizophrenia often causes cognitive impairments (e.g., concrete thinking, impaired information processing). The symptoms of schizophrenia adversely affect thinking, feeling, behavior, and social and occupational functioning. This illness is usually chronic, with a course encompassing a prodromal phase, an active phase, and a residual phase. The prodromal and residual phases are characterized by attenuated forms of active symptoms, such as odd beliefs and magical thinking, as well as deficits in self-care and interpersonal relatedness. Schizophrenia is well established as a brain disorder, with structural and functional abnormalities visible in neuroimaging studies and a genetic component as seen in twin studies.

II. History

1852—Schizophrenia was first formally described by Belgian psychiatrist Benedict Morel, who called it *démence précoce*.

1896—Emil Kraepelin, a German psychiatrist, applied the term *dementia praecox* to a group of illnesses beginning in adolescence that ended in dementia.

1911—Swiss psychiatrist Eugen Bleuler introduced the term *schizophrenia*. No signs or symptoms are pathognomonic; instead, a cluster of characteristic findings indicates the diagnosis. The diagnostic criteria in current use are from DSM-IV-TR (Table 8–2). The criteria formulated by Kraepelin, Bleuler (the four As), and Kurt Schneider (first-rank symptoms) are useful (Tables 8–3, 8–4, and 8–5); however, the DSM-IV-TR criteria are the most widely used and accepted.

III. Diagnosis, signs, and symptoms

See Table 8–2. Schizophrenia is a phenomenological diagnosis based on observation and description of the patient. Abnormalities are often present on most components of the mental status examination.

A. **Overall functioning.** The patient's level of functioning declines or fails to achieve the expected level.

B. **Thought content.** Abnormal (e.g., delusions, ideas of reference, poverty of content).

C. **Form of thought.** Illogical (e.g., derailment, loosening of associations, incoherence, circumstantiality, tangentiality, overinclusiveness, neologisms, blocking, echolalia—all incorporated as a thought disorder).

D. **Perception.** Distorted (e.g., hallucinations: visual, olfactory, tactile, and, most frequently, auditory).

E. **Affect.** Abnormal (e.g., flat, blunted, silly, labile, inappropriate).

F. **Sense of self.** Impaired (e.g., loss of ego boundaries, gender confusion, inability to distinguish internal from external reality).

TABLE 8–1
POSITIVE AND NEGATIVE SYMPTOMS

Positive Symptoms	Negative Symptoms
Delusions	Affective flattening
Hallucinations	Alogia
Disorganized behavior	Avolition
	Anhedonia

TABLE 8–2
DSM-IV-TR DIAGNOSTIC CRITERIA FOR SCHIZOPHRENIA

A. *Characteristic symptoms:* Two (or more) of the following, each present for a significant portion of time during a 1-month period (or less if successfully treated):

   (1) delusions
   (2) hallucinations
   (3) disorganized speech (e.g., frequent derailment or incoherence)
   (4) grossly disorganized or catatonic behavior
   (5) negative symptoms, i.e., affective flattening, alogia, or avolition

   Note: Only one criterion A symptom is required if delusions are bizarre or hallucinations consist of a voice keeping up a running commentary on the person's behavior or thoughts, or two or more voices conversing with each other.

B. *Social/occupational dysfunction:* For a significant portion of the time since the onset of the disturbance, one or more major areas of functioning, such as work, interpersonal relations, or self-care are markedly below the level achieved prior to the onset (or when the onset is in childhood or adolescence, failure to achieve expected level of interpersonal, academic, or occupational achievement).

C. *Duration:* Continuous signs of the disturbance persist for at least 6 months. This 6-month period must include at least 1 month of symptoms (or less if successfully treated) that meet criterion A (i.e., active-phase symptoms) and may include periods of prodromal or residual symptoms. During these prodromal or residual periods, the signs of the disturbance may be manifested by only negative symptoms or two or more symptoms listed in criterion A present in on attenuated form (e.g., odd beliefs, unusual perceptual experiences).

D. *Schizoaffective and mood disorder exclusion:* Schizoaffective disorder and mood disorder with psychotic features have been ruled out because either (1) no major depressive, manic, or mixed episodes have occurred concurrently with the active-phase symptoms, or (2) if mood episodes have occurred during active-phase symptoms, their total duration has been brief relative to the duration of the active and residual periods.

E. *Substance/general medical condition exclusion:* The disturbance is not due to the direct physiological effects of a substance (e.g., a drug of abuse, a medication) or a general medical condition.

F. *Relationship to a pervasive developmental disorder:* If there is a history of autistic disorder or another Pervasive Developmental disorder, the additional diagnosis of schizophrenia is made only if prominent delusions or hallucinations are also present for at least a month (or less if successfully treated.)

Classification of longitudinal course (can be applied only after at least 1 year has elapsed since the initial onset of active-phase symptoms):

   Episodic with interepisode residual symptoms (episodes are defined by the reemergence of prominent psychotic symptoms); *also specify if:* **with prominent negative symptoms.**
   Episodic with no interepisode residual symptoms
   Continuous (prominent psychotic symptoms are present throughout the period of observation); *also specify if:* **with prominent negative symptoms**
   Single episode in partial remission; *also specify if:* **with prominent negative symptoms**
   Single episode in full remission
   Other or unspecified pattern

TABLE 8-3
EMIL KRAEPELIN'S CRITERIA

- Disturbances of attention and comprehension
- Hallucinations, especially auditory (voices)
- *Gedankenlautwerden* (audible thoughts)
- Experiences of influenced thought
- Disturbances in the flow of thought, above all a loosening of associations
- Impairment of cognitive function and judgment
- Affective flattening
- Appearance of morbid behavior
  Reduced drive
    Automatic obedience
    Echolalia, echopraxia
    Acting out
    Catatonic frenzy
    Stereotypy
    Negativism
    Autism
    Disturbance of verbal expression

From World Psychiatric Association, with permission.

TABLE 8-4
EUGEN BLEULER'S SYMPTOM CRITERIA

Basic or fundamental disturbances
- Formal thought disorders[a]
- Disturbances of affect[a]
- Disturbances of the subjective experience of self
- Disturbances of volition and behavior
- Ambivalence[a]
- Autism[a]

Accessory symptoms
- Disorders of perception (hallucinations)
- Delusions
- Certain memory disturbances
- Modification of personality
- Changes in speech and writing
- Somatic symptoms
- Catatonic symptoms
- Acute syndrome (such as melancholic, manic, catatonic, and other states)

[a] Bleuler's four *A*s: association, affect, ambivalence, and autism.
From World Psychiatric Association, with permission.

TABLE 8-5
KURT SCHNEIDER'S CRITERIA, FIRST- AND SECOND-RANK SYMPTOMS

First-rank symptoms
- Audible thoughts
- Voices arguing or discussing
- Voices commenting
- Somatic passivity experiences
- Thought withdrawal and other experiences of influenced thought[a]
- Thought broadcasting
- Delusional perceptions
- All other experiences involving made volition, made affect, and made impulses

Second-rank symptoms
- Other disorders of perception
- Sudden delusional ideas
- Perplexity
- Depressive and euphoric mood changes
- Feelings of emotional impoverishment
- ". . . and several others as well"

[a] The symptom *thought insertion* was originally included under *other experiences of influenced thought*.
From World Psychiatric Association, with permission.

G. Volition.   Altered (e.g., inadequate drive or motivation and marked ambivalence).

H. Interpersonal functioning.   Impaired (e.g., social withdrawal and emotional detachment, aggressiveness, sexual inappropriateness).

I. Psychomotor behavior.   Abnormal or changed (e.g., agitation vs. withdrawal, grimacing, posturing, rituals, catatonia).

J. Cognition.   Impaired (e.g., concreteness, inattention, impaired information processing).

IV. Types

A. Paranoid
1. Preoccupation with systematized delusions or frequent auditory hallucinations related to a single theme, usually persecutory.
2. None of the following: incoherence, loosening of associations, flat or grossly inappropriate affect, catatonic behavior, grossly disorganized behavior.
3. Later onset and better prognosis than catatonic and disorganized types.

B. Disorganized
1. Incoherence, marked loosening of associations, regressed or grossly disorganized behavior.
2. Flat or grossly inappropriate affect.
3. Does not meet criteria for catatonic type.
4. Early onset, dilapidated appearance.

C. Catatonic
1. Stupor or mutism.
2. Negativism.
3. Rigidity.
4. Purposeless excitement with risk of injury to self or others.
5. Posturing.
6. Echolalia or echopraxia.
7. May need medical care for associated malnutrition or hyperpyrexia.

D. Undifferentiated type
1. Prominent delusions, hallucinations, incoherence, or grossly disorganized behavior.
2. Does not meet the criteria for paranoid, catatonic, or disorganized type.

E. Residual type
1. Absence of prominent delusions, hallucinations, incoherence, or grossly disorganized behavior.
2. Continuing evidence of the disturbance through two or more residual symptoms (e.g., emotional blunting, social withdrawal).

F. Type I and type II.
Another system proposes classification of schizophrenia into types I and II. The system is based on the presence of positive or negative symptoms. The negative symptoms include affective flattening or blunting, poverty of speech or speech content, blocking, poor grooming, lack of motivation, anhedonia, social withdrawal, cognitive defects, and attentional deficits. Positive symptoms include loose associations, hallucinations, bizarre behavior, and increased speech. Type I pa-

tients have mostly positive symptoms, and type II patients have mostly negative symptoms.

G. Paraphrenia. Sometimes used as a synonym for *paranoid schizophrenia*. The term also is used for either a progressively deteriorating course of illness or the presence of a well-systematized delusional system. These multiple meanings have reduced the usefulness of the term.

H. Simple schizophrenia. The term *simple schizophrenia* (called *simple deteriorative disorder* in DSM-IV-TR) was used when schizophrenia had a broad diagnostic conceptualization. Simple schizophrenia was characterized by a gradual, insidious loss of drive and ambition. Patients with the disorder were usually not overtly psychotic and did not experience persistent hallucinations or delusions. The primary symptom is the withdrawal of the patient from social and work-related situations.

V. Epidemiology

A. Incidence and prevalence. An estimated 2 million Americans suffer from schizophrenia. Worldwide, 2 million new cases appear each year. Lifetime prevalence is approximately 1–1.5%. Prevalence, morbidity, and severity of presentation are greater in urban than in rural areas. Furthermore, morbidity and severity of presentation are greater in industrialized than in nonindustrialized areas.

B. Sex ratio. The male-to-female ratio is 1:1.

C. Socioeconomic status. Increased prevalence in lower socioeconomic groups, but equal incidence across socioeconomic classes (reflects downward drift theory, which states that although those with the disorder originally may have been born into any socioeconomic class, they eventually tend to drift downward into the lower socioeconomic classes owing to their significant impairments).

D. Age of onset. Most common between ages 15 and 35 (50% below age 25). Rare before age 10 or after age 40. Earlier onset for men than for women.

E. Religion. Jews are affected less often than Protestants and Catholics.

F. Race. Prevalence is reported to be higher among blacks and Hispanics than among whites, but this assertion may reflect the bias of diagnosticians or a higher percentage of minority persons living in lower socioeconomic groups and in industrialized urban areas.

G. Seasonality. Higher incidence in both winter and early spring (January through April in the Northern Hemisphere, July through September in the Southern Hemisphere).

H. Inpatients versus outpatients. Since the 1970s (deinstitutionalization), the number of schizophrenia patients in hospitals has decreased by 40–50%. Currently, up to 80% of schizophrenic patients are treated as outpatients.

I. Cost. Direct and indirect costs in the United States are approximately $100 billion a year.

VI. Etiology

Owing to the heterogeneity of the symptomatic and prognostic presentations of schizophrenia, no single factor is considered causative. The stress diathesis model is most often used, which states that the person in whom schizophrenia develops has a specific biological vulnerability, or diathesis, that is triggered by stress and leads to schizophrenic symptoms. Stresses may be genetic, biological, and psychosocial or environmental.

A. Genetic. Both single-gene and polygenic theories have been proposed (Table 8–6). Although neither theory has been definitively substantiated, the polygenic theory appears to be more consistent with the presentation of schizophrenia.

   1. **Consanguinity.** Incidence in families is higher than in the general population, and monozygotic (MZ) twin concordance is greater than dizygotic (DZ) (Table 8–7).

   2. **Adoption studies.** Risk is secondary to biological parent, not adoptive parent.

      a. Risk to an adopted child (approximately 10–12%) is the same as if the child had been reared by his or her biological parents.

      b. The prevalence of schizophrenia is greater in the biological parents of schizophrenic adoptees than in adoptive parents.

      c. MZ twins reared apart have the same concordance rate as twins reared together.

      d. Rates of schizophrenia are not increased in children born to unaffected parents but raised by a schizophrenic parent.

B. Biological

   1. **Dopamine hypothesis.** Schizophrenic symptoms may result from increased limbic dopamine activity (positive symptoms) and decreased frontal dopamine activity (negative symptoms). Dopaminergic pathol-

---

TABLE 8–6
FEATURES CONSISTENT WITH POLYGENIC INHERITANCE[a]

- Disorder can be transmitted with two normal parents.
- Presentation of disorder ranges from very severe to less severe.
- More severely affected persons have a greater number of ill relatives than mildly affected persons do.
- Risk decreases as the number of shared genes decreases.
- Disorder present in both mother's and father's side of family.

[a] The number of affected genes determines a person's risk and symptomatic picture.

TABLE 8–7
PREVALENCE OF SCHIZOPHRENIA IN SPECIFIC POPULATIONS

Population	Prevalence (%)
General population	1–1.5
First-degree relative[a]	10–12
Second-degree relative	5–6
Child of two schizophrenic parents	40
Dizygotic twin	12–15
Monozygotic twin	45–50

[a] Schizophrenia is not a sex-linked disorder; it does not matter which parent has the disorder in terms of risk.

ogy may be secondary to abnormal receptor number or sensitivity, or abnormal dopamine release (too much or too little). The theory is based on psychotogenic effects of drugs that increase dopamine levels (e.g., amphetamines, cocaine) and the antipsychotic effects of dopamine receptor antagonists (e.g., haloperidol [Haldol]). Dopamine receptors D_1 through D_5 have been identified. The D_1 receptor may play a role in negative symptoms. Specific D_3 and D_4 receptor agonist and antagonist drugs are under development. Levels of the dopamine metabolite homovanillic acid may correlate with the severity and potential treatment responsiveness of psychotic symptoms. Limitations of the theory include the responsiveness of all types of psychoses to dopamine-blocking agents, which implicates dopaminergic abnormalities in psychoses of multiple causes. The complex interplay of different neurotransmitter systems, including serotonin–dopamine interactions, in addition to the effects of amino acid neurotransmitters on monoamines render single-neurotransmitter theories simplistic and incomplete.

2. **Norepinephrine hypothesis.** Increased norepinephrine levels in schizophrenia lead to increased sensitization to sensory input.

3. **γ-Aminobutyric acid (GABA) hypothesis.** Decreased GABA activity results in increased dopamine activity.

4. **Serotonin hypothesis.** Serotonin metabolism apparently is abnormal in some chronically schizophrenic patients, with both hyperserotoninemia and hyposerotoninemia being reported. Specifically, antagonism at the serotonin $5\text{-}HT_2$ receptor has been emphasized as important in reducing psychotic symptoms and in militating against the development of movement disorders related to D_2 antagonism. Research on mood disorders has implicated serotonin activity in suicidal and impulsive behavior, which schizophrenic patients also can exhibit.

5. **Hallucinogens.** It has been suggested that some endogenous amines act as substrates for abnormal methylation, resulting in endogenous hallucinogens. This hypothesis is not supported by reliable data.

6. **Glutamate hypothesis.** Hypofunction of the glutamate N-methyl-D-aspartate (NMDA)-type receptor is theorized to cause both positive and negative symptoms of schizophrenia based on the observed psychotogenic effects of the NMDA antagonists phencyclidine and ketamine (Ketalar), in addition to the observed therapeutic effects (in research settings) of the NMDA agonists glycine and D-cycloserine.

7. **Neurodevelopmental and neurodegenerative theories.** Evidence for abnormal neuronal migration during the second trimester of fetal development. Theories of abnormal neuronal functioning during adolescence leading to the emergence of symptoms. Glutamate receptor-mediated cell loss may occur. All the above could explain the cell loss without gliosis seen in schizophrenia, and the progressive nature of the disorder in some patients.

C. **Psychosocial and environmental**

1. **Family factors.** Patients whose families have high levels of expressed emotion (EE) have higher relapse rates than those whose families have low EE levels. EE has been defined as any overly involved,

intrusive behavior, be it hostile and critical or controlling and infantilizing. Relapse rates are better when family behavior is modified to lower EE. Most observers believe that family dysfunction is a consequence, rather than a cause, of schizophrenia.

2. **Other psychodynamic issues.** Understanding which psychosocial and environmental stressors may be specific to individual schizophrenic patients is crucial. Knowing what psychological and environmental stresses are most likely to trigger psychotic decompensation in a patient helps the clinician to address these issues supportively and, in the process, helps the patient to feel and remain more in control.

D. **Infectious theory.** Evidence for a slow virus etiology includes neuropathological changes consistent with past infections: gliosis, glial scarring, and antiviral antibodies in the serum and CSF of some schizophrenia patients. Increased frequency of perinatal complications and seasonality of birth data also can support an infectious theory.

VII. Laboratory and psychological tests

A. **EEG.** Most schizophrenic patients have normal EEG findings, but some have decreased alpha and increased theta and delta activity, paroxysmal abnormalities, and increased sensitivity to activation procedures (e.g., sleep deprivation).

B. **Evoked potential studies.** Initial hypersensitivity to sensory stimulation, with later compensatory blunting of information processing at higher cortical levels.

C. **Immunologic studies.** In some patients, atypical lymphocytes and decreased numbers of natural killer cells.

D. **Endocrinologic studies.** In some patients, decreased levels of luteinizing hormone and follicle-stimulating hormone; diminished release of prolactin and growth hormone following stimulation by gonadotropin-releasing hormone or thyrotropin-releasing hormone.

E. **Neuropsychological testing.** Thematic apperception test and Rorschach test usually reveal bizarre responses. When compared with the parents of normal controls, the parents of schizophrenic patients show more deviation from normal values in projective tests (may be a consequence of living with schizophrenic family member). Halstead-Reitan battery reveals impaired attention and intelligence, decreased retention time, and disturbed problem-solving ability in approximately 20–35% of patients. Schizophrenic patients have lower I.Q.s when compared with nonschizophrenic patients, although the range of I.Q. scores is wide. Decline in I.Q. occurs with progression of the illness.

VIII. Pathophysiology

A. **Neuropathology.** No consistent structural defects; changes noted include decreased number of neurons, increased gliosis, and disorganization of neuronal architecture. Degeneration in the limbic system, especially the amygdala, hippocampus, and cingulate cortex, and in the basal ganglia, especially the substantia nigra and dorsolateral prefrontal cortex.

B. Brain imaging

   1. **Computed tomography (CT).** Cortical atrophy in 10–35% of patients; enlargement of the lateral and third ventricle in 10–50% of patients; atrophy of the cerebellar vermis and decreased radiodensity of brain parenchyma. Abnormal CT findings may correlate with the presence of negative symptoms (e.g., flattened affect, social withdrawal, psychomotor retardation, lack of motivation, neuropsychiatric impairment, increased frequency of extrapyramidal symptoms resulting from antipsychotic medications, and poor premorbid history).

   2. **Magnetic resonance imaging (MRI).** Ventricles in MZ twins with schizophrenia are larger than those of unaffected siblings. Reduced volume of hippocampus, amygdala, and parahippocampal gyrus. Reduced limbic volume correlating with disease severity.

   3. **Magnetic resonance spectroscopy.** Decreased metabolism of the dorsolateral prefrontal cortex.

   4. **Positron emission tomography (PET).** In some patients, decreased frontal and parietal lobe metabolism, relatively high rate of posterior metabolism, and abnormal laterality.

   5. **Cerebral blood flow (CBF).** In some patients, decreased resting levels of frontal blood flow, increased parietal blood flow, and decreased whole-brain blood flow. When PET and CBF studies are considered together with CT findings, dysfunction of the frontal lobe is most clearly implicated. Frontal lobe dysfunction may be secondary, however, to disease elsewhere in the brain.

C. Physical findings. Minor (soft) neurological findings occur in 50–100% of patients: increased prevalence of primitive reflexes (e.g., grasp reflex), abnormal stereognosis and two-point discrimination, and dysdiadochokinesia (impairment in ability to perform rapidly alternating movements). Paroxysmal saccadic eye movements (inability to follow object through space with smooth eye movements) occur in 50–80% of schizophrenic patients and in 40–45% of first-degree relatives of schizophrenic patients (compared with an 8–10% prevalence in non-schizophrenic persons). This may be a neurophysiologic marker of a vulnerability to schizophrenia. Resting heart rates have been found to be higher in schizophrenic patients than in controls and may reflect a hyperaroused state.

IX. Psychodynamic factors

Understanding a patient's dynamics (or psychological conflicts and issues) is critical for complete understanding of the symbolic meaning of symptoms. A patient's internal experience is usually one of confusion and overwhelming sensory input, and defense mechanisms are the ego's attempt to deal with powerful affects. Three major primitive defenses interfere with reality testing: (1) Psychotic projection—attributing inner sensations of aggression, sexuality, chaos, and confusion to the outside world, as opposed to recognizing them as emanating from within; boundaries between inner and outer experience are confused. Projection is the major defense underlying paranoid delusions. (2) Reaction formation—turning a disturbing idea or impulse into its opposite.

(3) Psychotic denial—transforming confusing stimuli into delusions and hallucinations.

X. Differential diagnosis

A. Medical and neurological disorders. Present with impaired memory, orientation, and cognition; visual hallucinations; signs of CNS damage. Many neurological and medical disorders can present with symptoms identical to those of schizophrenia, including substance intoxication (e.g., cocaine, phencyclidine) and substance-induced psychotic disorder, CNS infections (e.g., herpes encephalitis), vascular disorders (e.g., systemic lupus erythematosus), complex partial seizures (e.g., temporal lobe epilepsy), and degenerative disease (e.g., Huntington's disease).

B. Schizophreniform disorder. Symptoms may be identical to those of schizophrenia but last for less than 6 months. Also, deterioration is less pronounced and the prognosis is better.

C. Brief psychotic disorder. Symptoms last less than 1 month and proceed from a clearly identifiable psychosocial stress.

D. Mood disorders. Both manic episodes and major depressive episodes of bipolar I disorder and major depressive disorder may present with psychotic symptoms. The differential diagnosis is particularly important because of the availability of specific and effective treatments for the mood disorders. DSM-IV-TR states that mood symptoms in schizophrenia must be brief relative to the essential criteria. Also, if hallucinations and delusions are present in a mood disorder, they develop in the context of the mood disturbance and do not persist. Other factors that help differentiate mood disorders from schizophrenia include family history, premorbid history, course (e.g., age at onset), prognosis (e.g., absence of residual deterioration following the psychotic episode), and response to treatment. Patients may experience postpsychotic depressive disorder of schizophrenia (i.e., a major depressive episode occurring during the residual phase of schizophrenia). True depression in these patients must be differentiated from medication-induced adverse effects, such as sedation, akinesia, and flattening of affect.

E. Schizoaffective disorder. Mood symptoms develop concurrently with symptoms of schizophrenia, but delusions or hallucinations must be present for 2 weeks in the absence of prominent mood symptoms during some phase of the illness. The prognosis of this disorder is better than that expected for schizophrenia and worse than that for mood disorders.

F. Psychotic disorder not otherwise specified. An atypical psychosis with a confusing clinical feature (e.g., persistent auditory hallucinations as the only symptom, many culture-bound psychoses).

G. Delusional disorders. Nonbizarre, systematized delusions that last at least 6 months in the context of an intact, relatively well-functioning personality in the absence of prominent hallucinations or other schizophrenic symptoms. Onset is in middle to late adult life.

H. Personality disorders. Generally no psychotic symptoms, but, if present, they tend to be transient and not prominent. The most important personality disorders in this differential diagnosis are schizotypal, schizoid, borderline, and paranoid.

I. Factitious disorder and malingering. No laboratory test or biological marker can objectively confirm the diagnosis of schizophrenia. Schizophrenic symptoms are therefore possible to feign for either clear secondary gain (malingering) or deep psychological motivations (factitious disorder).

J. Pervasive developmental disorders. Pervasive developmental disorders (e.g., autistic disorder) are usually recognized before 3 years of age. Although behavior may be bizarre and deteriorated, no delusions, hallucinations, or clear formal thought disorder is present (e.g., loosening of associations).

K. Mental retardation. Intellectual, behavioral, and mood disturbances that suggest schizophrenia. However, mental retardation involves no overt psychotic symptoms and involves a constant low level of functioning rather than a deterioration. If psychotic symptoms are present, a diagnosis of schizophrenia may be made concurrently.

L. Shared cultural beliefs. Seemingly odd beliefs shared and accepted by a cultural group are not considered psychotic.

XI. Course and prognosis

A. Course. Prodromal symptoms of anxiety, perplexity, terror, or depression generally precede the onset of schizophrenia, which may be acute or insidious. Prodromal symptoms may be present for months before a definitive diagnosis is made. Onset is generally in the late teens and early 20s; women generally are older at onset than men. Precipitating events (e.g., emotional trauma, use of drugs, a separation) may trigger episodes of illness in predisposed persons. Classically, the course of schizophrenia is one of deterioration over time, with acute exacerbations superimposed on a chronic picture. Vulnerability to stress is lifelong. Postpsychotic depressive episodes may occur in the residual phase. Other comorbidities include substance use disorders, obsessive-compulsive disorder, hyponatremia secondary to polydipsia, smoking, and HIV infection.

During the course of the illness, the more florid positive psychotic symptoms, such as bizarre delusions and hallucinations, tend to diminish in intensity, whereas the more residual negative symptoms, such as poor hygiene, flattened emotional response, and various oddities of behavior, may actually increase.

Relapse rates are approximately 40% in 2 years on medication and 80% in 2 years off medication. Suicide is attempted by 50% of patients; 10% are successful. Violence is a risk, particularly in untreated patients. Risk factors include persecutory delusions, a history of violence, and neurological deficits. The risk for sudden death and medical illness is increased, and life expectancy is shortened.

B. Prognosis. See Table 8–8. In terms of overall prognosis, some investigators have described a loose rule of thirds: approximately one third of patients lead somewhat normal lives, one third continue to experience significant symptoms but can function within society, and the remaining third

TABLE 8–8
FEATURES WEIGHTING TOWARD GOOD OR POOR PROGNOSIS IN SCHIZOPHRENIA

Good Prognosis	Poor Prognosis
Late onset	Early onset
Obvious precipitating factors	No precipitating factors
Acute onset	Insidious onset
Good premorbid social, sexual, and work histories	Poor premorbid social, sexual, and work histories
Mood disorder symptoms (especially depressive disorders)	Withdrawn, autistic behavior
Married	Single, divorced, or widowed
Family history of mood disorders	Family history of schizophrenia
Good support systems	Poor support systems
Positive symptoms	Negative symptoms
Female sex	Neurological signs and symptoms
	History of perinatal trauma
	No remissions in 3 years
	Many relapses
	History of assaultiveness

are markedly impaired and require frequent hospitalization. Approximately 10% of this final third of patients require long-term institutionalization. In general, women have a better prognosis than do men.

XII. Treatment

Clinical management of the schizophrenia patient may include hospitalization and antipsychotic medication in addition to psychosocial treatments, such as behavioral, family, group, individual, and social skills and rehabilitation therapies. Any of these treatment modalities can be given on an inpatient or outpatient basis. Indications for hospitalization include posing a danger to others, suicidality, severe symptomatology leading to poor self-care or risk for injury secondary to disorganization, diagnostic evaluation, failure to respond to treatment in less restrictive settings, complicating comorbidities, and the need to alter complex drug treatment regimens.

A. Pharmacological. See Table 8–9. The antipsychotics include the dopamine receptor antagonists and the serotonin-dopamine antagonists (SDAs), such as risperidone (Risperdal) and clozapine (Clozaril).

1. **Choice of drug.** See Table 8–10.

a. **Dopamine receptor antagonists (typical antipsychotics)**—the classic antipsychotic drugs, which are often effective in the treatment of positive symptoms of schizophrenia. High-potency agents (e.g., haloperidol) are most likely to cause extrapyramidal side effects such as akathisia, acute dystonia, and pseudoparkinsonism. Low-potency agents (e.g., chlorpromazine [Thorazine]) are more sedating, hypotensive, and anticholinergic. These agents can cause tardive dyskinesia at a rate of roughly 5% per year of exposure. A significant portion of patients are either unresponsive to or intolerant of these drugs.

b. **Serotonin-dopamine antagonists (atypical antipsychotics)**—the newer-generation antipsychotic drugs that provide potent $5-HT_2$ receptor blockade and varying degrees of D_2 receptor blockade, in addition to other receptor effects. In comparison with the dopamine receptor antagonists, these drugs cause fewer extrapyramidal side effects, do not elevate prolactin levels (with the exception of risperidone), and may be more effective in treating negative symptoms and less likely to cause tardive dyskinesia. Clozapine is the most atypical in that it causes minimal or no extrapyramidal side effects, regardless of dosage; seldom causes tardive dyskinesia; and is extremely effective in treating refractory patients despite weak D_2 receptor blockade. Risperidone is the least atypical in that it causes a significant, dosage-related increase in extrapyramidal side effects;

TABLE 8–9
SELECTED ANTIPSYCHOTIC DRUGS

Drug	Route of Administration	Usual Daily Oral Dose (mg)	Sedation	Autonomic	Extrapyramidal Adverse Effects
Phenothiazines					
Chlorpromazine	Oral, IM	200–600	+++	+++	++
Fluphenazine	Oral, IM, depot	2–20	+	+	+++
Trifluoperazine	Oral, IM	5–30	++	+	+++
Perphenazine	Oral, IM	8–64	++	+	+++
Thioridazine	Oral	200–600	+++	+++	++
Butyrophenones					
Haloperidol	Oral, IM, depot	5–20	+	+	+++
Thioxanthenes					
Thiothixene	Oral, IM	5–30	+	+	+++
Dihydroindolones					
Molindone	Oral	20–100	++	+	++
Dibenzoxazepine					
Loxapine	Oral, IM	20–100	++	+	++
Arylpiperidylindole					
Sertindole	Oral	12–24	+	++	0?
Thienobenzodiazepine					
Olanzapine	Oral	7.5–25	+	++	0?
Dibenzothiazepine					
Quetiapine	Oral	150–750	++	++	0?
Benzisoxazole					
Risperidone	Oral	2–16	+	++	+
Dibenzodiazepine					
Clozapine	Oral	150–900	+++	+++	0?

Table by Stephen R. Marder, M.D.

TABLE 8–10
FACTORS INFLUENCING ANTIPSYCHOTIC DRUG SELECTION

Factors	Considerations
Subjective response	A dyphoric subjective response to a particular drug predicts poor compliance with that drug
Sensitivity to extrapyrimidal adverse effects	A serotonin-dopamine antagonist (SDA)
Tardive dyskinesia	Clozapine (or possibly another SDA)
Poor medication compliance or high risk for relapse	Injectable form of a long-acting antagonist (haloperidol or fluphenazine)
Pregnancy	Probably haloperidol (most data supporting its safety)
Cognitive symptoms	Possibly an SDA
Negative symptoms	Possibly an SDA

Table by Stephen R. Marder, M.D.

is a potent D_2 blocker; and elevates prolactin levels. As a group, these agents can be highly sedating and cause weight gain in excess of that associated with the dopamine receptor antagonists (with the exception of risperidone). The atypical antipsychotics are generally better tolerated than typical antipsychotics. The serotonin-dopamine antagonists are widely prescribed as first-line treatment for patients with schizophrenia. Clozapine is not a first-line agent and is reserved for treatment-refractory patients.

2. **Dosage.** A moderate fixed dose that is maintained for 4 to 6 weeks (or longer in more chronic cases) is recommended for acute psychotic episodes. High dosages of antipsychotics (>1 g of chlorpromazine equivalents) and rapid neuroleptization are no longer recommended, as they increase side effects without enhancing efficacy. Typical therapeutic dosages are 4 to 6 mg of risperidone a day, 10 to 20 mg of olanzapine (Zyprexa) a day, and 6 to 20 mg of haloperidol a day. First-episode patients may respond well to lower dosages, whereas selected chronic or refractory patients may rarely require higher dosages. An antipsychotic response develops gradually. Agitation can be managed with benzodiazepines (e.g., 1 to 2 mg of lorazepam [Ativan] three or four times daily) on a standing or as-needed basis while an antipsychotic response is awaited. Patients who are noncompliant because of lack of insight may benefit from long-acting injectable antipsychotics (e.g., 25 mg of fluphenazine decanoate [Prolixin] intramuscularly every 2 weeks or 100 to 200 mg of haloperidol decanoate intramuscularly every 4 weeks). Patients should first be treated with oral preparations of these drugs to establish efficacy and tolerability. Patients who are treated with long-acting haloperidol must be converted to the depot drug via a loading-dose strategy or with oral supplementation until the depot preparation reaches steady-state levels (4 months).

3. **Maintenance.** Schizophrenia is usually a chronic illness, and long-term treatment with antipsychotic medication is usually required to decrease the risk for relapse. If a patient has been stable for approximately 1 year, then the medication can be gradually decreased to the minimum effective dosage, possibly at the rate of 10–20% per month. During dosage reduction, patients and their families must be educated to recognize and report warning signs of relapse, including insomnia, anxiety, withdrawal, and odd behavior. Strategies for dose reduction must be individualized based on the severity of past episodes, stability of symptoms, and tolerability of medication.

4. **Other drugs.** If standard antipsychotic medication alone is ineffective, several other drugs have been reported to cause varying degrees of improvement. The addition of lithium may be helpful in a significant percentage of patients; propranolol (Inderal), benzodiazepines, valproic acid (Depakene) or divalproex (Depakote), and carbamazepine (Tegretol) have been reported to lead to improvement in some cases.

B. Electroconvulsive therapy (ECT). Can be effective for acute psychosis and catatonic subtype. Patients in whom the illness has lasted less than 1 year are most responsive. ECT is a promising treatment for refractory positive symptoms. It has been shown to have synergistic efficacy with antipsychotic drugs.

C. Psychosocial. Antipsychotic medication alone is not as effective in treating schizophrenic patients as are drugs coupled with psychosocial interventions.

1. **Behavior therapy.** Desired behaviors are positively reinforced by rewarding them with specific tokens, such as trips or privileges. The intent is to generalize reinforced behavior to the world outside the hospital ward.

2. **Group therapy.** Focus is on support and social skills development (activities of daily living). Groups are especially helpful in decreasing social isolation and increasing reality testing.

3. **Family therapy.** Family therapy techniques can significantly decrease relapse rates for the schizophrenic family member. High-EE family interaction can be diminished through family therapy. Multiple family groups, in which family members of schizophrenic patients discuss and share issues, have been particularly helpful.

4. **Supportive psychotherapy.** Traditional insight-oriented psychotherapy is not usually recommended in treating schizophrenic patients because their egos are too fragile. Supportive therapy, which may include advice, reassurance, education, modeling, limit setting, and reality testing, is generally the therapy of choice. The rule is that as much insight as a patient desires and can tolerate is an acceptable goal. A type of supportive therapy called *personal therapy* involves a heavy reliance on the therapeutic relationship, with instillation of hope and imparting of information.

5. **Social skills training.** Attempts to improve social skills deficits, such as poor eye contact, lack of relatedness, inaccurate perceptions of others, and social inappropriateness, by means of supportive structurally based and sometimes manually based therapies (often in group settings), which utilize homework, videotapes, and role playing.

6. **Case management.** Responsible for the schizophrenia patient's concrete needs and coordination of care. Case managers participate in coordinating treatment planning and communication between various providers. They help patients to make appointments, obtain housing and financial benefits, and navigate the health care system (advocacy), and also provide outreach and crisis management to keep patients in treatment.

7. **Support groups.** The National Alliance for the Mentally Ill (NAMI), the National Mental Health Association (NMHA), and similar groups provide support, information, and education for patients and their families. NAMI-sponsored support groups are available in most states. NAMI can be contacted at 800-950-NAMI.

XIII. Interviewing techniques

A. **Understanding.** The most important task is to understand as well as possible what schizophrenic patients may be feeling and thinking. Schizophrenic patients are described as having extremely fragile ego structures, which leave them open to an unstable sense of self and others; primitive defenses; and a severely impaired ability to modulate external stress.

B. **Other critical tasks.** The other critical task for the interviewer is to establish contact with the patient in a manner that allows for a tolerable balance of autonomy and interaction.

   1. The patient has both a deep wish for and a terrible fear of interpersonal contact, called the *need–fear dilemma.*

   2. The fear of contact may represent the fear of a fundamental intrusion, resulting in delusional fears of personal and world annihilation in addition to loss of control, identity, and self.

   3. The wish for contact may represent fears that, without human interaction, the person is dead, nonhuman, mechanical, or permanently trapped.

   4. Schizophrenic patients may project their own negative, bizarre, and frightening self-images onto others, leading the interviewer to feel as uncomfortable, scared, or angry as the patient. Aggressive or hostile impulses are particularly frightening to these patients and may lead them to disorganization in thought and behavior.

   5. Offers of help may be experienced as coercion, attempts to force the person into helplessness, or a sense of being devoured.

C. **Dos and don'ts for the psychiatric and psychotherapeutic interview.** There is no one right thing to say to a schizophrenia patient. The most important task of the interviewer is to help to diminish the inner chaos, loneliness, and terror that the schizophrenic patient is feeling. The challenge is to convey empathy without being regarded as dangerously intrusive.

   1. *Don't* try to argue or rationally persuade the patient out of a delusion. Efforts to convince the patient that a delusion is not real generally lead to more tenacious assertions of delusional ideas.

   2. *Do* listen. How patients experience the world (e.g., dangerous, bizarre, overwhelming, invasive) is conveyed through their thought content and process. Listen for the feelings behind the delusional ideas—are they afraid, sad, angry, hopeless? Do they feel as though they have no privacy, no control? What is their image of themselves?

   3. *Do* acknowledge these feelings to the patient, simply and clearly. For example, when the patient says, "When I walk into a room, people can see inside my head and read my thoughts," the clinician might respond with, "What is that like for you?"

   4. *Don't* feel that anything must be said. Careful listening can convey that the clinician believes the person is human with something important to say.

5. *Do* be flexible about interview times, both the number of visits and how long each visit lasts. If a patient can tolerate only 10 minutes, tell him or her that the interview will resume later, and be clear and reliable about when; it can be an indicator of the clinician's trustworthiness.

6. *Do* be straightforward with a patient—*don't* pretend that a delusion is actually true, but convey that the delusion is true for the patient. Represent reality to the patient—the challenge is to be a consistent source of reality testing without making the patient feel humiliated or rejected. For example, if a patient says, "This song on the radio was written just for me, can't you hear the message?" one might respond, "I can hear that the song is about feeling sad after losing someone, and that you must be feeling like that yourself."

7. *Do* pay attention to how the patient makes you feel because this often reflects the patient's characteristic style of interaction. Be careful to sort out whether feelings are in direct response to the patient or to something unrelated (e.g., being annoyed because of an argument with a supervisor that morning or because the patient is making subtle, insulting remarks about doctors).

8. *Do* answer certain personal questions. Try to turn the interview back to the patient. Answering some personal questions may help patients talk more freely about themselves. For example, if the patient asks, "Are you married?" the clinician might respond, "Can you tell me why that is important to you?" *Patient:* "I just want to know; are you married?" *Interviewer:* "I will tell you, but let's talk a bit first about why that information is so important to you."

9. *Don't* automatically laugh at a patient when something is said that seems funny. Actively psychotic people will describe delusions that can sound absurd or humorous, but clearly the patient does not experience them as funny. Laughing at a patient can convey disrespect and a lack of understanding of the underlying terror and despair that many patients feel. Keeping this in mind can help to decrease the urge to laugh. Laughter can be appropriate, such as when a patient purposefully tells a joke. Humor can be an indication of health unless it is used excessively or inappropriately.

10. *Do* respect a paranoid patient's need for distance and control. Many paranoid patients feel more comfortable with a certain formality and respectful aloofness, as opposed to expressions of warmth and empathy.

For a more detailed discussion of this topic, see Schizophrenia, Ch 12, p 1096, in CTP/VII.

9

Schizoaffective, Delusional, and Other Psychotic Disorders

I. Introduction

The term *psychotic* refers to the loss of reality testing, usually with hallucinations, delusions, or thought disorder. A dynamic definition focuses on loss of ego boundaries. Psychotic symptoms are nonspecific and, like fever, have many causes. Clinicians must first rule out general medical conditions and substances as causative factors when evaluating psychotic patients. This chapter focuses on the psychotic syndromes that do not meet the criteria for schizophrenia or mood disorders with psychotic features. These include schizophreniform, schizoaffective, and delusional disorders, which require a comprehensive approach that includes pharmacologic, psychodynamic, and psychosocial management, with attention to precipitating environmental stressors, medical and psychiatric comorbidities, selection of an appropriate treatment setting, and awareness of high rates of treatment noncompliance.

II. Schizophreniform disorder

A. **Definition.** Symptoms identical to those of schizophrenia except that they resolve within 6 months and normal functioning returns.

B. **Diagnosis, signs, and symptoms.** See Table 9–1.

C. **Epidemiology.** Data are unavailable; however, the disorder may be less than half as common as schizophrenia.

D. **Etiology.** Related more to mood disorders than to schizophrenia. In general, schizophreniform patients have more mood symptoms and a better prognosis than do schizophrenic patients. Schizophrenia occurs more often in families of patients with mood disorder than in families of patients with schizophreniform disorder.

E. **Differential diagnosis.** Identical to that of schizophrenia. See Chapter 8.

F. **Course and prognosis.** Good prognostic features include absence of blunted or flat affect, good premorbid functioning, confusion and disorientation at the height of the psychotic episode, shorter duration, acute onset, and onset of prominent psychotic symptoms within 4 weeks of any first noticeable change in behavior.

G. **Treatment.** Antipsychotic medications should be used to treat psychotic symptoms. Consideration can be given to withdrawing or tapering the medication if the psychosis has been completely resolved for 6 months. The decision to discontinue medication must be individualized based on treatment response, side effects, and other factors. Recurrent episodes warrant a trial with lithium or anticonvulsants, or possibly ongoing maintenance therapy with antipsychotics. Psychotherapy is critical in helping patients to understand and deal with their psychotic experiences.

III. Schizoaffective disorder

A. Definition.   A disorder with concurrent features of both schizophrenia and mood disorder that cannot be diagnosed as either one separately.

B. Diagnosis, signs, and symptoms.   See Table 9–2.

C. Epidemiology.   Lifetime prevalence is less than 1%; it occurs equally in men and women.

D. Etiology.   Some patients may be misdiagnosed; they are actually schizophrenic with prominent mood symptoms or have a mood disorder with prominent psychotic symptoms. The prevalence of schizophrenia is not increased in schizoaffective families, but the prevalence of mood disorders is. See Etiology of Schizophrenia (Chapter 8) and Mood Disorders (Chapter 10) for additional data and theories.

TABLE 9–1
DSM-IV-TR DIAGNOSTIC CRITERIA FOR SCHIZOPHRENIFORM DISORDER

A. Criteria A, D, and E of schizophrenia are met.
B. An episode of the disorder (including prodromal, active, and residual phases) lasts at least 1 month but less than 6 months. (When the diagnosis must be made without waiting for recovery, it should be qualified as "provisional.")
Specify if:
   Without good prognostic features
   With good prognostic features: as evidenced by two (or more) of the following:
      (1) onset of prominent psychotic symptoms within 4 weeks of the first noticeable change in usual behavior or functioning
      (2) confusion or perplexity at the height of the psychotic episode
      (3) good premorbid social and occupational functioning
      (4) absence of blunted or flat affect

From American Psychiatric Association. *Diagnostic and Statistical Manual of Mental Disorders,* text revision, 4th ed. Washington, DC: American Psychiatric Association, Copyright 2000, with permission.

TABLE 9–2
DSM-IV-TR DIAGNOSTIC CRITERIA FOR SCHIZOAFFECTIVE DISORDER

A. An uninterrupted period of illness during which, at some time, there is either a major depressive episode, a manic episode, or a mixed episode concurrent with symptoms that meet criterion A for schizophrenia.
   Note: The major depressive episode must include criterion A1: depressed mood.
B. During the same period of illness, there have been delusions or hallucinations for at least 2 weeks in the absence of prominent mood symptoms.
C. Symptoms that meet criteria for a mood episode are present for a substantial portion of the total duration of the active and residual periods of the illness.
D. The disturbance is not due to the direct physiological effects of a substance (e.g., a drug of abuse, a medication) or a general medical condition.
Specify type:
   Bipolar type: if the disturbance includes a manic or a mixed episode (or a manic or a mixed episode and major depressive episodes)
   Depressive type: if the disturbance only includes major depressive episodes

From American Psychiatric Association. *Diagnostic and Statistical Manual of Mental Disorders,* text revision, 4th ed. Washington, DC: American Psychiatric Association, Copyright 2000, with permission.

   E. Differential diagnosis.   Any medical, psychiatric, or drug-related condition that causes psychotic or mood symptoms must be considered.

   F. Course and prognosis.   Poor prognosis is associated with positive family history of schizophrenia, early and insidious onset without precipitating factors, predominance of psychotic symptoms, and poor premorbid history. Schizoaffective patients have a better prognosis than schizophrenic patients and a worse prognosis than mood disorder patients. Schizoaffective patients respond more often to lithium and are less likely to have a deteriorating course than are schizophrenic patients.

   G. Treatment.   Antidepressant or antimanic treatments should be attempted, and antipsychotic medications should be used to control acute psychoses.

IV. Delusional disorder

   A. Definition.   Disorder in which the primary or sole manifestation is a nonbizarre delusion that is fixed and unshakable.

   B. Diagnosis, signs, and symptoms.   See Table 9–3. Delusions last at least 1 month and are well systematized as opposed to bizarre or fragmented. The patient's emotional response to the delusional system is congruent with and appropriate to the content of the delusion. The personality remains intact or deteriorates minimally. The fact that patients often are hypersensitive and hypervigilant may lead to social isolation despite their high-level functioning capacities. Under nonstressful circumstances, patients may be judged to be without evidence of mental illness.

TABLE 9–3
DSM-IV-TR DIAGNOSTIC CRITERIA FOR DELUSIONAL DISORDER

A. Nonbizarre delusions (i.e., involving situations that occur in real life, such as being followed, poisoned, infected, loved at a distance, or deceived by spouse or lover, or having a disease) of at least 1 month's duration.

B. Criterion A for schizophrenia has never been met. **Note:** Tactile and olfactory hallucinations may be present in delusional disorder if they are related to the delusional theme.

C. Apart from the impact of the delusion(s) or its ramifications, functioning is not markedly impaired and behavior is not obviously odd or bizarre.

D. If mood episodes have occurred concurrently with delusions, their total duration has been brief relative to the duration of the delusional periods.

E. The disturbance is not due to the direct physiologic effects of a substance (e.g., a drug of abuse, a medication) or a general medical condition.

Specify type (the following types are assigned based on the predominant delusional theme):
   Erotomanic type: delusions that another person, usually of higher status, is in love with the individual
   Grandiose type: delusions of inflated worth, power, knowledge, identity, or special relationship to a deity or famous person
   Jealous type: delusions that the individual's sexual partner is unfaithful
   Persecutory type: delusions that the person (or someone to whom the person is close) is being malevolently treated in some way
   Somatic type: delusions that the person has some physical defect or general medical condition
   Mixed type: delusions characteristics of more than one of the above types, but no one theme predominates
   Unspecified type

TABLE 9–4
EPIDEMIOLOGICAL FEATURES OF DELUSIONAL DISORDER

Incidence[a]	0.7–3.0
Prevalence[a]	24–30
Age at onset (range)	18–80 (mean, 34–45 years)
Type of onset	Acute or gradual
Sex ratio	Somewhat more frequently female
Prognosis	Best with early, acute onset
Associated features	Widowhood, celibacy often present, history of substance abuse, head injury not infrequent

[a] Incidence and prevalence figures represent cases per 100,000 population.
Adapted from Kendler KS. Demography of paranoid psychosis (delusional disorder). *Arch Gen Psychiatry* 1982;39:890, with permission.

C. **Epidemiology.**   See Table 9–4.

D. **Etiology**

1. **Genetic.** Genetic studies indicate that delusional disorder is neither a subtype nor an early or prodromal stage of schizophrenia or mood disorder. The risk for schizophrenia or mood disorder is not increased in first-degree relatives.

2. **Biological.** Patients may have discrete defects in the limbic system and basal ganglia.

3. **Psychosocial.** Delusional disorder is primarily psychosocial in origin. Common background characteristics include a history of physical or emotional abuse; cruel, erratic, and unreliable parenting; and an overly demanding or perfectionistic upbringing. Basic trust (Erik Erikson) does not develop, with the child believing that the environment is consistently hostile and potentially dangerous. Other psychosocial factors include a history of deafness, blindness, social isolation and loneliness, recent immigration or other abrupt environmental changes, and advanced age.

E. **Laboratory and psychological tests.**   No laboratory test can confirm the diagnosis. Projective psychological tests reveal a preoccupation with paranoid or grandiose themes and issues of inferiority, inadequacy, and anxiety.

F. **Pathophysiology.**   No known pathophysiology except when patients have discrete anatomic defects of the limbic system or basal ganglia.

G. **Psychodynamic factors.**   Defenses used: (1) denial, (2) reaction formation, (3) projection. Major defense is projection—symptoms are a defense against unacceptable ideas and feelings. Patients deny feelings of shame, humiliation, and inferiority; turn any unacceptable feelings into their opposites through reaction formation (inferiority into grandiosity); and project any unacceptable feelings outward onto others.

H. **Differential diagnosis**

1. **Psychotic disorder resulting from a general medical condition with delusions.** Conditions that may mimic delusional disorder include hypothyroidism and hyperthyroidism, Parkinson's disease, multiple sclerosis, Alzheimer's disease, tumors, and trauma to the basal ganglia. Many medical and neurologic illnesses can present with delusions (Table 9–5). The most common sites for lesions are the basal ganglia and the limbic system.

TABLE 9–5
NEUROLOGICAL AND MEDICAL CONDITIONS THAT CAN PRESENT WITH DELUSIONS

Basal ganglia disorders—Parkinson's disease, Huntington's disease
Deficiency states—B_{12}, folate, thiamine, niacin
Delirium
Dementia—Alzheimer's disease, Pick's disease
Drug-induced—amphetamines, anticholinergics, antidepressants, antihypertensives, antituberculosis
   drugs, anti-Parkinson agents, cimetidine, cocaine, disulfiram (Antabuse), hallucinogens
Endocrinopathies—adrenal, thyroid, parathyroid
Limbic system disorders—epilepsy, cerebrovascular diseases, tumors
Systemic—hepatic encephalopathy, hypercalcemia, hypoglycemia, porphyria, uremia

2. **Substance-induced psychotic disorder with delusions.** Intoxication with sympathomimetics (e.g., amphetamines, marijuana, or levodopa [Larodopa]) is likely to result in delusional symptoms.
3. **Paranoid personality disorder.** No true delusions are present, although overvalued ideas that verge on being delusional may be present. Patients are predisposed to delusional disorders.
4. **Paranoid schizophrenia.** More likely to present with prominent auditory hallucinations, personality deterioration, and more marked disturbance in role functioning. Age at onset tends to be younger in schizophrenia than in delusional disorder. Delusions are more bizarre.
5. **Major depressive disorder.** Depressed patients may have paranoid delusions secondary to major depressive disorder, but the mood symptoms and associated characteristics (e.g., vegetative symptoms, positive family history, response to antidepressants) are prominent.
6. **Bipolar I disorder.** Manic patients may have grandiose or paranoid delusions that are clearly secondary to the primary and prominent mood disorder; associated with such characteristics as euphoric and labile mood, positive family history, and response to lithium.

I. **Course and prognosis.**   Disorder tends to be chronic and unremitting in 30–50% of patients. Less satisfactory response to pharmacotherapy than in patients with delusional symptoms associated with schizophrenia or mood disorder. Psychotherapy is difficult because of lack of trust.

J. **Treatment.**   Patients rarely enter therapy voluntarily; rather, they are brought by concerned friends and relatives. Establishing rapport is difficult; patient's hostility is fear-motivated. Successful psychotherapy may enable the patient to improve social adaptation despite persistent delusions.

1. **Hospitalization.** Hospitalization is necessary if the patient is unable to control suicidal or homicidal impulses; if impairment is extreme (e.g., refusal to eat because of a delusion about food poisoning); or if a thorough medical workup is indicated.
2. **Psychopharmacotherapy.** Patients tend to refuse medications because of suspicion. Severely agitated patients may require intramuscular antipsychotic medication. Otherwise, oral antipsychotics may be tried. Delusional disorder may preferentially respond to pimozide (Orap). Delusional patients are more likely to react to drug side effects with delusional ideas; thus, a very gradual increase in dose is recom-

mended to diminish the likelihood of disturbing adverse effects. Antidepressants may be of use with severe depression. Selective serotonin reuptake inhibitors may be helpful in somatic type.

3. **Psychotherapy: dos and don'ts**

a. *Don't* argue with or challenge the patient's delusions. A delusion may become even more entrenched if the patient feels that it must be defended.

b. *Don't* pretend that the delusion is true because the clinician must represent reality to the patient. However, *do* listen to the patient's concerns about the delusion and try to understand what the delusion may mean, specifically in terms of the patient's self-esteem.

c. *Do* respond sympathetically to the fact that the delusion is disturbing and intrusive in the patient's life and offer to help the patient to develop ways to live more comfortably with the delusion.

d. *Do* understand that the delusional system may be a means of grappling with profound feelings of shame and inadequacy, and that the patient may be hypersensitive to any imagined slights or condescension.

e. *Do* be straightforward and honest in all dealings with the patient, as these patients are hypervigilant about being tricked or deceived. Explain side effects of medications and why you are giving medications (e.g., to help with anxiety, irritability, insomnia, anorexia); be reliable and on time for appointments; schedule regular appointments.

f. *Do* examine what particular stresses or experiences triggered the first appearance of the delusion and try to understand why they led to the patient's feelings of shame or inadequacy. Understand that other similar stresses or experiences in the patient's life may exacerbate delusional symptoms. Help the patient develop alternative means of responding to stressful situations.

V. Brief psychotic disorder

A. **Definition.** Symptoms last for less than 1 month and follow an obvious stress in the patient's life.

B. **Diagnosis, signs, and symptoms.** See Table 9–6. Similar to those of other psychotic disorders, but with an increase in volatility and lability, confusion, disorientation, and affective symptoms.

C. **Epidemiology.** No definitive data are available. More frequent in persons with preexisting personality disorders or who have previously experienced major stressors, such as disasters or dramatic cultural changes.

D. **Etiology.** Mood disorders are more common in the families of these patients. Psychosocial stress triggers the psychotic episode. Psychosis is understood as a defensive response in a person with inadequate coping mechanisms.

E. **Differential diagnosis.** Medical causes must be ruled out—in particular, drug intoxication and withdrawal. Seizure disorders must also be considered. Factitious disorders, malingering, schizophrenia, mood disorders, and transient psychotic episodes associated with borderline and schizotypal personality disorders must be ruled out.

F. Course and prognosis.   See Table 9–7.

G. Treatment.   Short-term hospitalization may be required; antipsychotic medications may not be necessary because often the symptoms resolve very quickly on their own. If medication is required, use as low a dose as possible and discontinue as soon as possible. Psychotherapy is extremely important to address the nature and significance of the specific social stress that triggered the psychotic episode. Patients must build more adaptive and less devastating means of coping with future stress.

VI. Shared psychotic disorder

A. Definition.   Delusional system shared by two or more persons; previously called *induced paranoid disorder* and *folie à deux*.

B. Diagnosis, signs, and symptoms.   Persecutory delusions are most common, and the key presentation is the sharing and blind acceptance of these delusions between two people. Suicide or homicide pacts may be present.

TABLE 9–6
DSM-IV-TR DIAGNOSTIC CRITERIA FOR BRIEF PSYCHOTIC DISORDER

A. Presence of one (or more) of the following symptoms:
   (1) delusions
   (2) hallucinations
   (3) disorganized speech (e.g., frequent derailment or incoherence)
   Note: Do not include a symptom if it is a culturally sanctioned response pattern.
B. Duration of an episode of the disturbance is at least 1 day but less than 1 month, with eventual full return to premorbid level of functioning.
C. The disturbance is not better accounted for by a mood disorder with psychotic features, schizoaffective disorder, or schizophrenia and is not due to the direct physiologic effects of a substance (e.g., a drug of abuse, a medication) or a general medical condition.
Specify if:
With marked stressor(s) (brief reactive psychosis): if symptoms occur shortly after and apparently in response to events that, singly or together, would be markedly stressful to almost anyone in similar circumstances in the person's culture
Without marked stressor(s): if psychotic symptoms do not occur shortly after, or are not apparently in response to, events that, singly or together, would be markedly stressful to almost anyone in similar circumstances in the person's culture
With postpartum onset: if onset within 4 weeks post partum

From American Psychiatric Association. *Diagnostic and Statistical Manual of Mental Disorders*, text revision, 4th ed. Washington, DC: American Psychiatric Association, Copyright 2000, with permission.

TABLE 9–7
GOOD PROGNOSTIC FEATURES FOR BRIEF PSYCHOTIC DISORDER

Good premorbid adjustment
Few premorbid schizoid traits
Severe precipitating stressor
Sudden onset of symptoms
Affective symptoms
Confusion and perplexity during psychosis
Little affective blunting
Short duration of symptoms
Absence of schizophrenic relatives

C. **Epidemiology.** The disorder is rare; more common in women and in persons with physical disabilities that make them dependent on another person. Family members, usually two sisters, are involved in 95% of cases.

D. **Etiology.** The cause is primarily psychological; however, a genetic influence is possible because the disorder most often affects members of the same family. The families of persons with this disorder are at risk for schizophrenia. Psychological or psychosocial factors include a socially isolated relationship in which one person is submissive and dependent and the other is dominant with an established psychotic system.

E. **Psychodynamic factors.** The dominant psychotic personality maintains some contact with reality through the submissive person, whereas the submissive personality is desperately anxious to be cared for and accepted by the dominant person. The two often have a strongly ambivalent relationship.

F. **Differential diagnosis.** Rule out personality disorders, malingering, and factitious disorders in the submissive patient. Medical causes must always be considered.

G. **Course and prognosis.** Recovery rates vary; some are as low as 10–40%. Traditionally, the submissive partner is separated from the dominant, psychotic partner, with the ideal outcome being a rapid diminution in the psychotic symptoms. If symptoms do not remit, the submissive person may meet the criteria for another psychotic disorder, such as schizophrenia or delusional disorder.

H. **Treatment.** Separate the persons and help the more submissive, dependent partner develop other means of support to compensate for the loss of the relationship. Antipsychotic medications are beneficial for both persons.

VII. Postpartum psychosis

A. **Definition.** Syndrome occurring after childbirth and characterized by severe depression and delusions. Most data suggest a close relation between postpartum psychosis and mood disorders.

B. **Diagnosis, signs, and symptoms.** Most cases occur 2 to 3 days postpartum. Initial complaints of insomnia, restlessness, and emotional lability progress to confusion, irrationality, delusions, and obsessive concerns about the infant. Thoughts of wanting to harm the baby or self are characteristic.

C. **Epidemiology.** Occurs with one to two deliveries per 1,000. Most episodes occur in primiparas.

D. **Etiology.** Usually secondary to underlying mental illness (e.g., schizophrenia, bipolar disorder).

  1. Sudden change in hormonal levels after parturition may contribute.
  2. Psychodynamic conflicts about motherhood—unwanted pregnancy, entrapment in unhappy marriage, fears of mothering.

E. **Differential diagnosis**

  1. **Postpartum blues.** Most women experience postpartum emotional lability. Clears spontaneously. No evidence of psychotic thinking.

2. **Substance-induced mood disorder.** Depression associated with postanesthetic states, such as after cesarean section or meperidine (Demerol)–scopolamine analgesia (twilight sleep).

3. **Psychotic disorder resulting from a general medical condition.** Rule out infection, hormonal imbalance (e.g., hypothyroidism), encephalopathy associated with toxemia of pregnancy, preeclampsia.

F. **Course and prognosis.** Risk for infanticide, suicide, or both is high in untreated cases. Supportive family network, good premorbid personality, and appropriate treatment are associated with good to excellent prognosis.

G. **Treatment.** Suicidal precautions in presence of suicidal ideation. Do not leave the infant alone with the mother if she has delusions or ruminates about the infant's health.

1. **Pharmacologic.** Medication for primary symptoms: antidepressants for suicidal ideation and depression; antianxiety agents for agitation, insomnia (e.g., 0.5 mg of lorazepam [Ativan] every 4 to 6 hours); lithium for manic behavior; antipsychotic agents for delusions (e.g., 0.5 mg of haloperidol every 6 hours).

2. **Psychological.** Psychotherapy, both individual and marital therapy, to deal with intrapsychic or interpersonal conflicts. Consider discharging mother and infant to home only after arrangements for temporary homemaker are in place to reduce environmental stresses associated with care of the newborn.

VIII. Psychotic disorder not otherwise specified

A. **Definition.** Patients whose psychotic presentation does not meet the diagnostic criteria for any established psychotic disorder; also known as *atypical psychosis*.

B. **Diagnosis, signs, and symptoms.** See Table 9–8. This diagnostic category includes disorders that present with various psychotic features (e.g., delusions, hallucinations, loosening of associations, catatonic be-

TABLE 9–8
DSM-IV-TR DIAGNOSTIC CRITERIA FOR PSYCHOTIC DISORDER NOT OTHERWISE SPECIFIED

This category includes psychotic symptomatology (i.e., delusions, hallucinations, disorganized speech, grossly disorganized or catatonic behavior) about which there is inadequate information to make a specific diagnosis or about which there is contradictory information, or disorders with psychotic symptoms that do not meet the criteria for any specific psychotic disorder.
Examples include:

1. Postpartum psychosis that does not meet criteria for mood disorder with psychotic features, brief psychotic disorder, psychotic disorder due to a general medical condition, or substance-induced psychotic disorder
2. Psychotic symptoms that have lasted for less than 1 month but that have not yet remitted, so that the criteria for brief psychotic disorder are not met
3. Persistent auditory hallucinations in the absence of any other features
4. Persistent nonbizarre delusions with periods of overlapping mood episodes that have been present for a substantial portion of the delusional disturbance
5. Situations in which the clinician has concluded that a psychotic disorder is present, but is unable to determine whether it is primary, due to a general medical condition, or substance induced

From American Psychiatric Association. *Diagnostic and Statistical Manual of Mental Disorders,* text revision, 4th ed. Washington, DC: American Psychiatric Association, Copyright 2000, with permission.

TABLE 9–9
CULTURE-BOUND SYNDROMES

Diagnosis	Country or Culture	Characteristics
Amok	Southeast Asia, Malaysia	Sudden rampage, usually including homicide and suicide; occurs in males; ends in exhaustion and amnesia.
Bouffée délirante	France	Transient psychosis with elements of trance or dream states.
Brain fag	Sub-Saharan Africa	Headache, agnosia, chronic fatigue, visual difficulties, anxiety; seen in male students.
Bulimia nervosa	North America	Food binges, self-induced vomiting; may occur with depression, anorexia nervosa, or substance abuse.
Colera	Mayan Indians (Guatemala)	Temper tantrums, violent outbursts, gasping, stuporousness, hallucinations, delusions.
Empacho	Mexican and Cuban American	Inability to digest and excrete recently ingested food.
Grisi siknis	Miskito of Nicaragua	Headache, anxiety, anger, aimless running.
Hi-Wa itck	Mohave American Indian	Anorexia nervosa, insomnia, depression, suicide associated with unwanted separation from loved one.
Involutional paraphrenia	Spain, Germany	Paranoid disorder occurring in midlife; distinct from schizophrenia but may have elements of both schizophrenia and paranoia.
Koro	Asia	Fear that the penis will withdraw into the abdomen, causing death.
Latah	Southeast Asia, Malaysia, Bantu of Africa, Ainu of Japan	Automatic obedience reaction with echopraxia and echolalia precipitated by a sudden minimal stimulus; occurs in females; also called a *startle reaction.*
Mal de ojo	Mediterranean	Vomiting, fever, restless sleep; caused by evil eye.
Nervios	Costa Rica and Latin America	Headache, insomnia, anorexia, fears, anger, diarrhea, despair.
Piblokto (Arctic hysteria, pibloktoq)	Eskimos of northern Greenland	Mixed anxiety and depression, confusion, depersonalization, derealization; occurs mainly in females; ends in stuporous sleep and amnesia.
Reactive psychosis	Scandinavia	Psychosis precipitated by psychosocial stress; sudden onset with good prognosis, premorbid personality intact.
Shinkeishitsu	Japan	Syndrome marked by obsessions, perfectionism, ambivalence, social withdrawal, neurasthenia, and hypochondriasis.
Susto	Latin America	Severe anxiety, restlessness, fear of black magic and evil eye.
Tabanka	Trinidad	Depression in men abandoned by their wives; high risk of suicide.
Taijin-Kyofusho	Japan	Anxiety, fear of rejection, easy blushing, fear of eye contact, concern about body odor.
Uqamairineq	Inuits	Paralysis associated with borderline sleep states, accompanied by agitation, anxiety, hallucinations.
Wihtigo or windigo	Native American Indians (Algonkian)	Fear of being turned into a cannibal through possession by supernatural monster, the windigo.

haviors) but that cannot be delineated as any specific disorder. The disorders may include postpartum psychoses and rare or exotic syndromes (e.g., specific culture-bound syndromes).

1. **Autoscopic psychosis.** Rare hallucinatory psychosis during which patient sees a phantom or specter of his or her own body. Usually psychogenic in origin, but consider irritable lesion of temporoparietal lobe. Responds to reassurance and antipsychotic medications.

2. **Capgras' syndrome.** Delusion that persons in the environment are not their real selves but are doubles imitating the patient or impostors imitating someone else. May be part of schizophrenia and cerebral dysfunction. Treat with antipsychotic medication. Psychotherapy is useful in understanding the dynamics of the delusional belief (e.g., distrust of certain real persons in the environment).

3. **Cotard's syndrome.** Delusions of nihilism (e.g., nothing exists, the body has disintegrated, the world is coming to an end). Usually seen as part of schizophrenia or severe bipolar disorder. May be early sign of Alzheimer's disease. May respond to antipsychotic or antidepressant medication.

IX. Culture-bound syndromes

See Table 9–9.

For a more detailed discussion of this topic, see Other Psychotic Disorders, Ch 13, p 1232, in CTP/VII.

10

Mood Disorders

I. Introduction

Mood is defined as a pervasive emotional tone that profoundly influences one's outlook and perception of self, others, and the environment in general. Mood disorders are common, potentially lethal, and highly treatable conditions in which patients experience abnormally depressed or elevated moods. Mood abnormalities are accompanied by multiple signs and symptoms affecting almost all areas of functioning. Vegetative symptoms include changes in sleep, appetite, libido, and energy. The mood disorders include major depressive disorders, the bipolar disorders (I and II), dysthymic disorder, cyclothymic disorder, mood disorders due to a general medical condition, substance-induced mood disorder, and the general categories of depressive and bipolar disorders not otherwise specified. Advances in treatment include a broadening array of pharmacological agents, a greater understanding of the need for combined biological and psychosocial interventions, a recognition of the often chronic nature of these disorders, and the resulting importance of long-term maintenance treatments.

II. Diagnosis, signs, and symptoms

A. Depression (major depressive episode). See Table 10–1.

1. Information obtained from history

a. Depressed mood—subjective sense of sadness, feeling "blue" or "down in the dumps" for a prolonged period of time.

b. Anhedonia—inability to experience pleasure.

c. Social withdrawal.

d. Lack of motivation, little tolerance of frustration.

e. Vegetative signs.

(1) Loss of libido.

(2) Weight loss and anorexia.

(3) Weight gain and hyperphagia.

(4) Low energy level; fatigability.

(5) Abnormal menses.

(6) Early morning awakening (terminal insomnia); approximately 75% of depressed patients have sleep difficulties, either insomnia or hypersomnia.

(7) Diurnal variation (symptoms worse in morning).

f. Constipation.

g. Dry mouth.

h. Headache.

TABLE 10-1
DSM-IV-TR DIAGNOSTIC CRITERIA FOR MAJOR DEPRESSIVE EPISODE

A. Five (or more) of the following symptoms have been present during the same 2-week period and represent a change from previous functioning; at least one of the symptoms is either (1) depressed mood or (2) loss of interest or pleasure

  Note: Do not include symptoms that are clearly due to a general medical condition, or mood-incongruent delusions or hallucinations.

  (1) depressed mood most of the day, nearly every day, as indicated by either subjective report (e.g., feels sad or empty) or observation made by others (e.g., appears fearful). **Note:** in children and adolescents, can be irritable mood

  (2) markedly diminished interest or pleasure in all, or almost all, activities most of the day, nearly every day (as indicated by either subjective account or observation made by others)

  (3) significant weight loss when not dieting or weight gain (e.g., a change of more than 5% of body weight in a month), or decrease or increase in appetite nearly every day. **Note:** in children, consider failure to make expected weight gains

  (4) Insomnia or hypersomnia nearly every day

  (5) psychomotor agitation or retardation nearly every day (observable by others, not merely subjective feelings of restlessness or being slowed down)

  (6) fatigue or loss of energy nearly every day

  (7) feelings of worthlessness or excessive or inappropriate guilt (which may be delusional) nearly every day (not merely self-reproach or guilt about being sick)

  (8) diminished ability to think or concentrate, or indecisiveness, nearly every day (either by subjective account or as observed by others)

  (9) recurrent thoughts of death (not just fear of dying), recurrent suicidal ideation without a specific plan, or a suicide attempt or a specific plan for committing suicide

B. The symptoms do not meet criteria for a mixed episode.

C. The symptoms cause clinically significant distress or impairment in social, occupational, or other important areas of functioning.

D. The symptoms are not due to the direct physiological effects of a substance (e.g., a drug of abuse, a medication) or a general medical condition (e.g., hypothyroidism).

E. The symptoms are not better accounted for by bereavement, i.e., after the loss of a loved one, the symptoms persist for longer than 2 months or are characterized by marked functional impairment, morbid preoccupation with worthlessness, suicidal ideation, psychotic symptoms, or psychomotor retardation.

From American Psychiatric Association. *Diagnostic and Statistical Manual of Mental Disorders*. Text revision, 4th ed. Washington, DC: American Psychiatric Association, Copyright 2000, with permission.

2. Information obtained from mental status examination

  a. General appearance and behavior—psychomotor retardation or agitation, poor eye contact, tearful, downcast, inattentive to personal appearance.

  b. Affect—constricted or labile.

  c. Mood—depressed, irritable, frustrated, sad.

  d. Speech—little or no spontaneity, monosyllabic, long pauses, soft, low, monotone.

  e. Thought content—suicidal ideation affects 60% of depressed patients, and 15% commit suicide; obsessive rumination; pervasive feelings of hopelessness, worthlessness, and guilt; somatic preoccupation; indecisiveness; poverty of thought content and paucity of speech; mood-congruent hallucinations and delusions.

  f. Cognition—distractible, difficulty concentrating, complaints of poor memory, apparent disorientation; abstract thought may be impaired.

  g. Insight and judgment—impaired because of cognitive distortions of personal worthlessness.

3. Associated features

a. Somatic complaints may mask depression—in particular, cardiac, gastrointestinal, and genitourinary symptoms; low back pain, other orthopedic complaints.

b. Content of delusions and hallucinations, when present, tends to be congruent with depressed mood; most common are delusions of guilt, poverty, and deserved persecution, in addition to somatic and nihilistic (end of the world) delusions. Mood-incongruent delusions are those with content not apparently related to the predominant mood (e.g., delusions of thought insertion, broadcasting, and control, or persecutory delusions unrelated to depressive themes).

4. Age-specific features. Depression can present differently at different ages.

a. **Prepubertal**—somatic complaints, agitation, single-voice auditory hallucinations, anxiety disorders, and phobias.

b. **Adolescence**—substance abuse, antisocial behavior, restlessness, truancy, school difficulties, promiscuity, increased sensitivity to rejection, poor hygiene.

c. **Elderly**—cognitive deficits (memory loss, disorientation, confusion); pseudodementia or the dementia syndrome of depression, apathy, and distractibility.

B. Mania (manic episode).   See Table 10–2.

1. Information obtained from history

a. Erratic and disinhibited behavior.

(1) Excessive spending or gambling.

(2) Impulsive travel.

(3) Hypersexuality, promiscuity.

TABLE 10–2
DSM-IV-TR DIAGNOSTIC CRITERIA FOR MANIC EPISODE

A. A distinct period of abnormally and persistently elevated, expansive, or irritable mood, lasting at least 1 week (or any duration if hospitalization is necessary).

B. During the period of mood disturbance, three (or more) of the following symptoms have persisted (four if the mood is only irritable) and have been present to a significant degree:

(1) inflated self-esteem or grandiosity

(2) decreased need for sleep (e.g., feels rested after only 3 hours of sleep)

(3) more talkative than usual or pressure to keep talking

(4) flight of ideas or subjective experience that thoughts are racing

(5) distractibility (i.e., attention too easily drawn to unimportant or irrelevant external stimuli)

(6) increase in goal-directed activity (either socially, at work or school, or sexually) or psychomotor agitation

(7) excessive involvement in pleasurable activities that have a high potential for painful consequences (e.g., engaging in unrestrained buying sprees, sexual indiscretions, or foolish business investments)

C The symptoms do not meet criteria for a mixed episode.

D. The mood disturbance is sufficiently severe to cause marked impairment in occupational functioning or in usual social activities or relationships with others, or to necessitate hospitalization to prevent harm to self or others, or there are psychotic features.

E. The symptoms are not due to the direct physiologic effects of a substance (e.g., a drug of abuse, a medication, or other treatment) or a general medical condition (e.g., hyperthyroidism).

Note: Manic-like episodes that are clearly caused by somatic antidepressant treatment (e.g., medication, electroconvulsive therapy, light therapy) should not count toward a diagnosis of bipolar I disorder.

b. Overextended in activities and responsibilities.

c. Low frustration tolerance with irritability, outbursts of anger.

d. Vegetative signs.

    (1) Increased libido.

    (2) Weight loss, anorexia.

    (3) Insomnia (expressed as no need to sleep).

    (4) Excessive energy.

2. Information obtained from mental status examination

a. General appearance and behavior—psychomotor agitation; seductive, colorful clothing; excessive makeup; inattention to personal appearance or bizarre combinations of clothes; intrusive; entertaining; threatening; hyperexcited.

b. Affect—labile, intense (may have rapid depressive shifts).

c. Mood—euphoric, expansive, irritable, demanding, flirtatious.

d. Speech—pressured, loud, dramatic, exaggerated; may become incoherent.

e. Thought content—highly elevated self-esteem, grandiose, extremely egocentric; delusions and less frequently hallucinations (mood-congruent themes of inflated self-worth and power, most often grandiose and paranoid).

f. Thought process—flight of ideas (if severe, can lead to incoherence); racing thoughts, neologisms, clang associations, circumstantiality, tangentiality.

g. Sensorium—highly distractible, difficulty concentrating; memory, if not too distracted, generally intact; abstract thinking generally intact.

h. Insight and judgment—extremely impaired; often total denial of illness and inability to make any organized or rational decisions.

C. Depressive disorders

1. Major depressive disorder. (Also known as *unipolar depression* and *unipolar disorder*.) Severe episodic depressive disorder. Symptoms must be present for at least 2 weeks and represent a change from previous functioning. More common in women than in men by 2:1. Precipitating event occurs in at least 25% of patients. Diurnal variation, with symptoms worse early in morning. Psychomotor retardation or agitation is present. Associated with vegetative signs. Mood-congruent delusions and hallucinations may be present. Median age of onset is 40 years, but can occur at any time. Genetic factor is present.

a. Melancholic—see Table 10–3. Severe and responsive to biological intervention.

b. Chronic—present for at least 2 years; more common in elderly men, especially alcohol and substance abusers, and responds poorly to medications. Accounts for the condition of 10–15% of those with major depressive disorder. Can also occur as part of depression bipolar I and II disorders.

c. Seasonal pattern—depression that develops with shortened daylight in winter and fall and disappears during spring and summer; also known as *seasonal affective disorder*. Characterized by hyper-

TABLE 10–3
DSM-IV-TR DIAGNOSTIC CRITERIA FOR MELANCHOLIC FEATURES SPECIFIED

Specify if:
  With melancholic features (can be applied to the current or most recent major depressive episode in major depressive disorder and to a major depressive episode in bipolar I or bipolar II disorder only if it is the most recent type of mood episode)
A. Either of the following, occurring during the most severe period of the current episode:
  (1) loss of pleasure in all, or almost all, activities
  (2) lack of reactivity to usually pleasurable stimuli (does not feel much better, even temporarily, when something good happens)
B. Three (or more) of the following:
  (1) distinct quality of depressed mood (i.e., the depressed mood is experienced as distinctly different from the kind of feeling experienced after the death of a loved one)
  (2) depression regularly worse in the morning
  (3) early morning awakening (at least 2 hours before usual time of awakening)
  (4) marked psychomotor retardation or agitation
  (5) significant anorexia or weight loss
  (6) excessive or inappropriate guilt

From American Psychiatric Association. *Diagnostic and Statistical Manual of Mental Disorders*, text revision, 4th ed. Washington, DC: American Psychiatric Association, Copyright 2000, with permission.

somnia, hyperphagia, and psychomotor slowing. Related to abnormal melatonin metabolism. Treated with exposure to bright, artificial light for 2 to 6 hours daily. May also occur as part of bipolar I and II disorders.

  d. **Postpartum onset**—severe depression beginning within 4 weeks of giving birth. Most often occurs in women with underlying or preexisting mood or other psychiatric disorder. Symptoms range from marked insomnia, lability, and fatigue to suicide. Homicidal and delusional beliefs about the baby may be present. Can be psychiatric emergency, with both mother and baby at risk. Also applies to manic or mixed episodes or to brief psychotic disorder (Chapter 9).

  e. **Atypical features**—sometimes called *hysterical dysphoria*. Major depressive episode characterized by weight gain and hypersomnia rather than weight loss and insomnia. More common in women than in men by 2:1 to 3:1. Common in major depressive disorder with seasonal pattern. May also occur as part of depression in bipolar I or II disorder and dysthymic disorder.

  f. **Pseudodementia**—major depressive disorder presenting as cognitive dysfunction resembling dementia. Occurs in elderly persons, and more often in patients with previous history of mood disorder. Depression is primary and preeminent, antedating cognitive deficits. Responsive to electroconvulsive therapy (ECT) or antidepressant medication.

  g. **Depression in children**—not uncommon. Signs and symptoms similar to those in adults. Masked depression seen in running away from home, school phobia, substance abuse. Suicide may occur.

  h. **Double depression**—development of superimposed major depressive disorder in dysthymic patients (about 10–15%).

  i. **Depressive disorder not otherwise specified**—depressive features that do not meet the criteria for a specific mood disorder (e.g., minor depressive disorder, recurrent brief depressive disorder, and premenstrual dysphoric disorder).

2. Dysthymic disorder. (Previously known as *depressive neurosis.*) Less severe than major depressive disorder. More common and chronic in women than in men. Insidious onset. Occurs more often in persons with history of long-term stress or sudden losses; often coexists with other psychiatric disorders (e.g., substance abuse, personality disorders, obsessive-compulsive disorder). Symptoms tend to be worse later in the day. Onset generally between ages of 20 and 35, although an early-onset type begins before age 21. More common among first-degree relatives with major depressive disorder. Symptoms should include at least two of the following: poor appetite, overeating, sleep problems, fatigue, low self-esteem, poor concentration or difficulty making decisions, and feelings of hopelessness.

D. Bipolar disorders

   1. Bipolar I disorder. Patient has met the criteria for a full manic or mixed episode, usually sufficiently severe to require hospitalization. May occur with major depressive or hypomanic episodes.

   2. Bipolar II disorder. Patient has had at least one major depressive episode and at least one hypomanic episode (Table 10–4), but no manic episode.

   3. Rapid-cycling bipolar disorder. Four or more depressive, manic, or mixed episodes within 12 months. Bipolar disorder with mixed or rapid cycling episodes appears to be more chronic than bipolar disorder without alternating episodes.

   4. Adolescent mania. Signs of mania masked by substance abuse, alcoholism, and antisocial behavior.

TABLE 10–4
DSM-IV-TR CRITERIA FOR HYPOMANIC EPISODE

A. A distinct period of persistently elevated, expansive, or irritable mood, lasting throughout 4 days, that is clearly different from the usual nondepressed mood.

B. During the period of mood disturbance, three (or more) of the following symptoms have persisted (four if the mood is only irritable) and have been present to a significant degree:
   (1) inflated self-esteem or grandiosity
   (2) decreased need for sleep (e.g., feels rested after only 3 hours of sleep)
   (3) more talkative than usual or pressure to keep talking
   (4) flight of ideas or subjective experience that thoughts are racing
   (5) distractibility (i.e., attention too easily drawn to unimportant or irrelevant external stimuli)
   (6) increase in goal-directed activity (either socially, at work or school, or sexually) or psychomotor agitation
   (7) excessive involvement in pleasurable activities that have a high potential for painful consequences (e.g., the person engages in unrestrained buying sprees, sexual indiscretions, or foolish business investments)

C. The episode is associated with an unequivocal change in functioning that is uncharacteristic of the person when not symptomatic.

D. The disturbance in mood and the change in functioning are observable by others.

E. The episode is not severe enough to cause marked impairment in social or occupational functioning, or to necessitate hospitalization, and there are no psychotic features.

F. The symptoms are not due to the direct physiologic effects of a substance (e.g., a drug of abuse, a medication, or other treatment) or a general medical condition (e.g., hyperthyroidism).

From American Psychiatric Association. *Diagnostic and Statistical Manual of Mental Disorders,* text revision, 4th ed. Washington, DC: American Psychiatric Association, Copyright 2000, with permission.

5. **Cyclothymic disorder.** Less severe disorder, with alternating periods of hypomania and moderate depression. The condition is chronic and nonpsychotic. Symptoms must be present for at least 2 years. Equally common in men and women. Onset usually is insidious and occurs in late adolescence or early adulthood. Substance abuse is common. Major depressive disorder and bipolar disorder are more common among first-degree relatives than among the general population. Recurrent mood swings may lead to social and professional difficulties. May respond to lithium.

III. Epidemiology

See Tables 10–5 and 10–6.

IV. Etiology

A. Biological

1. **Biogenic amines.** Heterogeneous dysregulation of biogenic amines, based on findings of abnormal levels of monoamine metabolites homovanillic acid (HVA) (from dopamine), 5-hydroxyindoleacetic acid (5-HIAA) (from serotonin), and 3-methoxy-4-hydroxyphenylgycol

TABLE 10–5
EPIDEMIOLOGY OF MAJOR DEPRESSIVE DISORDER AND BIPOLAR I DISORDER

	Major Depressive Disorder	Bipolar I Disorder
Incidence (new cases per year)	1/100 men 3/100 women	1.2/100 men 1.8/100 women
Prevalence (existing cases)	2–3/100 men 5–10/100 women	1/100 men and women
Sex	2:1 women/men	Men or women (may be slightly higher in women)
Age	40—mean age men/women 10% occur after age 60 Small peak in adolescence 50% occur before age 40	30—mean age men/women
Race	No difference	No difference
Sociocultural	↑ risk with family history of alcohol/depression/parental loss before age 13 Slightly ↑ risk in lower socioeconomic groups	↑ risk with family history of mania/bipolar illness No difference urban/rural Slightly increased in higher socioeconomic groups
Family history	(Evidence for heritability stronger for bipolar disorder than for depression) Approximately 10–13% risk for first-degree relatives MZ concordance rate higher than DZ, but ratio not as high as seen in bipolar disorder	20–25% risk for first-degree relatives 50% of bipolar patients have parent with mood disorder Child with one bipolar parent has 25% risk of developing disorder Child with two bipolar parents has 50–75% risk Bipolar MZ concordance rate = 40–70% Bipolar DZ concordance rate = 20%

Data from American Psychiatric Assocation. *Diagnostic and Statistical Manual of Mental Disorders*, text revision, 4th ed. Washington, DC: American Psychiatric Association, Copyright 2000, with permission.

TABLE 10–6
LIFETIME PREVALENCE OF SOME DSM-IV-TR MOOD DISORDERS

Mood Disorder	Lifetime Prevalence
Depressive disorders	
Major depressive disorder (MDD)	10–25% for women; 5–12% for men
Recurrent, with full interepisode recovery, superimposed on dysthymic disorder	Approximately 3% of persons with MDD
Recurrent, without full interepisode recovery, superimposed on dysthymic disorder (double depression)	Approximately 25% of persons with MDD
Dysthymic disorder	Approximately 6%
Bipolar disorders	
Bipolar I disorder	0.4–1.6%
Bipolar II disorder	Approximately 0.5%
Bipolar I disorder or bipolar II disorder, with rapid cycling	5–15% of persons with bipolar disorder
Cyclothymic disorder	0.4–1.0%

Data from American Psychiatric Association. *Diagnostic and Statistical Manual of Mental Disorders,* text revision, 4th ed. Washington, DC: American Psychiatric Association, Copyright 2000, with permission.

(MHPG) (from norepinephrine) in blood, urine, and CSF fluid of patient with mood disorders. Serotonin depletion is associated with depression, whereas serotoninergic agents are effective treatments for depression. Low levels of 5-HIAA are associated with violence and suicide. Dopamine activity may be reduced in depression and increased in mania.

2. **Neuroendocrine regulation.** In general, neuroendocrine abnormalities probably reflect disruptions in biogenic amine input to the hypothalamus. Hyperactivity of the hypothalamic–pituitary–adrenal axis in depression leads to increased cortisol secretion. Also in depression—decreased release of thyroid-stimulating hormone (TSH), growth hormone (GH), follicle-stimulating hormone (FSH), luteinizing hormone (LH), and testosterone; decreased nocturnal secretion of melatonin. Immune functions are decreased in both mania and depression.

3. **Sleep.** In depression, abnormalities include delayed sleep onset, shortened rapid eye movement (REM) latency (the time between falling asleep and the first REM period), increased length of first REM period, and abnormal delta sleep. Multiple awakenings and decreased total sleep time are common in mania. Sleep deprivation has been found to have antidepressant effects.

4. **Kindling.** A process by which repeated subthreshold stimulation of a neuron generates an action potential. This stimulation leads to a seizure at an organ level. The effectiveness of anticonvulsants such as mood stabilizers and the periodic nature of some mood disorders has led to the theory that the mood disorders may be a consequence of kindling in the temporal lobes.

5. **Genetic.** Both bipolar disorders and depressive disorders run in families, but evidence for heritability is higher in bipolar disorder.

One parent with bipolar I disorder, 25% chance of mood disorder in child. Two parents with bipolar I disorder, 50–75% chance of mood disorder in child. One parent with major depressive disorder, 10–13%

chance of mood disorder in child. One monozygotic (MZ) twin with bipolar I disorder, 33–90% chance of bipolar I in other twin (dizygotic [DZ] twin, 5–25%). One MZ twin with major depressive disorder, about 50% chance of major depressive disorder in other twin (DZ twins, 10–25%).

No genetic association has been consistently replicated. Associations between the mood disorders, particular bipolar I disorder, and genetic markers have been reported for chromosomes 5, 11, and X.

6. **Neuroanatomic.** Limbic system, hypothalamus, and basal ganglia are involved.

B. **Psychosocial**

1. **Psychoanalytic.** Symbolic or real loss of loved person (love object) perceived as rejection. Mania and elation viewed as defense against underlying depression. Rigid superego serves to punish person with feelings of guilt about unconscious sexual or aggressive impulses. Freud described internalized ambivalence toward love object, which can produce a pathological form of mourning if the object is lost or perceived as lost. This mourning takes the form of severe depression with feelings of guilt and worthlessness and suicidal ideation.

2. **Cognitive.** Cognitive triad of Aaron Beck: (1) negative self-view ("things are bad because I'm bad"); (2) negative interpretation of experience ("everything has always been bad"); (3) negative view of future (anticipation of failure). **Learned helplessness** is a theory that attributes depression to a person's inability to control events. Theory is derived from observed behavior of animals experimentally given unexpected random shocks from which they cannot escape.

3. **Stressful life events.** Often precede first episodes of mood disorders. Such events may cause permanent neuronal changes that predispose a person to subsequent episodes of a mood disorder. Losing a parent before age 11 is the life event most associated with later development of depression.

V. **Laboratory and psychological tests**

A. **Dexamethasone suppression test.** Nonsuppression (positive test result) represents hypersecretion of cortisol secondary to hyperactivity of hypothalamic–pituitary–adrenal axis. Abnormal in 50% of patients with major depression. Of limited clinical usefulness owing to frequency of false-positives and false-negatives. Diminished release of TSH in response to thyrotropin-releasing hormone (TRH) reported in both depression and mania. Prolactin release decreased in response to tryptophan. Tests are not definitive.

B. **Psychological tests**

1. **Rating scales.** Can be used to assist in diagnosis and assessment of treatment efficacy. The Beck Depression Inventory (BDI) and Zung Self-rating Scale are scored by patients. The Hamilton Rating Scale for Depression (HAM-D), Montgomery Asberg Depression Rating Scale (MADRS), and Young Manic Rating Scale are scored by the examiner.

2. **Rorschach test.** Standardized set of 10 inkblots scored by examiner—few associations, slow response time in depression.

3. **Thematic apperception test (TAT).** Series of 30 pictures depicting ambiguous situations and interpersonal events. Patient creates a story about each scene. Depressives will create depressed stories, manics more grandiose and dramatic ones.

C. **Brain imaging.**   No gross brain changes. Enlarged cerebral ventricles on computed tomography (CT) in some patients with mania or psychotic depression; diminished basal ganglia blood flow in some depressive patients. Magnetic resonance imaging (MRI) studies have also indicated that patients with major depressive disorder have smaller caudate nuclei and smaller frontal lobes than do control subjects. Magnetic resonance spectroscopy (MRS) studies of patients with bipolar I disorder have produced data consistent with the hypothesis that the pathophysiology of the disorder may involve an abnormal regulation of membrane phospholipid metabolism.

VI. Psychodynamics

In depression, introjection of ambivalently viewed lost objects leads to an inner sense of conflict, guilt, rage, pain, and loathing; a pathological mourning becomes depression as ambivalent feelings meant for the introjected object are directed at the self. In mania, feelings of inadequacy and worthlessness are converted by means of denial, reaction formation, and projection to grandiose delusions.

VII. Differential diagnosis

Table 10–7 lists the clinical differences between depression and mania.

A. **Mood disorder resulting from general medical condition.**   Depressive, manic, or mixed features or major depressive-like episode secondary to medical illness (e.g., brain tumor, metabolic illness, HIV disease, Parkinson's disease, Cushing's syndrome) (Table 10–8). Cognitive deficits are common.

1. **Myxedema madness.** Hypothyroidism associated with fatigability, depression, and suicidal impulses. May mimic schizophrenia, with thought disorder, delusions, hallucinations, paranoia, and agitation. More common in women.

2. **Mad hatter's syndrome.** Chronic mercury intoxication (poisoning) produces manic (and sometimes depressive) symptoms.

B. **Substance-induced mood disorder.**   See Table 10–9. Mood disorders caused by a drug or toxin [e.g., cocaine, amphetamine, propranolol (Inderal), steroids]. Must always be ruled out when patient presents with depressive or manic symptoms. Mood disorders often occur simultaneously with substance abuse and dependence.

C. **Schizophrenia.** Schizophrenia can look like a manic, major depressive, or mixed episode with psychotic features. To differentiate, rely on such factors as family history, course, premorbid history, and response to medication. Depressive-like or manic-like episode with presence of

TABLE 10–7
CLINICAL DIFFERENCES BETWEEN DEPRESSION AND MANIA

	Depressive Syndrome	Mania Syndrome
Mood	Depressed, irritable, or anxious (the patient may, however, smile or deny subjective mood change and instead complain of pain or other somatic distress)	Elated, irritable, or hostile
	Crying spells (the patient may, however, complain of inability to cry or experience emotions)	Momentary tearfulness (as part of mixed state)
Associated psychological manifestations	Lack of self-confidence; low self-esteem; self-reproach	Inflated self-esteem; boasting; grandiosity
	Poor concentration; indecisiveness	Racing thoughts; clang associations (new thoughts triggered by word sounds rather than meaning); distractibility
	Reduction in gratification; loss of interest in usual activities; loss of attachments; social withdrawal	Heightened interest in new activities, people, creative pursuits; increased involvement with people (who are often alienated because of the patient's intrusive and meddlesome behavior); buying sprees; sexual indiscretions; foolish business investment
	Negative expectations; hopelessness; helplessness; increased dependency	
	Recurrent thoughts of death and suicide	
Somatic manifestations	Psychomotor retardation; fatigue	Pyschomotor acceleration;
	Agitation	eutonia (increased sense of physical well-being)
	Anorexia and weight loss, or weight gain	Possible weight loss from increased activity and inattention to proper dietary habits
	Insomnia, or hypersomnia	Decreased need for sleep
	Menstrual irregularities; amenorrhea	
	Anhedonia; loss of sexual desire	Increased sexual desire
Psychotic symptoms	Delusions of worthlessness and sinfulness	Grandiose delusions of exceptional talent
	Delusions of reference and persecution	Delusions of assistance; delusions of reference and persecution
	Delusion of ill health (nihilistic, somatic, or hypochondriacal)	Delusions of exceptional mental and physical fitness
	Delusions of poverty	Delusions of wealth, aristocratic ancestry, or other grandiose identity
	Depressive hallucinations in the auditory, visual, and (rarely) olfactory spheres	Fleeting auditory or visual hallucinations

From Berkow R, ed. *Merck Manual*, 15ᵗʰ ed. Rahway, NJ: Merck Sharp & Dohme Research Laboratories, 1987:1518, with permission.

mood-incongruent psychotic features suggests schizophrenia. Thought insertion and broadcasting, loose associations, poor reality testing, or bizarre behavior may also suggest schizophrenia. Bipolar disorder with depression or mania more often is associated with mood-congruent hallucinations or delusions.

TABLE 10–8
NEUROLOGIC AND MEDICAL CAUSES OF DEPRESSIVE (AND MANIC) SYMPTOMS

Neurologic	
Cerebrovascular diseases	
Dementias (including dementia of the Alzheilmer's type with depressed mood)	Postpartum[a]
	Thyroid disorders (hypothyroidism and apathetic hyperthyroidism)[a]
Epilepsy[a]	
Fahr's disease[a]	*Infectious and inflammatory*
Huntington's disease[a]	AIDS[a]
Hydrocephalus	Chronic fatigue syndrome
Infections (including HIV and neurosyphilis)[a]	Mononucleosis
Migraines[a]	Pneumonia—viral and bacterial
Multiple sclerosis[a]	Rheumatoid arthritis
Narcolepsy	Sjögren's arteritis
Neoplasms[a]	Systemic lupus erythematosus[a]
Parkinson's disease	Temporal arthritis
Progressive supranuclear palsy	Tuberculosis
Sleep apnea	
Trauma[a]	*Miscellaneous medical*
Wilson's disease[a]	Cancer (especially pancreatic and other gastrointestinal)
	Cardiopulmonary disease
Endocrine	Porphyria
Adrenal (Cushing's, Addison's diseases)	Uremia (and other renal diseases)[a]
Hyperaldosteronism	Vitamin deficiencies (B$_{12}$, folate, niacin, thiamine)[a]
Menses-related[a]	
Parathyroid disorders (hyper- and hypo-)	

[a] These conditions are also associated with manic symptoms.

D. Grief. Not a true disorder. Known as *bereavement* in DSM-IV-TR. Profound sadness secondary to major loss. Presentation may be similar to that of major depressive disorder, with anhedonia, withdrawal, and vegetative signs. Remits with time. Differentiated from major depressive disorder by absence of suicidal ideation or profound feelings of hopelessness and worthlessness. Usually resolves within a year. May develop into major depressive episode in predisposed persons.

E. Personality disorders. Lifelong behavioral pattern associated with rigid defensive style; depression may occur more readily after stressful life event because of inflexibility of coping mechanisms. Manic episode may also occur more readily in predisposed people with preexisting personality disorder. A mood disorder may be diagnosed on Axis I simultaneously with a personality disorder on Axis II.

F. Schizoaffective disorder. Signs and symptoms of schizophrenia accompany prominent mood symptoms. Course and prognosis are between those of schizophrenia and mood disorders.

G. Adjustment disorder with depressed mood. Moderate depression in response to clearly identifiable stress, which resolves as stress diminishes. Considered a maladaptive response resulting from either impairment in functioning or excessive and disproportionate intensity of symptoms. Persons with personality disorders or cognitive deficits may be more vulnerable.

H. Primary sleep disorders. Can cause anergy, dyssomnia, irritability. Distinguish from major depression by assessing for typical signs and symptoms of depression and occurrence of sleep abnormalities only in the

TABLE 10-9
PHARMACOLOGICAL CAUSES OF DEPRESSION AND MANIA

Pharmacological Causes of Depression		Pharmacological Causes of Mania
Cardiac and antihypertensive drugs		Amphetamines
Bethanidine	Digitalis	Antidepressants
Clonidine	Prazosin	Baclofen
Guanethidine	Procainamide	Bromide
Hydralazine	Veratrum	Bromocriptine
Methyldopa	Lidocaine	Captopril
Propranolol	Oxprenolol	Cimetidine
Reserpine	Methoserpidine	Cocaine
Sedatives and hypnotics		Corticosteroids (including corticotropin)
Barbiturates	Benzodiazepines	Cyclosporine
Chloral hydrate	Chlormethiazole	Disulfiram
Ethanol	Chlorazepate	Hallucinogens (intoxication and flashbacks)
Steroids and hormones		Hydralazine
Corticosteroids	Triamcinolone	Isoniazid
Oral contraceptives	Norethisterone	Levodopa
Prednisone	Danazol	Methylphenidate
Stimulants and appetite suppressants		Metrizamide (following myelography)
Amphetamine	Diethylpropion	Opioids
Fenfluramine	Phenmetrazine	Phencyclidine
Psychotropic drugs		Procarbazine
Butyrophenones	Phenothiazines	Procyclidine
Neurologic agents		Yohimbine
Amantadine	Baclofen	
Bromocriptine	Carbamazepine	
Levodopa	Methosuximide	
Tetrabenazine	Phenytoin	
Analgesics and antiinflammatory drugs		
Fenoprofen	Phenacetin	
Ibuprofen	Phenylbutazone	
Indomethacin	Pentazocine	
Opioids	Benzydamine	
Antibacterial and antifungal drugs		
Ampicillin	Griseofulvin	
Sulfamethoxazole	Metronidazole	
Clotrimazole	Nitrofurantoin	
Cycloserine	Nalidixic acid	
Dapsone	Sulfonamides	
Ethionamide	Streptomycin	
Tetracycline	Thiocarbanilide	
Antineoplastic drugs		
C-Asparaginase	6-Azauridine	
Mithramycin	Bleomycin	
Vincristine	Trimethoprim	
	Zidovudine	
Miscellaneous drugs		
Acetazolamide	Anticholinesterases	
Choline	Cimetidine	
Cyproheptadine	Diphenoxylate	
Disulfiram	Lysergide	
Methysergide	Mebeverine	
Meclizine	Metoclopramide	
Pizotifen	Salbutamol	

Adapted from Cummings JL. *Clinical Neuropsychiatry.* Orlando, FL: Grune & Stratton, 1985:187, with permission.

context of depressive episodes. Consider obtaining a sleep laboratory evaluation in cases of refractory depression.

I. **Other mental disorders.** Eating disorders, somatoform disorders, and anxiety disorders are all commonly associated with depressive symptoms and must be considered in the differential diagnosis of a patient with depressive symptoms. Perhaps the most difficult differential is that between anxiety disorders with depression and depressive disorders with marked anxiety. The difficulty of making this differentiation is reflected in the inclusion of the research category of mixed anxiety–depressive disorder in DSM-IV-TR (Chapter 11).

VIII. Course and prognosis

Fifteen percent of depressed patients eventually commit suicide. An untreated, average depressed episode lasts about 10 months. At least 75% of affected patients have a second episode of depression, usually within the first 6 months after the initial episode. The average number of depressive episodes in a lifetime is five. The prognosis generally is good: 50% recover, 30% partially recover, 20% have a chronic course. About 20–30% of dysthymic patients develop, in descending order of frequency, major depressive disorder (called *double depression*), bipolar II disorder, or bipolar I disorder. A major mood disorder, usually bipolar II disorder, develops in about one third of patients with cyclothymic disorder. Forty-five percent of manic episodes recur. Untreated, manic episodes last 3 to 6 months, with a high rate of recurrence (average of 10 recurrences). Some 80–90% of manic patients eventually experience a full depressive episode. The prognosis is fair: 15% recover, 50–60% partially recover (multiple relapses with good interepisodic functioning), and one third have some evidence of chronic symptoms and social deterioration.

IX. Treatment

A. **Depressive disorders.**   Major depressive episodes are treatable in 70–80% of patients. The physician must integrate pharmacotherapy with psychotherapeutic interventions. If physicians view mood disorders as fundamentally evolving from psychodynamic issues, their ambivalence about the use of drugs may result in a poor response, noncompliance, and probably inadequate dosing for too short a treatment period. Conversely, if physicians ignore the psychosocial needs of the patient, the outcome of pharmacotherapy may be compromised.

1. **Biological.** Almost always indicated in major depressive disorder and dysthymic disorder. Clinicians now have a large number of effective drugs from which to choose. The selective serotonin reuptake inhibitors (SSRIs) have become the most widely prescribed first-line agents for the treatment of depression owing to their safety, efficacy, and tolerability. Tricyclics, tetracyclics, and other mixed reuptake inhibitors (including atypical antipsychotic medication) are also effective in the treatment of severe depression. Prior personal or family history of a good response to a particular agent are indications to use that particular drug for the current episode. If no such information is available,

then the drug should be chosen based on its adverse effects profile or potential for drug–drug interactions (Table 10–10). The most common clinical mistake leading to an unsuccessful trial of an antidepressant drug is the use of too low a dosage for too short a time. Unless adverse events prevent it, the dosage should be raised to the maximum recommended level and maintained for at least 4 or 5 weeks before another drug is tried.

a. Most clinicians begin treatment with an SSRI. Early transient side effects include anxiety, gastrointestinal upset, and headache. Educating patients about the self-limited nature of these effects can enhance compliance. Sexual dysfunction is often a persistent, common side effect that may respond to a change in drug or dosage, or adjunctive therapy with an agent such as bupropion (Wellbutrin) or buspirone (BuSpar). The early anxiogenic effects of SSRIs can be managed by either reducing the dose or adding an anxiolytic (e.g., 0.5 mg of clonazepam [Klonopin] in the morning and at night). Insomnia can be managed with a benzodiazepine, zolpidem (Am-

TABLE 10–10
SELECTED DRUGS USED TO TREAT DEPRESSION

Drug	Starting Dose (mg)	Dosage[a] (mg/d)	Therapeutic Plasma Concentration (ng/mL)
Amitriptyline (Elavil, Endep)	25 hs to 25 tid	50–300	60–200[b]
Amoxapine (Asendin)	50 bid[b]–50 tid	100–600	180–600[b]
Bupropion (Wellbutrin)	50–75 bid	150–450	50–100[b]
	SR:150[d]	150–400	50–100[b]
Citalopram (Celexa)	10–20	20–80	—
Clomipramine (Anafranil)	25 tid	100–250	200–300[b]
Desipramine (Norpramin, Pertofrane)	25 hs to 25 tid	50–300	125–250[c]
Doxepin (Adapin, Sinequan)	25 hs to 25 bid	75–300	110–250
Fluoxetine (Prozac)	20 qam	10–80	—
Fluvoxamine (Luvox)	50–100 qam	100–300	—
Imipramine (Janimine, Tofranil)	25 hs to 25 tid	50–300	>180[b,c]
Maprotiline (Ludiomil)	25 hs to 25 tid	50–225	200–400[b]
Mirtazapine (Remeron)	15	15–45	—
Nefazodone (Serzone)	100 mg tid	100–600	—
Nortriptyline (Aventyl, Pamelor)	25 hs to 25 tid	50–200	50–150[c]
Paroxetine (Paxil)	20 qam	10–50	—
Phenelzine (Nardil)	15 qam	15–90	80% inhibition of platelet MAO activity
Protriptyline (Vivactyl)	10 qam	15–60	100–200
Sertraline (Zoloft)	50 qam	50–200	—
Trazodone (Desyrel)	50 tid	50–600	800–1600
Trimipramine (Surmontil)	25 hs to 25 tid	75–300	—
Tranylcypromine (Parnate)	10 qam	10–60	80% inhibition of platelet MAO activity
Venlafaxine (Effexor)	37.5 bid	75–375	—
	XR:37.5 qd[e]	75–225	

[a] In geriatric patients, the appropriate dose is widely variable but in general is one-half the young adult dosage range for tricyclic antidepressants and for those compounds with significant cardiovascular toxicity.
[b] Parent and metabolite.
[c] Therapeutic drug monitoring well established.
[d] Sustained-release formulation.
[e] Extended-release formulation.
Reprinted from *Prim Psychiatry* 1995;2:41, with permission.

bien), trazodone (Desyrel), or mirtazapine (Remeron). Patients who do not respond to or who cannot tolerate one SSRI may respond to another. Some clinicians switch to an agent with a different mechanism of action, such as bupropion, venlafaxine (Effexor), mirtazapine, nefazodone (Serzone), a tricyclic, or a monoamine oxidase inhibitor (MAOI). Any of the above drugs can be used as first-line agents. However, the tricyclics and MAOIs are generally well considered as second- or third-line agents because of their side effects and potential lethality in overdose.

b. Bupropion is a noradrenergic, dopaminergic drug with stimulant-like properties. It is generally well tolerated and may be particularly useful for depression marked by anergy and psychomotor retardation. It is also devoid of sexual side effects. It may exacerbate anxiety and agitation. Its dopaminergic properties have the potential to exacerbate psychosis. Prior concerns about its tendency to cause seizures have been mitigated by the availability of a sustained-release formulation that carries the same risk for seizure as the SSRIs (0.1%).

c. Venlafaxine is a serotonin-norepinephrine reuptake inhibitor that may be particularly effective in severe or refractory cases of depression. Response rates increase with higher doses. Side effects are similar to those of SSRIs.

d. Nefazodone is a drug with serotoninergic properties. Its main mechanism of action is postsynaptic 5-HT$_2$ blockade. As a result, it produces beneficial effects on sleep and has a low rate of sexual side effects. It can cause hypotension and sedation. Gradual dose titration is required. It has anxiolytic properties.

e. Mirtazapine has antihistamine, noradrenergic, and serotoninergic actions. It specifically blocks 5-HT$_2$ and 5-HT$_3$ receptors, so that the anxiogenic, sexual, and gastrointestinal side effects of serotoninergic drugs are avoided. At low doses, it can be highly sedating and cause weight gain. At higher dosages, it becomes more noradrenergic relative to its antihistamine effects and so a more activating drug.

f. Reboxetine (Vestra) is a selective norepinephrine reuptake inhibitor that is reported to be well tolerated. It may be particularly useful in cases of depression characterized by psychomotor retardation and cognitive impairment. It may also be effective in severe or refractory depression.

g. The tricyclics are highly effective but require dose titration. Side effects include anticholinergic effects in addition to potential cardiac conduction delay and orthostasis. The secondary amines, such as nortriptyline, are often better tolerated than the tertiary amines, such as amitriptyline (Elavil). Blood levels can be helpful in determining optimal dosage and adequacy of a therapeutic trial. Lethality in overdose remains a concern.

h. Augmentation strategies in treatment-resistant or partially responsive patients include liothyronine (Cytomel), lithium, amphetamines, buspirone, or antidepressant combinations such as bupropion added to an SSRI.

i. If symptoms still do not improve, try an MAOI. An MAOI is safe with reasonable dietary restriction of tyramine-containing substances. Major depressive episodes that have atypical features or psychotic features or that are related to bipolar I disorder may preferentially respond to MAOIs. MAOIs must not be administered for 2 to 5 weeks after discontinuation of an SSRI or other serotoninergic drugs (e.g., 5 weeks for fluoxetine [Prozac], 2 weeks for paroxetine [Paxil]). An SSRI or other serotoninergic drug (e.g., clomipramine [Anafranil]) must not be administered for 2 weeks after discontinuation of an MAOI (Table 10–11). Serotonergic-dopamine antagonists are also of use in depression with psychotic features.

j. Maintenance treatment for at least 5 months with antidepressants helps to prevent relapse. Long-term treatment may be indicated in patients with recurrent major depressive disorder. The antidepressant dosage required to achieve remission should be continued during maintenance treatment.

k. ECT is useful in refractory major depressive disorder and major depressive episodes with psychotic features; ECT also is indicated when a rapid therapeutic response is desired or when side effects of antidepressant medications must be avoided. (ECT is underused as a first-line antidepressant treatment.)

l. Lithium can be a first-line antidepressant in treating the depression of bipolar disorder. A heterocyclic antidepressant or MAOI may be added as necessary, but monitor the patient carefully for emergence of manic symptoms.

TABLE 10–11
DRUGS TO BE AVOIDED DURING TREATMENT WITH MONOAMINE OXIDASE INHIBITORS

Never use
Antiasthmatics
Antihypertensives (methyldopa, guanethidine, reserpine)
Buspirone
Levodopa
Opioids (especially meperidine, dextromethorphan, propoxyphene, tramadol; morphine or codeine may be less dangerous)
Cold, allergy, or sinus medications containing dextromethorphan or sympathomimetics
SSRIs, clomipramine, venlafaxine, sibutramine
Sympathomimetics (amphetamines, cocaine, methylphenidate, dopamine, metaraminol, epinephrine, norepinephrine, isoproterenol, ephedrine, pseudoephedrine, phenylpropanolamine)
L−tryptophan
Use carefully
Anticholinergics (propranolol)
Antihistamines
Disulfiram
Bromocriptine
Hydralazine
Sedative-hypnotics
Terpin hydrate with codeine
Tricyclics and tetracyclics (avoid clomipramine)

m. Repetitive transcranial magnetic stimulation (rTMS) is currently experimental. Shows promise as a treatment for depression. rTMS uses magnetic fields to stimulate specific brain regions (e.g., left prefrontal cortex) believed to be involved in the pathophysiology of specific disorders.

n. An experimental treatment of vagus nerve stimulation with implanted electrodes is being studied.

2. **Psychological.** Psychotherapy in conjunction with antidepressants is more effective than either treatment alone in the management of major depressive disorder.

a. **Cognitive**—short-term treatment with interactive therapist and assigned homework aimed at testing and correcting negative cognitions and the unconscious assumptions that underlie them; based on correcting chronic distortions in thinking that lead to depression, in particular the cognitive triad of feelings of helplessness and hopelessness about one's self, one's future, and one's past.

b. **Behavioral**—based on learning theory (classic and operant conditioning). Generally short-term and highly structured; aimed at specific, circumscribed undesired behaviors. The operant conditioning technique of positive reinforcement may be an effective adjunct in the treatment of depression.

c. **Interpersonal**—developed as a specific short-term treatment for nonbipolar, nonpsychotic depression in outpatients. Emphasis on ongoing, current interpersonal issues as opposed to unconscious, intrapsychic dynamics.

d. **Psychoanalytically oriented**—insight-oriented therapy of indeterminate length aimed at achieving understanding of unconscious conflicts and motivations that may be fueling and sustaining depression.

e. **Supportive**—therapy of indeterminate length with the primary aim of providing emotional support. Indicated particularly in acute crisis, such as grief, or when the patient is beginning to recover from a major depressive episode but cannot yet engage in more demanding, interactive therapy.

f. **Group**—not indicated for acutely suicidal patients. Other depressed patients may benefit from support, ventilation, and positive reinforcement of groups, and from interpersonal interaction and immediate correction of cognitive and transference distortions by other group members.

g. **Family**—particularly indicated when patient's depression is disrupting family stability, when depression is related to family events, or when it is supported or maintained by family patterns.

B. Bipolar disorders
1. Biological
a. Lithium, divalproex (Depakote), and olanzapine (Zyprexa) are the only FDA-approved treatments for the manic phase of bipolar disorder, but carbamazepine (Tegretol) is also a well-established treatment. Gabapentin (Neurontin) and lamotrigine (Lamictal) are

promising treatments for refractory or treatment-intolerant patients. The efficacy of the latter two agents is not well established, but their clinical use is expanding. Topiramate (Topamax) is another anticonvulsant showing benefit in bipolar patients. ECT is highly effective in all phases of bipolar disorder. Carbamazepine, divalproex, and valproic acid (Depakene) appear more effective than lithium in the treatment of mixed or dysphoric mania, rapid cycling, and psychotic mania, and in the treatment of patients with a history of multiple manic episodes or comorbid substance abuse.

b. Treatment of acute manic episodes often requires adjunctive use of potent sedative drugs. Drugs commonly used at the start of treatment include clonazepam (1 mg every 4 to 6 hours) and lorazepam (Ativan) (2 mg every 4 to 6 hours). Haloperidol (Haldol) (2 to 10 mg/d), olanzapine (2.5 to 10 mg/d), and risperidone (Risperdal) (0.5 to 6 mg/d) are also of use. Bipolar patients may be particularly sensitive to the side effects of typical antipsychotics. The atypical antipsychotics (e.g., olanzapine [Zyprexa] [10 to 15 mg/d]) are often used as monotherapy for acute control and may have intrinsic antimanic properties. Physicians should attempt to taper these adjunctive agents when the patient stabilizes.

c. Lithium remains a mainstay of treatment in bipolar disorders. A blood level of 0.8 to 1.2 mEq/L is usually needed to control acute symptoms. A complete trial should last at least 4 weeks, with 2 weeks at therapeutic levels. Prelithium workup includes a complete blood cell count, ECG, thyroid function tests, measurement of blood urea nitrogen and serum creatinine, and a pregnancy test. Lithium has a narrow therapeutic index, and levels can become toxic quickly when a patient is dehydrated. A level of 2.0 mEq or higher is toxic. Lithium treatment can be initiated at 300 mg three times per day. A level should be checked after 5 days and the dose titrated accordingly. The clinical response may take 4 days after a therapeutic level has been achieved. Typical side effects include thirst, polyuria, tremor, metallic taste, cognitive dulling, and gastrointestinal upset. Lithium can induce hypothyroidism and, in rare cases, renal toxicity. Lithium is a first-line treatment for bipolar depression and achieves an antidepressant response in 50% of patients. Lithium is most effective for prophylaxis of further mood episodes at levels of 0.8 to 1.2 mEq/L. However, in many patients, remission can be maintained at lower levels, which are better tolerated and thereby promote enhanced compliance. Patients with depressive breakthrough on lithium should be assessed for lithium-induced hypothyroidism. Lithium is excreted unchanged by the kidneys and must be used with caution in patients with renal disease. Because lithium is not metabolized by the liver, it may be the best choice for treating bipolar disorder in patients with hepatic impairment.

d. Valproic acid and divalproex have a broad therapeutic index and appears effective at levels of 50 to 125 μg/mL. Pretreatment workup includes a complete blood cell count and liver function tests. A pregnancy test is needed because this drug can cause neural tube defects in developing fetuses. It can cause thrombocytopenia and increased transaminase levels, both of which are usually benign and self-limited but require increased blood monitoring. Fatal hepatic toxicity has been reported only in children under 10 who received multiple anticonvulsants. Typical side effects include hair loss (which can be treated with zinc and selenium), tremor, weight gain, and sedation. Gastrointestinal upset is common but can be minimized by using enteric-coated tablets (Depakote) and titrating gradually. Valproic acid can be loaded for acute symptom control by administering at 20 mg/kg in divided doses. This strategy also produces a therapeutic level and may improve symptoms within 7 days. For outpatients, more physically brittle patients, or less severely ill patients, medication can be started at 250 to 750 mg/d and gradually titrated to a therapeutic level. Blood levels can be checked after 3 days at a particular dosage.

e. Carbamazepine is usually titrated to response rather than blood level, although many clinicians titrate to reach levels of 4 to 12 μg/mL. Pretreatment evaluation should include liver function tests and a complete blood cell count as well as ECG, electrolytes, reticulocytes, and pregnancy test. Side effects include nausea, sedation, and ataxia. Hepatic toxicity, hyponatremia, or bone marrow suppression may rarely occur. Rash occurs in 10% of patients. Exfoliative rashes (Stevens-Johnson syndrome) are rare but potentially fatal. The drug can be started at 200 to 600 mg/d, with adjustments every 5 days based on clinical response. Improvement may be seen 7 to 14 days after a therapeutic dose has been achieved. Drug interactions complicate carbamazepine use and probably relegate it to second-line status. It is a potent enzyme inducer and can lower levels of other psychotropics, such as haloperidol. Carbamazepine induces its own metabolism (autoinduction), and the dosage often needs to be increased during the first few months of treatment to maintain a therapeutic level and clinical response.

f. Lamotrigine and gabapentin are anticonvulsants that may have antidepressant, antimanic, and mood-stabilizing properties. They do not require blood monitoring. Gabapentin is excreted exclusively by the kidneys. It has a benign side effect profile that can include sedation or activation, dizziness, and fatigue. It does not interact with other drugs. Dose reduction in patients with renal insufficiency is required. Gabapentin can be titrated aggressively, and therapeutic response has been reported at dosages of 300 to 3,600 mg/day. It has a short half-life, and dosing to three times a day is required. Lamotrigine requires gradual titration to decrease the risk for rash, which occurs in 10% of patients. Stevens-Johnson syndrome occurs in 0.1% of patients treated with lamotrigine. Other side effects include nausea, sedation, ataxia, and insomnia. Dosage can be initiated at 25 to 50 mg/day for 2 weeks and then increased slowly to

150 to 250 mg twice daily. Valproate raises lamotrigine levels. In the presence of valproate, lamotrigine titration should be slower and dosages lower (e.g., 25 mg orally four times daily for 2 weeks, with 25-mg increases every 2 weeks to a maximum of 150 mg/day).

Topiramate has shown preliminary efficacy in bipolar disorders. Its side effects include fatigue and cognitive dulling. This drug has the unique property of causing weight loss. One series of overweight patients with bipolar disorder lost an average of 5% of their body weight while taking topiramate as an adjunct to other medications. The starting dosage is usually 25 to 50 mg/day to a maximum of 400 mg/day.

g. Maintenance treatment is required in patients with recurrent illness. During long-term treatment, laboratory monitoring is required for lithium, valproic acid, and carbamazepine. These requirements are outlined in Chapter 25.

h. Patients who do not respond adequately to one mood stabilizer may do well with combination treatment. Lithium and valproic acid are commonly used together. Increased neurotoxicity is a risk, but the combination is safe. Other combinations include lithium plus carbamazepine, carbamazepine plus valproic acid (requires increased laboratory monitoring for drug interactions and hepatic toxicity), and combinations with the newer anticonvulsants.

i. Other agents used in bipolar disorder include verapamil (Isoptin, Calan), nimodipine (Nimotop), clonidine (Catapres), clonazepam, and levothyroxine (Levoxyl, Levothroid, Synthroid) (Chapter 25). Clozapine (Clozaril) has also been shown to have potent antimanic and mood-stabilizing properties in treatment-refractory patients.

j. ECT should be considered in refractory or emergent cases. See Chapter 25 for further discussion.

2. **Psychological.** Psychotherapy in conjunction with antimanic drugs (e.g., lithium) is more effective than either treatment alone. Psychotherapy is not indicated when a patient is experiencing a manic episode. In this situation, the safety of the patient and others must be paramount, and pharmacologic and physical steps must be taken to protect and calm the patient.

a. **Cognitive**—has been studied in relation to increasing compliance with lithium therapy among patients with bipolar disorder.

b. **Behavioral**—can be most effective during inpatient treatment of manic patients. Helps to set limits on impulsive or inappropriate behavior through such techniques as positive and negative reinforcement and token economies.

c. **Psychoanalytically oriented**—can be beneficial in the recovery and stabilization of manic patients if patient is capable of and desires insight into underlying conflicts that may trigger and fuel manic episodes. Can also help patients understand resistance to medication and thus increase compliance.

d. **Supportive**—indicated particularly during acute phases and in early recompensation. Some patients can tolerate only supportive therapy, whereas others can tolerate insight-oriented therapy. Supportive therapy more often is indicated for patients with chronic bipolar disorder, who may have significant interepisodic residual symptoms and experience social deterioration.

e. Group—can be helpful in challenging denial and defensive grandiosity of manic patients. Useful in addressing such common issues among manic patients as loneliness, shame, inadequacy, fear of mental illness, and loss of control. Helpful in reintegrating patients socially.

f. Family—particularly important with bipolar patients because their disorder is strongly familial (22–25% of first-degree relatives) and because manic episodes are so disruptive to patients' interpersonal relationships and jobs. During manic episodes, patients may spend huge amounts of family money or act with sexual inappropriateness; residual feelings of anger, guilt, and shame among family members must be addressed. Ways to help with compliance and recognizing triggering events can be explored.

For more detailed discussion of this topic, see Mood Disorders, Ch 14, p 1284, in CTP/VII.

11

Anxiety Disorders

I. Definition

Anxiety is a state characterized by a feeling of dread and accompanied by somatic signs that indicate a hyperactive autonomic nervous system. It is differentiated from fear, which is an appropriate response to a known threat; anxiety is a response to a threat that is unknown, vague, or conflictual.

II. Diagnosis, signs, and symptoms

See Table 11–1.

A. Panic disorder and agoraphobia. See Table 11–2. Panic disorder is characterized by spontaneous panic attacks (Table 11–3). It may occur alone or be associated with agoraphobia (fear of being in open spaces, outside the home alone, or in a crowd). Panic may evolve in stages: subclinical attacks, full panic attacks, hypochondriacal fears, anticipatory anxiety, phobic avoidance of specific situations, and agoraphobia. It can lead to alcohol or drug abuse, depression, and occupational and social restrictions. Agoraphobia can occur alone, although patients usually have associated panic attacks. Anticipatory anxiety is characterized by the fear that panic, with helplessness or humiliation, will occur. Agoraphobic patients may become housebound and never leave the home or go outside only with a companion.

B. Generalized anxiety disorder. See Table 11–4. Involves excessive worry about actual circumstances, events, or conflicts. The symptoms may fluctuate. Occurs in children and adults.

C. Specific phobia. See Table 11–5. A phobia is an irrational fear of an object (e.g., horses, heights, needles). The person experiences massive anxiety when exposed to the feared object and tries to avoid it at all costs.

D. Social phobia. See Table 11–6. Social phobia is an irrational fear of public situations [e.g., speaking in public, eating in public, using public bathrooms (shy bladder)]. In the generalized type, most social situations are avoided.

E. Obsessive-compulsive disorder. See Table 11–7. Obsessive-compulsive disorder involves recurrent intrusive ideas, images, ruminations, impulses, thoughts (obsessions), or repetitive patterns of behavior or actions (compulsions). Both obsessions and compulsions are ego-alien and produce anxiety if resisted.

F. Posttraumatic and acute stress disorders. See Table 11–8. In these disorders, anxiety is produced by an extraordinarily stressful event. The event is relived in dreams and waking thoughts (flashbacks). The

TABLE 11-1
SIGNS AND SYMPTOMS OF ANXIETY DISORDERS

Physical Signs	Psychological Symptoms
Trembling, twitching, feeling shaky	Feeling of dread
Backache, headache	Difficulty concentrating
Muscle tension	Hypervigilance
Shortness of breath, hyperventilation	Insomnia
Fatigability	Decreased libido
Startle response	"Lump in the throat"
Autonomic hyperactivity	Upset stomach ("butterflies")
Flushing and pallor	
Tachycardia, palpitations	
Sweating	
Cold hands	
Diarrhea	
Dry mouth (xerostomia)	
Urinary frequency	
Paresthesia	
Difficulty swallowing	

TABLE 11-2
DSM-IV-TR DIAGNOSTIC CRITERIA FOR PANIC DISORDER WITHOUT AGORAPHOBIA

A. Both (1) and (2):
   (1) recurrent unexpected panic attacks
   (2) at least one of the attacks has been followed by 1 month (or more) of one (or more) of the following:
      (a) persistent concern about having additional attacks
      (b) worry about the implications of the attack or its consequences (e.g., losing control, having a heart attack, "going crazy")
      (c) a significant change in behavior related to the attacks
B. Absence agoraphobia
C. The panic attacks are not due to the direct physiological effects of a substance (e.g., or a drug of abuse, a medication) or a general medical condition (e.g., hyperthyroidism).
D. The panic attacks are not better accounted for by another mental disorder, such as social phobia (e.g., occurring on exposure to feared social situations), specific phobia (e.g., on exposure to a specific phobic situation), obsessive-compulsive disorder (e.g., on exposure to dirt in someone with an obsession about contamination), posttraumatic stress disorder (e.g., in response to stimuli associated with a severe stressor), or separation anxiety disorder (e.g., in response to being away from home or close relatives).

From American Psychiatric Association. *Diagnostic and Statistical Manual of Mental Disorders*, text revision, 4th ed. Washington, DC: American Psychiatric Association, Copyright 2000, with permission.

TABLE 11-3
DSM-IV-TR DIAGNOSTIC CRITERIA FOR PANIC ATTACK

Note: A panic attack is not a codable disorder. Code the specific diagnosis in which the panic attack occurs (e.g., panic disorder with agoraphobia).
A discrete period of intense fear or discomfort, in which four (or more) of the following symptoms developed abruptly and reached a peak within 10 minutes:
   (1) palpitations, pounding heart, or accelerated heart rate
   (2) sweating
   (3) trembling or shaking
   (4) sensations of shortness of breath or smothering
   (5) feeling of choking
   (6) chest pain or discomfort
   (7) nausea or abdominal distress
   (8) feeling dizzy, unsteady, lightheaded, or faint
   (9) derealization (feelings of unreality) or depersonalization (being detached from oneself)
   (10) fear of losing control or going crazy
   (11) fear of dying
   (12) paresthesias (numbness or tingling sensations)
   (13) chills or hot flushes

From American Psychiatric Association. *Diagnostic and Statistical Manual of Mental Disorders*, text revision, 4th ed. Washington, DC: American Psychiatric Association, Copyright 2000, with permission.

TABLE 11–4
DSM-IV-TR DIAGNOSTIC CRITERIA FOR GENERALIZED ANXIETY DISORDER

A. Excessive anxiety and worry (apprehensive expectation), occurring more days than not for at least 6 months, about a number of events or activities (such as work or school performance).
B. The person finds it difficult to control the worry.
C. The anxiety and worry are associated with three (or more) of the following six symptoms (with at least some symptoms present for more days than not for the past 6 months). **Note:** Only one item is required in children.
   (1) restlessness or feeling keyed up or on edge
   (2) being easily fatigued
   (3) difficulty concentrating or mind going blank
   (4) irritability
   (5) muscle tension
   (6) sleep disturbance (difficulty falling or staying asleep, or restless, unsatisfying sleep)
D. The focus of the anxiety and worry is not confined to features of an Axis I disorder, e.g., the anxiety or worry is not about having a panic attack (as in panic disorder), being embarrassed in public (as in social phobia), being contaminated (as in obsessive-compulsive disorder), being away from home or close relatives (as in separation anxiety disorder), gaining weight (as in anorexia nervosa), having multiple physical complaints (as in somatization disorder), or having a serious illness (as in hypochondriosis), and the anxiety and worry do not occur exclusively during posttraumatic stress disorder.
E. The anxiety, worry, or physical symptoms cause clinically significant distress or impairment in social, occupational, or other important areas of functioning.
F. The disturbance is not due to the direct physiologic effects of a substance (e.g., drug of abuse, a medication) or a general medical condition (e.g., hyperthyroidism) and does not occur exclusively during a mood disorder, a psychotic disorder, or a pervasive development disorder.

From American Psychiatric Association. *Diagnostic and Statistical Manual of Mental Disorders,* text revision, 4th ed. Washington, DC: American Psychiatric Association, Copyright 2000, with permission.

TABLE 11–5
DSM-IV-TR DIAGNOSTIC CRITERIA FOR SPECIFIC PHOBIA

A. Marked and persistent fear that is excessive or unreasonable, cued by the presence or anticipation of a specific object or situation (e.g., flying, heights, animals, receiving an injection, seeing blood).
B. Exposure to the phobic stimulus almost invariably provokes an immediate anxiety response, which may take the form of a situationally bound or situationally predisposed panic attack. **Note:** in children, the anxiety may be expressed by crying, tantrums, freezing, or clinging.
C. The person recognizes that the fear is excessive or unreasonable. **Note:** In children, this feature may be absent.
D. The phobic situation(s) is avoided or else is endured with intense anxiety or distress.
E. The avoidance, anxious anticipation, or distress in the feared situation(s) interferes significantly with the person's normal routine, occupational (or academic) functioning, or social activities or relationships, or there is marked distress about having the phobia.
F. In individuals under age 18 years, the duration is at least 6 months.
G. The anxiety, panic attacks, or phobic avoidance associated with the specific object or situation is not better accounted for by another mental disorder, such as obsessive-compulsive disorder (e.g., fear of dirt in someone with an obsession about contamination), posttraumatic stress disorder (e.g., avoidance of stimuli associated with a severe stressor), separation anxiety disorder (e.g., avoidance of school), social phobia (e.g., avoidance of social situations because of fear of embarrassment), panic disorder with agoraphobia, or agoraphobia without history of panic disorder.
Specify type:
   Animal type.
   Natural environment type (e.g., heights, storms, water)
   Blood-injection-injury type
   Situational type (e.g., airplanes, elevators, enclosed places)
   Other type (e.g., phobic avoidance or situations that may lead to choking, vomiting, or contracting an illness; in children, avoidance of loud sounds or costumed characters)

From American Psychiatric Association. *Diagnostic and Statistical Manual of Mental Disorders,* text revision, 4th ed. Washington, DC: American Psychiatric Association, Copyright 2000, with permission.

TABLE 11–6
DSM-IV DIAGNOSTIC CRITERIA FOR SOCIAL PHOBIA

A. A marked and persistent fear of one or more social or performance situations in which the person is exposed to unfamiliar people or to possible scrutiny by others. The individual fears that he or she will act in a way (or show anxiety symptoms) that will be humiliating or embarrassing. **Note:** In children, there must be evidence of the capacity for age-appropriate social relationships with familiar people and the anxiety must occur in peer settings, not just in interactions with adults.
B. Exposure to the feared social situation almost invariably provokes anxiety, which may take the form of a situationally bound or situationally predisposed panic attack. **Note:** In children, the anxiety may be expressed by crying, tantrums, freezing, or shrinking from social situations with unfamiliar people.
C. The person recognizes that the fear is excessive or unreasonable. **Note:** In children, this feature may be absent.
D. The feared social or performance situations are avoided or else are endured with intense anxiety or distress.
E. The avoidance, anxious anticipation, or distress in the feared social or performance situation(s) interferes significantly with the person's normal routine, occupational (academic) functioning, or social activities or relationships, or there is marked distress about having the phobia.
F. In individuals under age 18 years, the duration is at least 6 months.
G. The fear or avoidance is not due to the direct physiologic effects of a substance (e.g., a drug of abuse, a medication) or a general medical condition and is not better accounted for by another mental disorder (e.g., panic disorder with or without agoraphobia, separation anxiety disorder, body dysmorphic disorder, a pervasive developmental disorder, or schizoid personality disorder).
H. If a general medical condition or another mental disorder is present, the fear in Criterion A is unrelated to it, e.g., the fear is not of stuttering, trembling in Parkinson's disease, or exhibiting abnormal eating behavior in anorexia nervosa or bulimia nervosa.
Specify if:
   Generalized: if the fears include most social situations (also consider the additional diagnosis of avoidant personality disorder).

From American Psychiatric Association. *Diagnostic and Statistical Manual of Mental Disorders,* text revision, 4th ed. Washington, DC: American Psychiatric Association, Copyright 2000, with permission.

symptoms of repeated experience, avoidance, and hyperarousal last more than 1 month. For patients in whom symptoms have been present less than 1 month, the appropriate diagnosis is acute stress disorder.
   G. **Anxiety disorder due to a general medical condition.** A wide range of medical conditions can cause anxiety symptoms. See Table 11–9.
   H. **Substance-induced anxiety disorder.** A wide range of substances can cause anxiety symptoms. See Table 11–10.
   I. **Mixed anxiety–depressive disorder.** This disorder describes patients with both anxiety and depressive symptoms that do not meet the diagnostic criteria for either an anxiety disorder or a mood disorder. The diagnosis is sometimes used in primary care settings and is used in Europe; sometimes called *neurasthenia.*
   J. **Other anxiety states**
      1. **Adjustment disorder with anxiety.** This applies to the patient with an obvious stressor in whom excessive anxiety develops within 3 months and is expected to last no longer than 6 months.
      2. **Anxiety secondary to another psychiatric disorder.** Seventy percent of depressed patients have anxiety. Patients with psychoses—schizophrenia, mania, or brief psychotic disorder—often exhibit anxiety (psychotic anxiety). Anxiety is common in delirium and in dementia (catastrophic reaction).

TABLE 11–7
DSM-IV-TR DIAGNOSTIC CRITERIA FOR OBSESSIVE-COMPULSIVE DISORDER

A. Other obsessions or compulsions:
   Obsessions as defined by (1), (2), (3), and (4):
   (1) recurrent and persistent thoughts, impulses, or images that are experienced, at some time during the disturbance, as intrusive and inappropriate and that cause marked anxiety or distress
   (2) the thoughts, impulses, or images are not simply excessive worries about real-life problems
   (3) the person attempts to ignore or suppress such thoughts, impulses, or images, or to neutralize them with some other thought or action
   (4) the person recognizes that the obsessional thoughts, impulses, or images are a product of his or her own mind (not imposed from without, as in thought insertion)
   Compulsions as defined by (1) and (2):
   (1) repetitive behaviors (e.g., hand washing, ordering, checking) or mental acts (e.g., praying, counting, repeating words silently) that the person feels driven to perform in response to an obsession, or according to rules that must be applied rigidly
   (2) the behaviors or mental acts are aimed at preventing or reducing distress or preventing some dreaded event or situation; however, these behaviors or mental acts either are not connected in a realistic way with what they are designed to neutralize or prevent or are clearly excessive
B. At some point during the course of the disorder, the person has recognized that the obsessions or compulsions are excessive or unreasonable. **Note:** This does not apply to children.
C. The obsessions or compulsions cause marked distress, are time consuming (take more than 1 hour a day), or significantly interfere with the person's normal routine, occupational (or academic) functioning, or usual social activities or relationships.
D. If another Axis I disorder is present, the content of the obsessions or compulsions is not restricted to it (e.g., preoccupation with food in the presence of an eating disorder; hair pulling in the presence of trichochotillomania; concern with appearance in the presence of body dysmorphic disorder; preoccupation with drugs in the presence of a substance use disorder; preoccupation with having a serious illness in the presence of hypochondriasis; preoccupations with sexual urges or fantasies in the presence of a paraphilia; or guilty ruminations in the presence of major depressive disorder).
E. The disturbance is not caused by the direct physiologic effects of a substance (e.g., a drug of abuse, a medication) or a general medical condition.
Specify if:
   With poor insight: If, for most of the time during the current episode, the person does not recognize that the obsessions and compulsions are excessive or unreasonable

From American Psychiatric Association. *Diagnostic and Statistical Manual of Mental Disorders.* Text revisions, 4th ed. Washington, DC: American Psychiatric Association, Copyright 2000, with permission.

3. **Situational anxiety.** Effects of a stressful situation temporarily overwhelm the ability to cope. This may occur in minor situations if it brings to mind past overwhelming stress.

4. **Death anxiety.** This typically involves fears of helplessness, physical changes, loss of control, and loss of others in addition to guilt and shame.

5. **Separation anxiety and stranger anxiety.** Regressed adults, including some who are medically ill, may manifest anxiety related to these childhood phenomena when separated from loved ones or when having to react to staff in a hospital.

6. **Anxiety related to loss of self-esteem.** This may be a reaction to illness, rejection, or loss of a job, especially if it is experienced as a defeat or failure.

7. **Anxiety related to loss of self-control.** In circumstances in which control must be surrendered, such as medical illness or hospitalization, patients with a need to feel in control may be very threatened.

TABLE 11–8
DSM-IV-TR DIAGNOSTIC CRITERIA FOR POSTTRAUMATIC STRESS DISORDER

A. The person has been exposed to a traumatic event in which both of the following were present:
   (1) the person experienced, witnessed, or was confronted with an event or events that involved actual or threatened death or serious injury, or a threat to the physical integrity of self or others
   (2) the person's response involved intense fear, helplessness, or horror. **Note:** in children, this may be expressed instead by disorganized or agitated behavior
B. The traumatic event is persistently reexperienced in one (or more) of the following ways:
   (1) recurrent and intrusive distressing recollections of the event, including images, thoughts, or perceptions. **Note:** in young children, repetitive play may occur in which themes or aspects of the trauma are expressed.
   (2) recurrent distressing dreams of the event. **Note:** in children, there may be frightening dreams without recognizable content.
   (3) acting or feeling as if the traumatic event were recurring (includes a sense of reliving the experience, illusions, hallucinations, and dissociative flashback episodes, including those that occur on awakening or when intoxicated). **Note:** In young children, trauma-specific reenactment may occur.
   (4) intense psychological distress at exposure to internal or external cues that symbolize or resemble an aspect of the traumatic event
   (5) physiological reactivity on exposure to internal or external cues that symbolize or resemble an aspect of the traumatic event
C. Persistent avoidance of stimuli associated with the trauma and numbing of general responsiveness (not present before the trauma), as indicated by three (or more) of the following:
   (1) efforts to avoid thoughts, feelings, or conversations associated with the trauma
   (2) efforts to avoid activities, places, or people that arouse recollections of the trauma
   (3) inability to recall an important aspect of the trauma
   (4) markedly diminished interest or participation in significant activities
   (5) feeling of detachment or estrangement from others
   (6) restricted range of affect (e.g., unable to have loving feelings)
   (7) sense of a foreshortened future (e.g., does not expect to have a career, marriage, children, or a normal life span)
D. Persistent symptoms of increased arousal (not present before the trauma), as indicated by two (or more) of the following:
   (1) difficulty falling or staying asleep
   (2) irritability or outbursts of anger
   (3) difficulty concentrating
   (4) hypervigilance
   (5) exaggerated startle response
E. Duration of the disturbance (symptoms in Criteria B, C, and D) is more than 1 month.
F. The disturbance causes clinically significant distress or impairment in social, occupational, or other important areas of functioning.
Specify if:
   Acute: if symptoms last less than 3 months
   Chronic: if symptoms last 3 months or more
Specify if:
   With delayed onset: if symptoms begin at least 6 months after the stressor

From American Psychiatric Association. *Diagnostic and Statistical Manual of Mental Disorders*, text revision, 4th ed. Washington, DC: American Psychiatric Association, Copyright 2000, with permission.

8. **Anxiety related to dependence or intimacy.** If past dependency needs were not met or resolved, a patient can resist situations, such as medical care or a close relationship, that involve some dependence.
9. **Anxiety related to guilt and punishment.** If a patient expects punishment for imagined or real misdeeds, he or she may feel anxiety and the punishment may be actively sought or even self-inflicted.

10. Signal anxiety. Sigmund Freud's term to describe anxiety not consciously experienced but that triggers defense mechanisms used by the person to deal with a potentially threatening situation.

III. Epidemiology

The anxiety disorders make up the most common group of psychiatric disorders. Generally, women are more affected than men (Table 11–11).

TABLE 11–9
MEDICAL AND NEUROLOGICAL CAUSES OF ANXIETY

Neurological disorders
Cerebral neoplasms
Cerebral trauma and postconcussive syndromes
Cerebrovascular disease
Subarachnoid hemorrhage
Migraine
Encephalitis
Cerebral syphilis
Multiple sclerosis
Wilson's disease
Huntington's disease
Epilepsy

Systemic conditions
Hypoxia
Cardiovascular disease
Pulmonary insufficiency
Anemia

Endocrine disturbances
Pituitary dysfunction
Thyroid dysfunction
Parathyroid dysfunction
Adrenal dysfunction
Pheochromocytoma
Female virilization disorders

Inflammatory disorders
Lupus erythematosus
Rheumatoid arthritis
Polyarteritis nodosa
Temporal arteritis

Deficiency states
Vitamin B_{12} deficiency
Pellagra

Miscellaneous conditions
Hypoglycemia
Carcinoid syndrome
Systemic malignancies
Premenstrual syndrome
Febrile illnesses and chronic infections
Porphyria
Infectious mononucleosis
Posthepatitis syndrome
Uremia

Toxic conditions
Alcohol and drug withdrawal
Vasopressor agents
Penicillin
Sulfonamides
Mercury
Arsenic
Phosphorus
Organophosphates
Carbon disulfide
Benzene
Aspirin intolerance

Adapted from Cummings JL. *Clinical Neuropsychiatry.* Orlando, FL: Grune & Stratton, 1985:214, with permission.

TABLE 11–10
SOME SUBSTANCES THAT MAY CAUSE ANXIETY

Intoxication	Withdrawal
Amphetamines and other sympathomimetics	Alcohol
Amyl nitrite	Antihypertensives
Anticholinergics	Caffeine
Caffeine	Opioids
Cannabis	Sedative-hypnotics
Cocaine	
Hallucinogens	
Theophylline	
Yohimbine	

TABLE 11-11
EPIDEMIOLOGY OF ANXIETY DISORDERS

	Panic Disorder	Phobia	Obsessive Compulsive Disorder	Generalized Anxiety Disorder	Post-traumatic Stress Disorder
Lifetime prevalence	1.5–4% of population	Most common anxiety disorder: 10% of population	2–3% of population	3–8% of population	1–3% of population; 30% of Vietnam veterans
Male-to-female ratio	1:1 (without agoraphobia) 1:2 (with agaraphobia)	1:2	1:1	1:2	1:2
Age at onset	Late 20s	Late childhood	Adolescence or early adulthood	Variable; early adulthood	Any age, including childhood
Family history	20% of first-degree relatives of agoraphobic patients have agoraphobia	May run in families, especially blood injection, injury type	35% in first-degree relatives	25% of first-degree relatives affected	—
Twin studies	Higher concordance in monozygotic (MZ) twins than in dizygotic (DZ) twins	—	Higher concordance in MZ twins than in DZ twins	80–90% concordance in MZ twins; 10–15% in DZ twins	—

IV. Etiology

A. Biological

1. Anxiety involves an excessive autonomic reaction with increased sympathetic tone.
2. The release of catecholamines is increased.
3. Increased production of norepinephrine metabolites (e.g., 3-methoxy-4-hydroxyphenylglycol). Experimental infusion of lactate increases norepinephrine levels and produces anxiety in patients with panic disorder.
4. Decreased rapid eye movement (REM) latency and stage IV sleep (similar to depression) may develop.
5. Decreased levels of γ-aminobutyric acid (GABA) cause CNS hyperactivity (GABA inhibits CNS irritability).
6. Serotonin decrease causes anxiety; increased dopaminergic activity is associated with anxiety.
7. Activity in the temporal cerebral cortex is increased.
8. The locus ceruleus, a brain center of noradrenergic neurons, is hyperactive in anxiety states, especially panic attacks.

B. Psychoanalytic.
According to Freud, unconscious impulses (e.g., sex or aggression) threaten to burst into consciousness and produce anxiety. Anxiety is related developmentally to childhood fears of disintegration that derive from the fear of loss of a loved object or fear of castration.

C. Learning theory

1. Anxiety is produced by continued or severe frustration or stress. The anxiety then becomes a conditioned response to other situations that are less severely frustrating or stressful.
2. It may be learned through identification and imitation of anxiety patterns in parents (social learning theory).
3. Anxiety is associated with a naturally frightening stimulus (e.g., accident). Subsequent displacement or transference to another stimulus through conditioning produces a phobia to a new and different object or situation.
4. Anxiety disorders involve faulty, distorted, or counterproductive patterns of cognitive thinking.

D. Genetic studies

1. Half of patients with panic disorder have one affected relative.
2. About 5% have a variant of the gene associated with serotonin metabolism and have high levels of anxiety.

V. Psychological tests

A. Rorschach test

1. Anxiety responses include animal movements, unstructured forms, and heightened color.
2. Phobic responses include anatomic forms or bodily harm.
3. Obsessive-compulsive responses include over-attention to detail.

B. Thematic apperception test

1. Increased fantasy productions may be present.
2. Themes of aggression and sexuality may be prominent.
3. Feelings of tension may be evident.

C. Bender-Gestalt

1. No changes indicative of brain damage are apparent.
2. Use of small area may be manifested in obsessive-compulsive disorder.
3. Productions may spread out on the page in anxiety states.

D. Draw-a-Person

1. Attention to head and general detailing may be noted in obsessive-compulsive disorder.
2. Body image distortions may be present in phobias.
3. Rapid drawing may be evident in anxiety disorders.

E. Minnesota Multiphasic Personality Inventory-II.   High hypochondriasis, psychasthenia, hysteria scales in anxiety.

VI. Laboratory tests

No specific laboratory tests for anxiety.

VII. Pathophysiology

A. No pathognomonic changes.
B. In obsessive-compulsive disorder, positron emission tomography reveals decreased metabolism in the orbital gyrus, caudate nuclei, and cingulate gyrus.

C. Positron emission tomography reveals increased blood flow in the right parahippocampus in panic and in the frontal lobe in anxiety.

D. Mitral valve prolapse is present in 50% of patients with panic disorder.

E. Nonspecific EEG changes may be noted.

F. Dexamethasone suppression test does not suppress cortisol in some obsessive-compulsive patients.

G. Panic-inducing substances include carbon dioxide, sodium lactate, methylchlorophenylpiperazine (mCPP), carbolines, $GABA_B$ receptor antagonists, caffeine, isoproterenol, and yohimbine (Yocon).

H. Right temporal atrophy is seen in some panic disorder patients, and cerebral vasoconstriction is often present in anxiety.

VIII. Psychodynamics

Defense mechanisms ward off anxiety. A breakdown of repression produces anxiety (Table 11–12).

IX. Differential diagnosis

Anxiety is a major feature in psychological, medical, and neurological disorders.

A. Depressive disorders.   Fifty percent to seventy percent of depressed patients exhibit anxiety or obsessive brooding; 20–30% of primarily anxious patients also experience depression.

B. Schizophrenia.   Schizophrenic patients may be anxious and have severe obsessions in addition to or preceding the outbreak of hallucinations or delusions.

C. Bipolar I disorder.   Massive anxiety may occur during a manic episode.

D. Atypical psychosis (psychotic disorder not otherwise specified).   Massive anxiety is present, in addition to psychotic features.

TABLE 11–12
PSYCHODYNAMICS OF ANXIETY DISORDERS

Disorder	Defense	Comment
Phobia	Displacement Symbolization	Anxiety detached from idea or situation and displaced on some other symbolic object or situation.
Agoraphobia	Projection Displacement	Repressed hostility, rage, or sexuality projected on environment, which is seen as dangerous.
Obsessive-compulsive disorder	Undoing Isolation Reaction formation	Severe superego acts against impulses about which patient feels guilty; anxiety controlled by repetitious act or thought.
Anxiety	Regression	Repression of forbidden sexual, aggressive, or dependency strivings breaks down.
Panic	Regression	Anxiety overwhelms personality and is discharged in panic state. Total breakdown of repressive defense and regression occurs.
Posttraumatic stress disorder	Regression Repression Denial Undoing	Trauma reactivates unconscious conflicts; ego relives anxiety and tries to master it.

TABLE 11–13
DIFFERENTIAL DIAGNOSIS OF COMMON MEDICAL CONDITIONS MIMICKING ANXIETY

Angina pectoris/myocardial infarction (MI)	Electrocardiogram with ST depression in angina; cardiac enzymes in MI. Crushing chest pain usually associated with angina/MI. Anxiety pains usually sharp and more superficial.
Hyperventilation syndrome	History of rapid, deep respirations; circumoral pallor; carpopedal spasm; responds to rebreathing in paper bag.
Hypoglycemia	Fasting blood sugar usually under 50 mg/dl; signs of diabetes mellitus—polyuria, polydypsia, polyphagia.
Hyperthyroidism	Elevated triiodothyronine (T_1), thyroxine (T_4); exophthalmos in severe cases.
Carcinoid syndrome	Hypertension accompanies anxiety; elevated urinary catecholamines (5-hydroxyindoleacetic acid (5-HIAA)).

E. **Adjustment disorder with anxiety.**   Patient has a history of a psychosocial stressor within 3 months of onset.

F. **Medical and neurological conditions.**   A secondary psychotic disorder is caused by a specific medical or biological factor (Tables 11–9 and 11–13); cognitive impairment may be present.

G. **Substance-related disorders.**   Panic or anxiety is often associated with intoxication (especially caffeine, cocaine, amphetamines, hallucinogens) and withdrawal states (Table 11–10).

X. **Course and prognosis**

A. **Panic disorder**
    1. Panic attacks tend to recur two to three times a week.
    2. The course is chronic, with remissions and exacerbations.
    3. The prognosis is excellent with therapy.

B. **Phobic disorder**
    1. The course is chronic.
    2. Phobias may worsen or spread if untreated.
    3. Prognosis is a good to excellent with therapy.
    4. Agoraphobia is the most resistant of all phobias.

C. **Obsessive-compulsive disorder**
    1. Course is chronic, with waxing and waning of symptoms.
    2. Prognosis with therapy is fair, but some cases are intractable.

D. **Generalized anxiety disorder**
    1. Course is chronic; symptoms may diminish as the patient gets older.
    2. With time, secondary depression may develop. This is not uncommon if the condition is left untreated.

E. **Posttraumatic stress disorder**
    1. Course is chronic.
    2. The trauma is reexperienced periodically for several years.
    3. The prognosis is worse with preexisting psychopathology.

XI. Treatment

Some anxiety disorders, such as posttraumatic stress disorder, are treated primarily with psychotherapy; others, such as phobias, generalized anxiety, panic disorder, and obsessive-compulsive disorder, are treated with medication or with combined drug therapy and psychotherapy.

A. Pharmacologic.   Table 11–14 lists some drugs used to treat anxiety and the dosages for panic disorder.

1. Benzodiazepines

a. Diazepam (Valium)

(1) The dosage is 2 to 10 mg orally two to four times a day, or 2 to 10 mg intramuscularly or intravenously for acute agitation.

(2) Indications include generalized anxiety disorder, panic attacks, posttraumatic stress disorder, and other acute anxiety states.

(3) Common adverse effects include drowsiness and fatigue. Paradoxical excitement may occur rarely.

(4) **Cautions:** Long-term use can cause physical dependence (i.e., withdrawal symptoms on abrupt discontinuation, most often in patients with history of alcoholism or drug abuse).

b. Alprazolam (Xanax)

(1) The dosage is 0.25 to 0.5 mg orally three times a day; it may be increased to 6 to 8 mg/d.

TABLE 11–14
RECOMMENDED DOSAGES FOR ANTIPANIC DRUGS (DAILY UNLESS INDICATED OTHERWISE)

	Starting (mg)	Maintenance (mg)
SSRIs		
Paroxetine	5–10	20–60
Fluoxetine	2–5	20–60
Sertraline	12.5–25	50–200
Fluvoxamine	12.5	100–150
Citalopram	10	20–40
Tricyclic antidepressants		
Clomipramine	5–12.5	50–125
Imipramine	10–25	150–500
Desipramine	10–25	150–200
Benzodiazepines		
Alprazolam	0.25–0.5 tid	0.5–2 tid
Clonazepam	0.25–0.5 bid	0.5–2 bid
Diazepam	2–5 bid	5–30 bid
Lorazepam	0.25–0.5 bid	0.5–2 bid
MAOIs		
Phenelzine	15 bid	15–45 bid
Tranylcypromine	10 bid	10–30 bid
RIMAs		
Moclobemide	50	300–600
Brofaromine	50	150–200
Atypical antidepressants		
Venlafaxine	6.25–25	50–150
Nefazodone	50 bid	100–300 bid
Other agents		
Valproic acid	125 bid	500–750 bid
Inositol	6000 bid	6000 bid

(2) Indications: This is a rapidly acting, short-term treatment for panic disorder and agoraphobia.

(3) Common adverse effects include drowsiness, cognitive impairment, and hypotension. Alprazolam may be associated with a more severe discontinuation syndrome than other benzodiazepines.

c. Clonazepam (Klonopin)

(1) The dosage is 0.5 mg twice daily; it may be increased to 2 to 6 mg/d.

(2) Psychiatric indications include generalized anxiety disorder, panic disorder, and posttraumatic stress disorder.

(3) Adverse effects include drowsiness and ataxia.

d. Lorazepam (Ativan)

(1) The dosage is 0.5 to 2 mg two to four times a day, and 0.5 to 2 mg intravenously for acute agitation.

(2) Indications include generalized anxiety disorder, panic attacks and acute anxiety states, and posttraumatic stress disorder.

(3) Adverse effects include drowsiness and ataxia.

2. Selective serotonin reuptake inhibitors (SSRIs)

a. Table 11–14 provides SSRI dosages for use in anxiety.

b. Indications include obsessive-compulsive disorder, panic disorder, social phobia, generalized anxiety disorder, and posttraumatic stress disorder, as well as depression and premenstrual dysphoric disorder.

3. Tricyclics. See Chapter 25 for other tricyclic drugs useful for anxiety disorders.

a. Imipramine (Tofranil)

(1) The dosage is 50–75 mg/day orally to start; it may be increased to 150 to 300 mg. **Note:** In elderly or adolescent patients, start with 25 to 50 mg/day and increase to 75 to 150 mg/day.

(2) Indications are primarily for mood disorder, but imipramine is useful in panic disorder, social phobia, and posttraumatic stress disorder.

(3) Common adverse effects include drowsiness and anticholinergic effects (confusion, dry mouth, tachycardia, arrhythmias, constipation, delayed micturition). **Note:** Obtain an ECG in patients over age 40 to test cardiac function. Do not prescribe monoamine oxidase inhibitors (MAOIs) until 14 days after imipramine therapy has been discontinued.

b. Clomipramine (Anafranil)

(1) The dosage is 150 to 250 mg/day.

(2) The chief indication is obsessive-compulsive disorder.

(3) Adverse effects are similar to those of imipramine.

4. Buspirone (BuSpar)

a. The dosage is 5 mg twice daily; it may be increased to 15 to 60 mg/day in divided doses.

b. The chief indication is generalized anxiety disorder.

c. Common adverse effects include headache and dizziness. **Note:** Buspirone is not cross-tolerant with benzodiazepines.

5. MAOIs

a. The dosage for tranylcypromine (Parnate) is 10 mg orally in the morning and 10 mg in the afternoon; it may be increased to 30 to 50 mg/day in divided doses. See Table 11–14 for dosages of MAOIs and reversible inhibitors of MAO_A RIMAs).

b. Indications are primarily depressive disorders, but MAOIs are useful in panic disorder and social phobia. **Note:** Use in elderly persons with caution. Do not use with narcotics (i.e., opioids) (especially meperidine [Demerol]); coadministration may be fatal. Note the need for dietary precautions and avoidance of a number of other medications and over-the-counter preparations.

c. The major adverse effect is a hypertensive crisis caused by foods containing tryptophan or tyramine, sympathomimetic agents, other MAOIs, tricyclics, and narcotics; all may produce fatal intracranial bleeding secondary to an acute hypertensive episode.

6. β-Adrenergic receptor antagonists (beta blockers)

a. Propranolol (Inderal).

(1) The dosage is 10 mg orally twice daily; it may be increased to 80 to 160 mg/day in divided doses; the patient may take a dose of 20 to 40 mg 30 minutes before phobic situation (e.g., public speaking). A long-acting form is available.

(2) The main indication is social phobia.

(3) Adverse effects include bradycardia, hypotension, and drowsiness. **Note:** Do not use if the patient has a history of asthma, congestive heart failure, or diabetes. It is not useful in chronic anxiety unless caused by a hypersensitive adrenergic state.

b. Other beta blockers (e.g., pindolol [Visken]) may be useful.

7. Venlafaxine (Effexor)

a. The dosage is 50 to 375 mg/day.

b. The major indication is depression, but venlafaxine is also indicated for generalized anxiety disorder and other anxiety disorders.

8. Nefazodone (Serzone)

a. The dosage is 300 to 600 mg/day.

b. The primary indication is depression, but it is sometimes useful for panic disorder and other anxiety disorders.

B. Psychological. The following information can be viewed as an introduction to the topic discussed in greater detail in Chapter 24.

1. **Supportive psychotherapy.** This approach involves the use of psychodynamic concepts and a therapeutic alliance to promote adaptive coping. Adaptive defenses are encouraged and strengthened, and maladaptive ones are discouraged. The therapist assists in reality testing and may offer advice regarding behavior.

2. **Insight-oriented psychotherapy.** The goal is to increase the patient's development of insight into psychological conflicts that, if unresolved, can manifest as symptomatic behavior (e.g., anxiety, phobias, obsessions and compulsions, and posttraumatic stress reactions). This modality is particularly indicated if (1) anxiety symptoms are clearly secondary to an underlying unconscious conflict, (2) anxiety

continues after behavioral or pharmacologic treatments are instituted, (3) new anxiety symptoms develop after the original symptoms have resolved (symptom substitution), or (4) the anxieties are more generalized and less specific.

3. **Behavior therapy.** The basic assumption is that change can occur without the development of psychological insight into underlying causes. Techniques include positive and negative reinforcement, systematic desensitization, flooding, implosion, graded exposure, response prevention, stop-thought, relaxation techniques, panic control therapy, self-monitoring, and hypnosis.

   a. Behavior therapy is indicated for clearly delineated, circumscribed, maladaptive behaviors (e.g., panic attacks, phobias, compulsions, obsessions). Compulsive behavior generally is more responsive than obsessional thinking.

   b. Most current strategies for the treatment of anxiety disorders include a combination of pharmacologic and behavioral interventions.

   c. Current thinking generally maintains that although drugs can reduce anxiety early, treatment with drugs alone leads to equally early relapse. The response of patients who are also treated with cognitive and behavioral therapies appears to be significantly and consistently better than the response of those who receive drugs alone.

4. **Cognitive therapy.** This is based on the premise that maladaptive behavior is secondary to distortions in how people perceive themselves and in how others perceive them. Treatment is short-term and interactive, with assigned homework and tasks to be performed between sessions that focus on correcting distorted assumptions and cognitions. The emphasis is on confronting and examining situations that elicit interpersonal anxiety and associated mild depression.

5. **Group therapy.** Groups range from those that provide only support and an increase in social skills to those that focus on relief of specific symptoms to those that are primarily insight-oriented. Groups may be heterogeneous or homogeneous in terms of diagnosis. Homogeneous groups are commonly used in the treatment of such diagnoses as post-traumatic stress disorder, in which therapy is aimed at education about dealing with stress.

For more detailed discussion of this topic, see Anxiety Disorders, Ch 15, p 1441 in CTP/VII.

12

Somatoform Disorders, Factitious Disorders, and Malingering

I. Somatoform disorders

The somatoform disorders are distinguished by physical symptoms suggesting a medical condition, yet the symptoms are not fully explained by the medical condition, substance use, or another mental disorder. The symptoms are severe enough to cause the patient significant distress or functional impairment. Five specific somatoform disorders are recognized in DSM-IV-TR: somatization disorder, conversion disorder, hypochondriasis, body dysmorphic disorder, and pain disorder. Two residual diagnostic categories in DSM-IV-TR are undifferentiated somatoform disorder and somatoform disorder not otherwise specified. Table 12–1 summarizes the clinical features of somatoform disorders.

A. Somatization disorder

1. **Diagnosis, signs, and symptoms.** See Table 12–2.
2. **Epidemiology**
   a. Lifetime prevalence in the general population is 0.1–0.5%.
   b. Affects more women than men.
   c. Affects 1–2% of all women.
   d. More common in less well-educated persons and persons of low socioeconomic status.
   e. Usual onset is in adolescence and young adulthood.
3. **Etiology**
   a. **Psychosocial**—suppression or repression of anger toward others, with turning of anger toward self, can account for symptoms. Punitive personality organization with strong superego. Low self-esteem is common. Identification with parent who models sick role. Some dynamic similarity to depression.
   b. **Genetic**—positive family history; present in 10–20% of mothers and sisters of affected patients; twins—concordance rate of 29% in monozygotic and 10% in dizygotic twins.
4. **Laboratory and psychological tests.** Minor neuropsychological abnormality in some patients (e.g., faulty assessment of somatosensory input).
5. **Pathophysiology.** None. Prolonged use of medications may cause adverse effects unrelated to somatization complaint.
6. **Psychodynamics.** Repression of wish or impulse expressed through body complaints. Superego conflicts, partially expressed by symptom. Anxiety converted into specific symptom.

TABLE 12–1
CLINICAL FEATURES OF SOMATOFORM DISORDERS

Diagnosis	Clinical Presentation	Demographic and Epidemiological Features	Diagnostic Features	Management Strategy	Prognosis	Associated Disturbances	Primary Differential Presentation	Psychologic Processes Contributing to Symptoms	Motivation for Symptom Production
Somatization disorder	Polysymptomatic Recurrent and chronic Sickly by history	Young age Female predominance 20:1 Familial pattern 5–10% incidence in primary care populations	Review of systems profusely positive Multiple clinical contacts Polysurgical	Therapeutic alliance Regular appointments Crisis intervention	Poor to fair	Histrionic personality disorder Antisocial personality disorder Alcohol and other substance abuse Conversion disorder	Physical disease Depression	Unconscious Cultural and developmental	Unconscious psychological factors
Conversion disorder	Monosymptomatic Mostly acute Simulates disease	Highly prevalent Female predominance Young age Rural and low social class Little-educated and psychologically unsophisticated	Simulation incompatible with known physiologic mechanisms or anatomy	Suggestion and persuasion Multiple techniques	Excellent except in chronic conversion disorder	Alcohol and other substance dependence Antisocial personality Somatization disorder Histrionic personality disorder	Depression Schizophrenia Neurological disease	Unconscious Psychological stress or conflict may be present	Unconscious psychological factors
Hypochondriasis	Disease concern or preoccupation	Previous physical disease Middle or old age Male–female ratio equal	Disease conviction amplifies symptoms Obsessional	Document symptoms Psychosocial review Psychotherapeutic	Fair to good Waxes and wanes	Obsessive-compulsive personality disorder Depressive and anxiety disorders	Depression Physical disease Personality disorder Delusional disorder	Unconscious Stress— bereavement Developmental factors	Unconscious psychological factors

Body dysmorphic disorder	Subjective feelings of ugliness or concern with body defect	Adolescence or young adult ? Female predominance Largely unknown	Pervasive bodily concerns	Therapeutic alliance Stress management Psycho-therapies Anti-depressant medications	Unknown	Anorexia nervosa Psychosocial distress Avoidant or obsessive-compulsive personality disorder	Delusional disorder Depressive disorders Somatization disorder	Unconscious Self-esteem factors	Unconscious psychological factors
Pain disorder	Pain syndrome simulated	Female pre-dominance 2:1 Older: 4th or 5th decade Familial Up to 40% of pain populations	Simulation or intensity incompatible with known physiologic mechanisms or anatomy	Therapeutic alliance Redefine goals of treatment Anti-depressant medications	Guarded, variable	Depressive disorders Alcohol and other substance abuse Dependent or histrionic personality disorder	Depression Psycho-physiologic Physical disease Malingering and disability syndrome	Unconscious Acute stressor and developmental Physical trauma may predispose	Unconscious psychological factors

Adapted from Folks DG, Ford CV, Houck CA. Somatoform disorders, factitious disorders, and malingering: In: Stoudemire A, ed. *Clinical Psychiatry for Medical Students*. Philadelphia: Lippincott, 1990:233.

TABLE 12–2
DSM-IV-TR DIAGNOSTIC CRITERIA FOR SOMATIZATION DISORDER

A. A history of many physical complaints beginning before age 30 years that occur over a period of several years and result in treatment being sought or significant impairment in social, occupational, or other important areas of functioning.

B. Each of the following criteria must have been met, with individual symptoms occurring at any time during the course of the disturbance:

(1) *four pain symptoms:* a history of pain related to at least four different sites or functions (e.g., head, abdomen, back, joints, extremities, chest, rectum, during menstruation, during sexual intercourse, or during urination)

(2) *two gastrointestinal symptoms:* a history of at least two gastrointestinal symptoms other than pain (e.g., nausea, bloating, vomitting other than during pregnancy, diarrhea, or intolerance of several different foods)

(3) *one sexual symptom:* a history of at least one sexual or reproductive symptom other than pain (e.g., sexual indifference, erectile or ejaculatory dysfunction, irregular menses, excessive menstrual bleeding, vomitting throughout pregnancy)

(4) *one pseudoneurological symptom:* a history of at least one symptom or deficit suggesting a neurological condition not limited to pain (conversion symptoms such as impaired coordination or balance, paralysis or localized weakness, difficulty swallowing or lump in throat, aphonia, urinary retention, hallucinations, loss of touch or pain sensation, double vision, blindness, deafness, seizures; dissociative symptoms such as amnesia; or loss of consciousness other than fainting)

C. Either (1) or (2):

(1) after appropriate investigation, each of the symptoms in criterion B cannot be fully explained by a known general medical condition or the direct effects of a substance (e.g., a drug of abuse, a medication)

(2) when there is a related general medical condition, the physical complaints or resulting social or occupational impairment are in excess of what would be expected from the history, physical examination, or laboratory findings

D. The symptoms are not intentionally feigned or produced (as in factitious disorder or malingering).

From American Psychiatric Association. *Diagnostic and Statistical Manual of Mental Disorders,* text revision, 4th ed. Washington, DC: American Psychiatric Association, Copyright 2000, with permission.

7. Differential diagnosis

a. Rule out organic cause for somatic symptom.

b. Multiple sclerosis for weakness.

c. Epstein-Barr virus for chronic fatigue syndrome.

d. Porphyria for abdominal pain.

e. Somatic delusion occurs in schizophrenia.

f. The cardiovascular symptoms of panic attacks are intermittent, episodic.

g. Conversion disorder causes fewer symptoms with clearer symbolic meaning.

h. Factitious disorder—conscious faking of symptoms to achieve role of patient; usually eager to be in hospital.

i. Pain disorder—pain is usually only complaint.

8. Course and prognosis

a. Chronic course with few remissions; however, severity of complaints can fluctuate. Complications include unnecessary surgery, repeated medical workups, substance dependence, and adverse effects of unnecessary prescribed drugs.

b. Depression is frequent.

9. Treatment

a. **Pharmacologic**—avoid psychotropics, except during period of acute anxiety or depression, because patients tend to become psy-

chologically dependent. Antidepressants are useful in secondary depression.

   b. Psychological—long-term insight or supportive psychotherapy is required to provide understanding of dynamics, support through distressing life events, or both; also to follow patient to prevent substance abuse, doctor shopping, unnecessary procedures and
   diagnostic tests.

B. Undifferentiated somatoform disorder

  1. Definition. Residual category used to describe a partial picture of somatoform disorder.

  2. Diagnosis, signs, and symptoms. See Table 12–3. The patient may
  have multiple somatic complaints that are not severe enough or that are
  too vague to warrant a diagnosis of full somatoform disorder. General
  fatigue is the most common syndrome.

  3. Course and prognosis. Unpredictable. Frequently, another mental
  disorder or medical condition is ultimately diagnosed.

  4. Differential diagnosis. See Table 12–4.

C. Conversion disorder

  1. Definition. Characterized by one or more neurological symptoms associated with psychological conflict or need; not physical, neurological, or substance-related disorder.

  2. Diagnosis, signs, and symptoms

   a. Motor abnormalities—paralysis, ataxia, dysphagia, vomiting,
   aphonia.

   b. Disturbances of consciousness—pseudoseizures, unconsciousness.

TABLE 12–3
DSM-IV-TR DIAGNOSTIC CRITERIA FOR UNDIFFERENTIATED SOMATOFORM DISORDER

A. One or more physical complaints (e.g., fatigue, loss of appetite, gastrointestinal or urinary complaints).
B. Either (1) or (2):
   (1) after appropriate investigation, the symptoms cannot be fully explained by a known general med-
       ical condition or the direct effects of a substance (e.g., a drug of abuse, a medication)
   (2) when there is a related general medical condition, the physical complaints or resulting social or
       occupational impairment is in excess of what would be expected from the history, physical ex-
       amination, or laboratory findings
C. The symptoms cause clinically significant distress or impairment in social, occupational, or other im-
   portant areas of functioning.
D. The duration of the disturbance is at least 6 months.
E. The disturbance is not better accounted for by another mental disorder (e.g., another somatoform dis-
   order, sexual dysfunction, mood disorder, anxiety disorder, sleep disorder, or psychotic disorder).
F. The symptom is not intentionally produced or feigned (as in factitious disorder or malingering).

From American Psychiatric Association. *Diagnostic and Statistical Manual of Mental Disorders*, text revision, 4th ed. Washington, DC: American Psychiatric Association, Copyright 2000, with permission.

TABLE 12–4
DIFFERENTIAL DIAGNOSIS FOR UNDIFFERENTIATED SOMATOFORM DISORDER

Somatoform disorder—multiple symptoms, several years' duration, onset before 30 years of age
Somatoform disorder NOS—symptoms for less than 6 months
Major depressive disorder, anxiety disorders, adjustment disorder—frequently include unexplained
symptoms
Factitious disorder and malingering—symptoms intentionally produced or fabricated

c. Sensory disturbances or alterations—blindness, deafness, anosmia, anesthesia, analgesia, diplopia, glove-and-stocking anesthesia (does not follow known sensory pathways).

d. Close temporal relationship between symptom and stress or intense emotion.

e. Left-sided symptoms more common than right-sided symptoms.

f. The person is not conscious of intentionally producing the symptom.

g. The symptom is not a culturally sanctioned response pattern and after appropriate investigation cannot be explained by a known physical disorder.

3. Epidemiology

a. Incidence and prevalence—10% of hospital inpatients and 5–15% of all psychiatric outpatients.

b. Age—early adulthood, but can occur in middle or old age.

c. The male-to-female ratio is 1:2.

d. Family history—more frequent in family members.

e. More common in persons of low socioeconomic status and less well-educated persons.

4. Etiology

a. Biological

(1) Symptom depends on activation of inhibitory brain mechanisms.

(2) Excessive cortical arousal triggers inhibitory CNS mechanisms at synapses, brainstem, reticular activating system.

(3) Increased susceptibility in patients with frontal lobe trauma or other neurological deficits.

b. Psychological

(1) Expression of unconscious psychological conflict that is repressed.

(2) Premorbid personality disorder—avoidant, histrionic.

(3) Impulse (e.g., sex or aggression) is unacceptable to ego and is disguised through symptom.

(4) Identification with family member who has same symptoms caused by real disease.

5. Laboratory and psychological tests

a. Evoked potential shows disturbed somatosensory perception; diminished or absent on side of defect.

b. Mild cognitive impairment, attentional deficits, and visuoperceptive changes on Halstead-Reitan Battery.

c. Minnesota Multiphasic Personality Inventory-2 (MMPI-2), Rorschach test show increased instinctual drives, sexual repression, inhibited aggression.

6. Pathophysiology. No changes.

7. Psychodynamics

a. *La belle indifférence* is a lack of concern about illness present in some patients.

b. *Primary gain* refers to the reduction of anxiety by repression of unacceptable impulse. Symbolization of impulse onto symptom (e.g., paralysis of arm prevents expression of aggressive impulse).

c. Other defense mechanisms—reaction formation, denial, displacement.

d. *Secondary gain* refers to benefits of illness (e.g., compensation from lawsuit [compensation neurosis], avoidance of work, dependence on family). Patient usually lacks insight about this dynamic.

8. **Differential diagnosis.** Major task is to distinguish from organically based disorder. Eventually, a physical or medical disorder is diagnosed in 25–50% of patients.

a. **Paralysis**—in conversion, paralysis is inconsistent; it does not follow motor pathways. No pathological reflexes (e.g., Babinski's sign) are present. Spastic paralysis, clonus, cogwheel rigidity absent in conversion disorder.

b. **Ataxia**—bizarre character in conversion disorder. Leg may be dragged and not circumducted as in organic lesion. *Astasia–abasia* is an unsteady gait that does not cause the patient with conversion disorder to fall or sustain injury.

c. **Blindness**—no pupillary response is seen in neurological blindness (except that occipital lobe lesions produce cortical blindness with intact pupillary response). Tracking movements are absent in true blindness. Monocular diplopia, triplopia, and tunnel vision can be conversion complaints. Ophthalmologists use tests with distorting prisms and colored lenses to detect hysterical blindness.

d. **Deafness**—loud noise will awaken sleeping patient with conversion disorder but not patient with organic deafness. Audiometric tests reveal varying responses in conversion.

e. **Sensory**—sensory loss does not follow dermatomes; hemisensory loss, which stops at midline, or glove-and-stocking anesthesia occurs in conversion disorder.

f. **Hysterical**—pain most often relates to head, face, back, and abdomen. Look for organic findings—muscular spasm, osteoarthritis.

g. **Pseudoseizures**—incontinence, loss of motor control, and tongue biting are rare in pseudoseizures; an aura usually is present in organic epilepsy. Look for abnormal electroencephalogram (EEG); however, EEG results are abnormal in 10–15% of the normal adult population. Babinski's sign occurs in organic seizure and postictal state but not in conversion seizures.

h. **Differentiate conversion from the following:**

(1) **Schizophrenia**—thought disorder.

(2) **Mood disorder**—depression or mania.

(3) **Malingering and factitious disorder with physical symptoms**—difficult to distinguish, but malingerers are aware that they are faking symptoms and have insight into what they are doing; patients with factitious disorder also are aware that they are faking, but they do so because they want to be patients and be in a hospital.

i. **Drug-assisted interview**—intravenous amobarbital (Amytal) (100 to 500 mg) in slow infusion often causes conversion symptoms to abate. For example, patient with hysterical aphonia will begin to talk. Test can be used to aid in diagnosis but is not always reliable.

9. **Course and prognosis.** Tends to be recurrent, episodes separated by asymptomatic periods. Major concern is not to miss early neurological symptom that subsequently progresses into full-blown syndrome (e.g., multiple sclerosis may begin with spontaneously remitting diplopia or hemiparesis). Table 12–5 lists factors associated with good and bad prognoses.

10. **Treatment**

   a. **Pharmacologic.** Benzodiazepines for anxiety and muscular tension; antidepressants or serotonergic agents for obsessive rumination about symptoms.

   b. **Psychological**

      (1) Insight-oriented therapy is useful in helping the patient to understand the dynamic principles and conflicts behind symptoms. Patient learns to accept sexual or aggressive impulses and not to use conversion disorder as a defense.

      (2) Behavior therapy is used to induce relaxation.

      (3) Hypnosis and reeducation are useful in uncomplicated situations.

      (4) Do not accuse the patient of trying to get attention or of not wanting to get better.

      (5) Narcoanalysis sometimes removes symptoms.

D. **Pain disorder**

1. **Definition.** Somatoform pain disorder is a preoccupation with pain in the absence of physical disease to account for its intensity. It does not follow a neuroanatomic distribution. Stress and conflict may closely correlate with the initiation or exacerbation of the pain.

2. **Diagnosis, signs, and symptoms.** See Table 12–6. Pain may be accompanied by localized sensorimotor symptoms, such as anesthesia, paresthesia. Symptoms of depression are common.

3. **Epidemiology.** Onset can be at any age, but especially the 30s and 40s. More common in women than in men. Some evidence of first-de-

TABLE 12–5
FACTORS ASSOCIATED WITH GOOD AND POOR PROGNOSES IN CONVERSION DISORDER

Good prognosis
Sudden onset
Clearly identifiable stress at onset
Short time between onset and treatment
Above-average I.Q.
Symptoms of paralysis, aphonia, blindness
Poor prognosis
Comorbid mental disorders
Ongoing litigation
Symptoms of tremor, seizures

TABLE 12–6
DSM-IV-TR DIAGNOSTIC CRITERIA FOR PAIN DISORDER

A. Pain in one or more anatomical sites is the predominant focus of the clinical presentation and is of sufficient severity to warrant clinical attention.

B. The pain causes clinically significant distress or impairment in social, occupational, or other important areas of functioning.

C. Psychological factors are judged to have an important role in the onset, severity, exacerbation, or maintenance of the pain.

D. The symptom or deficit is not intentionally produced or feigned (as in factitious disorder or malingering).

E. The pain is not better accounted for by a mood, anxiety, or psychotic disorder and does not meet criteria for dyspareunia.

Code as follows:

Pain disorder associated with psychological factors: psychological factors are judged to have the major role in the onset, severity, exacerbation, or maintenance of the pain. (If a general medical condition is present, it does not have a major role in the onset, severity, exacerbation, or maintenance of the pain.) This type of pain disorder is not diagnosed if criteria are also met for somatization disorder.

Specify if:

Acute: duration of less than 6 months

Chronic: duration of 6 months or longer

Pain disorder associated with both psychological factors and a general medical condition: both psychological factors and a general medical condition are judged to have important roles in the onset, severity, exacerbation, or maintenance of the pain. The associated general medical condition or anatomical site of the pain is coded on Axis III.

Specify if:

Acute: duration of less than 6 months

Chronic: duration of 6 months or longer

From American Psychiatric Association. *Diagnostic and Statistical Manual of Mental Disorders,* text revision, 4th ed. Washington, DC: American Psychiatric Association, Copyright 2000, with permission.

gree biological relatives having a high incidence of pain, depression, and alcoholism.

4. **Etiology**

a. **Behavioral**—pain behaviors are reinforced when rewarded (e.g., pain symptoms may become intense when followed by attentive behavior from others or avoidance of disliked activity).

b. **Interpersonal**—pain is a way to manipulate and gain advantage in a relationship (e.g., to stabilize a fragile marriage).

c. **Biological**—some patients may have pain disorder, rather than another mental disorder, because of sensory and limbic structural or chemical abnormalities that predispose them to pain.

5. **Psychodynamics.** Patients may be symbolically expressing an intrapsychic conflict through the body. Persons may unconsciously regard emotional pain as weak and displace it to the body. Pain can be a method to obtain love or can be used as a punishment. Defense mechanisms involved in the disorder include displacement, substitution, and repression.

E. **Hypochondriasis**

1. **Definition.** Morbid fear or belief that one has a serious disease even though none exists.

2. **Diagnosis, signs, and symptoms**

a. Any organ or functional system can be affected; gastrointestinal and cardiovascular systems most commonly affected.

    b. Patient believes that disease or malfunction is present.

    c. Negative physical examination or laboratory test results reassure patient, but only briefly; symptoms then return. (In somatic delusion, patient cannot be reassured.)

    d. Disturbance lasts at least 6 months.

    e. The belief is not of delusional intensity.

3. Epidemiology

    a. Prevalence—10% of all medical patients.

    b. Men and women are affected equally.

    c. Occurs at all ages; peaks in 30s for men and 40s for women.

    d. Seen in monozygotic twins and first-degree relatives.

4. Etiology

    a. Psychogenic, but patient may have congenital hypersensitivity to bodily functions and sensations and low threshold for pain or physical discomfort.

    b. Aggression toward others is turned against the self through a particular body part.

    c. Affected organ may have important symbolic meaning.

5. Laboratory and psychological tests

    a. Results of repeated physical examinations to rule out medical illness are negative.

    b. MMPI-2 shows elevated hysterical scale.

    c. Many color responses on Rorschach test.

6. Psychodynamics.
Repression of anger toward others; displacement of anger toward physical complaints; pain and suffering used as punishment for unacceptable guilty impulses; undoing.

7. Differential diagnosis.
Diagnosis is made by inclusion, *not* by exclusion. Physical disorders must be ruled out; however, 15–30% of patients with hypochondriacal disorder have physical problems. Workup for medical disease may aggravate the condition by placing too much emphasis on the physical complaint.

    a. Depression—patient may have a somatic complaint, or somatic complaint can be part of a depressive syndrome. Look for signs of depression (e.g., apathy, anhedonia, feelings of worthlessness).

    b. Anxiety disorder—manifested by marked anxiety or obsessive-compulsive signs or symptoms; *la belle indifférence* is not present.

    c. Somatization disorder—multiple organ systems involved; vague complaints.

    d. Pain disorder—pain is major and usually sole complaint.

    e. Malingering and factitious disorders—history is associated with frequent hospitalizations, marked secondary gain; symptoms lack symbolic value and are under conscious control. *La belle indifférence* is not present.

    f. Sexual dysfunction—if sex is complaint, diagnose as sexual disorder.

8. Course and prognosis.
Chronic course with remissions. Exacerbations are usually associated with identifiable life stress. Good prognosis is associated with minimal premorbid personality, poor prognosis with antecedent or superimposed physical disorder.

9. Treatment

a. Pharmacologic. Pharmacological targeting of symptoms; antianxiety drugs and antidepressant drugs for anxiety and depression. Serotonergic drugs useful for depression and obsessive-compulsive disorder. Drug-assisted interview can induce catharsis and potential removal of symptoms; however, such relief usually is only temporary.

b. Psychological

(1) Insight-oriented dynamic psychotherapy uncovers symbolic meaning of symptom and is useful. Do not confront patient with such statements as, "It's all in your head." Long-term relationship with physician or psychiatrist is valuable, with reassurance that no physical disease is present.

(2) Hypnosis and behavior therapy are useful to induce relaxation. Prolonged conversion disorder can produce physical deterioration (e.g., muscle atrophy or contractures, osteoporosis), so attention to these issues is necessary.

F. Body dysmorphic disorder

1. **Definition.** Imagined belief (not of delusional proportions) that a defect in the appearance of all or a part of the body is present.

2. **Diagnosis, signs, and symptoms.** Patient complains of defect (e.g., wrinkles, hair loss, too small breasts or penis, age spots, stature). Complaint is out of proportion to any minor objective physical abnormality. If a slight physical anomaly is present, the person's concern is grossly excessive; however, the belief is not of delusional intensity, as in delusional disorder, somatic type (i.e., the person can acknowledge the possibility that he or she may be exaggerating the extent of the defect or that there may be no defect at all).

3. **Epidemiology.** Onset from adolescence through early adulthood. Men and women are affected equally.

4. **Etiology.** Unknown.

   a. Biological—responsiveness to serotonergic agents suggests involvement of serotonin or relation to another mental disorder.

   b. Psychological—look for unconscious conflict relating to a distorted body part.

5. **Laboratory and psychological tests.** Draw-a-Person test shows exaggeration, diminution, or absence of affected body part.

6. **Pathophysiology.** No known pathological abnormalities. Minor body deficits may actually exist upon which imagined belief develops.

7. **Psychodynamics.** Defense mechanisms include repression (of unconscious conflict), distortion and symbolization (of body part), and projection (belief that other persons also see imagined deformity).

8. **Differential diagnosis.** Distorted body image occurs in schizophrenia, mood disorders, medical disorders, anorexia nervosa, bulimia nervosa, obsessive-compulsive disorder, gender identity disorder, *koro* (worry that penis is shrinking into abdomen).

9. **Course and prognosis.** Chronic course with repeated visits to doctors, plastic surgeons, or dermatologists. Secondary depression may

occur. In some cases, imagined body distortion progresses to delusional belief.

10. Treatment

a. **Pharmacological**—serotoninergic drugs (e.g., fluoxetine [Prozac], clomipramine [Anafranil]) effectively reduce symptoms in at least 50% of patients. Treatment with surgical, dermatological, and dental procedures is rarely successful.

b. **Psychological**—psychotherapy is useful; uncovers conflicts relating to symptoms, feelings of inadequacy.

II. Factitious disorders

A. Definition.   In factitious disorders, patients deliberately produce physical or psychological symptoms with the goal of assuming the sick role. In these disorders, patients intentionally produce signs of medical or mental disorders and misrepresent their histories and symptoms. The only apparent objective is to assume the role of a patient without an external incentive. Hospitalization is often a primary objective and a way of life. The disorders have a compulsive quality, but the behaviors are deliberate and voluntary, even if they cannot be controlled.

B. Diagnosis, signs, and symptoms

1. **With predominantly physical signs and symptoms.** Also known as *Munchausen syndrome*. Intentional production of physical symptoms—nausea, vomiting, pain, seizures. Patients may intentionally put blood in feces or urine, artificially raise body temperature, take insulin to lower blood sugar. Gridiron abdomen sign is the result of scars from multiple surgical operations.

2. **With predominantly psychological signs and symptoms.** Intentional production of psychiatric symptoms—hallucinations, delusions, depression, bizarre behavior. Patients may make up a story that they suffered major life stress to account for symptoms. *Pseudologia fantastica* consists of making up extravagant lies that the patient believes. Substance abuse, especially of opioids, is common in both types.

3. **With combined physical and psychological signs and symptoms.** Intentional production of both physical and psychological symptoms.

4. **Factitious disorder not otherwise specified.** Includes disorders that do not meet criteria for factitious disorder (e.g., factitious disorder by proxy—intentionally feigning symptoms in another person who is under the person's care so as to assume the sick role indirectly).

C. Epidemiology.   Unknown. More common in men than in women. Usually adult onset. Factitious illness, especially feigned fever, accounts for 5–10% of all hospital admissions. More common in health care workers.

D. Etiology.   Early real illness coupled with parental abuse or rejection is typical. Patient recreates illness as an adult to gain loving attention from doctors. Masochistic gratification for some patients who want to undergo surgical procedures. Others identify with important past figure who had psychological or physical illness.

E. **Psychodynamics.** Repression, identification with the aggressor, regression, symbolization.

F. **Differential diagnosis**

1. **Physical illness.** Physical examination and laboratory workup should be performed; results will be negative. The nursing staff should observe carefully for deliberate elevation of temperature, alteration of body fluids.

2. **Somatoform disorder.** Symptoms are voluntary in factitious disorder and not caused by unconscious or symbolic factors. *La belle indifférence* is not present in factitious disorder. Hypochondriacs do not want to undergo extensive tests or surgery.

3. **Malingering.** Most difficult differential diagnosis. Malingerers have specific goals (e.g., insurance payments, avoidance of jail term).

4. **Ganse's syndrome.** Found in prisoners who give approximate answers to questions and talk past the point. Classified as a dissociative disorder not otherwise specified.

G. **Course and prognosis.** Course is usually chronic. Begins in adulthood, but onset may be earlier. Frequent consultation with doctors and history of hospitalizations as patient seeks repeated care. High risk for substance abuse over time. Prognosis improves if associated depression or anxiety is present that responds to pharmacotherapy. Risk for death if patient undergoes multiple life-threatening surgical procedures.

H. **Treatment**

1. Avoid unnecessary laboratory tests or medical procedures. Confront patient with diagnosis of factitious disorder and feigned symptoms. Patients rarely enter psychotherapy because of poor motivation; however, working alliance with doctor is possible over time, and patient may gain insight into behavior. Good management, however, is more likely than a cure. A data bank of patients with repeated hospitalizations for factitious illness is available in some areas of the United States.

2. Psychopharmacological therapy is useful for associated anxiety or depression. Substance abuse should be treated if present.

3. Contact child welfare services if a child is at risk (e.g., with factitious disorder by proxy).

III. **Malingering**

A. **Definition.** Voluntary production of physical or psychological symptoms to accomplish specific goal (e.g., to receive insurance payments, avoid jail term or punishment).

B. **Diagnosis, signs, and symptoms.** Patients have many vague or poorly localized complaints that are presented in great detail; they are easily irritated if a doctor is skeptical of the history. Psychosocial history reveals a need to avoid some situation or obtain money, presence of legal problems. Look for defined goal (secondary gain).

C. **Epidemiology.** Unknown. Malingering occurs most frequently in settings with a preponderance of men—the military, prisons, factories, and other industrial settings—although the condition also occurs in women.

    D. Etiology.   Unknown. May be associated with antisocial personality disorder.

    E. Differential diagnosis

       1. Factitious disorders. No obvious secondary gain.

       2. Somatoform disorder. Symbolic or unconscious component to symptom. Symptoms are not voluntarily and willfully produced.

    F. Treatment.   Result of physical and laboratory workups often are negative. Patient should be monitored as if real disease were present, but no treatment should be offered. At some time, identify areas of secondary gain and encourage patient to ventilate. Help provide ways of managing stress. Patient may then be willing to give up symptoms.

For more detailed discussion of this topic, see Somatoform Disorders, Factitious Disorders, and Malingering, Ch 16, p 1504, in CTP/VII.

13

Dissociative Disorders

I. General introduction

Dissociative disorders are defined in DSM-IV-TR as having the essential feature of disrupted "consciousness, memory, identity, or perception of the environment." Patients with these disorders can demonstrate dissociative phenomena ranging from normal (hypnotizability) to pathological (multiple personalities). Dissociation is a defense against trauma that helps persons remove themselves from the trauma as it occurs and delays the working through of the trauma. DSM-IV-TR recognizes four specific dissociative disorders: dissociative amnesia, dissociative fugue, dissociative identity disorder, and depersonalization disorder. Dissociative disorder not otherwise specified is a residual category.

II. Dissociative amnesia

A. Definition. Loss of important personal memory, usually stressful or traumatic, with preserved capacity to learn new material; not caused by a medical condition or drug.

B. Diagnosis, signs and symptoms. See Table 13–1. Patient is usually alert and aware of loss of memory. Most common type of loss is localized amnesia in which the events of a short period of time are lost to memory. Apparent indifference to memory loss may be seen; mild clouding of consciousness may occur.

C. Epidemiology. See Table 13–2.

D. Etiology. See Table 13–2.

E. Laboratory and psychological tests. Must rule out medical disease as indicated. Drug-assisted interview (e.g., amobarbital [Amytal]) can help in distinguishing between amnestic disorder resulting from a general medical condition and dissociative amnesia; organically amnestic patients tend to worsen under amobarbital, whereas memory may return to psychogenically amnestic patients.

F. Psychodynamics. Memory loss is secondary to painful psychological conflict in which the patient has limited emotional resources. Defenses include repression (unconscious blocking of disturbing impulses from awareness), denial (external reality is ignored), and dissociation (separation and independent functioning of one group of mental processes from others). Similar defenses are used in all the dissociative disorders.

G. Differential diagnosis. See Table 13–3.

H. Course and prognosis. See Table 13–2.

I. Treatment. Recovery generally is spontaneous without treatment.

1. Hypnosis. Patient relaxes sufficiently to recall forgotten information.

TABLE 13–1
DSM-IV-TR DIAGNOSTIC CRITERIA FOR DISSOCIATIVE AMNESIA

A. The predominant disturbance is one or more episodes of inability to recall important personal information, usually of a traumatic or stressful nature, that is too extensive to be explained by ordinary forgetfulness.
B. The disturbance does not occur exclusively during the course of dissociative identity disorder, dissociative fugue, posttraumatic stress disorder, acute stress disorder, or somatization disorder and is not due to the direct physiologic effects of a substance (e.g., a drug of abuse, a medication) or a neurological or other general medical condition (e.g., amnestic disorder due to head trauma).
C. The symptoms cause clinically significant distress or impairment in social, occupational, or other important areas of functioning.

From American Psychiatric Association. *Diagnostic and Statistical Manual of Mental Disorders,* text revision, 4th ed. Washington, DC: American Psychiatric Association, Copyright 2000, with permission.

 2. **Drug-assisted interview.** Intermediate and short-acting barbiturates (e.g., thiopental [Pentothal] and sodium amobarbital [Amytal]) or benzodiazepines, given intravenously, may be used to help patients recover their forgotten memories.
 3. **Psychotherapy.** Helps patients to incorporate the memories into their conscious state.

III. Dissociative fugue

 A. **Definition.** Unexpected, sudden travel away from customary home or work and failure to remember important aspects of previous identity (name, family, occupation). A new identity often is assumed.
 B. **Diagnosis, signs, and symptoms.** See Table 13–4. Sudden loss of memory associated with purposeful, unconfused travel, often for extended periods of time. Partial or complete loss of memory for past life, often without awareness of the loss. Assumption of apparently normal, nonbizarre new identity. However, perplexity and disorientation may occur.
 C. **Epidemiology.** See Table 13–2.
 D. **Etiology.** See Table 13–2.
 E. **Laboratory and psychological tests.** Hypnosis and drug-assisted interviews help in clarifying the diagnosis if patient regains memory.
 F. **Differential diagnosis**
  1. **Cognitive disorder.** Wandering is not as purposeful or complex.
  2. **Temporal lobe epilepsy.** Generally no new identity is assumed.
  3. **Dissociative amnesia.** No purposeful travel or new identity.
  4. **Malingering.** Difficult to distinguish. Clear secondary gain should raise suspicion.
 G. **Course and prognosis.** See Table 13–2.
 H. **Treatment.** Recovery generally is spontaneous without treatment.
  1. **Hypnosis and drug-assisted interviews.** May help reveal precipitating stressor.
  2. **Psychotherapy.** To help patients incorporate the precipitating stressors into their psyches in a healthy and integrated manner. Expressive-supportive psychodynamic psychotherapy is the treatment of choice.

TABLE 13–2
SUMMARY OF DISSOCIATIVE DISORDERS

	Dissociative Amnesia	Dissociative Fugue	Dissociative Identity Disorder	Depersonalization Disorder
Signs and symptoms	Loss of memory, usually with abrupt onset Patient aware of loss Alert before and after loss	Purposeful wandering, often long distances Amnesia for past life Often unaware of loss of memory Often assumes new identity Normal behavior during fugue	More than one distinct personality within one person, each of which dominates person's behavior and thinking when it is present Sudden transition from one personality to another Generally amnesia for other personalities	Persistent sense of unreality about one's body and self Intact reality testing Ego-dynamic
Epidemiology	Most common dissociative disorder More common following disasters or during war Female > male Adolescence, young adulthood	Rare More common following disasters or during war Variable sex ratio and age of onset	Not nearly as rare as once thought Affects as many as 5% of psychiatric patients Adolescence–young adulthood (although may begin much earlier) Female > male Increased in first-degree relatives	Although pure disorder rare, intermittent episodes of depersonalization common Rare over age 40 May be more common in women
Etiology	Precipitating emotional trauma (e.g., domestic violence) Rule out medical causes	Precipitating emotional trauma Heavy alcohol abuse may predispose Borderline, histrionic, schizoid personality disorders predispose Rule out medical causes	Severe sexual and psychological abuse in childhood Lack of support from significant others Epilepsy may be involved Rule out medical causes	Severe stress, anxiety, depression predispose Rule out medical causes
Course and prognosis	Abrupt termination Few recurrences	Usually brief, hours or days Can last months and involve extensive travel Recovery generally spontaneous and rapid Recurrences rare	Most severe and chronic of dissociative disorders Incomplete recovery	Onset usually sudden Tends to be chronic

IV. Dissociative identity disorder (multiple personality disorder)

A. Definition. Distinct personalities or identities within the same person, each of which when present may dominate the person's attitudes, behavior, and self-view, as though no other personality existed.

B. Diagnosis, signs, and symptoms. See Table 13–5. Original personality is generally amnestic for and unaware of other personalities. Transition from one personality to another tends to be abrupt. Some personalities may be aware of aspects of other personalities; each personality may have its own set of memories and associations, and each generally has its own name or description. Different personalities may have different physiologic characteristics (e.g., different eyeglass prescriptions) and different responses to psychometric testing (e.g., different I.Q. scores). Personalities may be of different sexes, ages, or races. One or more of the personalities may exhibit signs of a coexisting psychiatric disorder (e.g., mood disorder, personality disorder). Signs of dissociative identity disorder are listed in Table 13–6.

TABLE 13–3
DIFFERENTIAL DIAGNOSTIC CONSIDERATIONS IN DISSOCIATIVE AMNESIA

Dementia
Delirium
Amnestic disorder due to a general medical condition
  Anoxic amnesia
  Cerebral infections (e.g., herpes simplex affecting temporal lobes)
  Cerebral neoplasms (especially limbic and frontal)
  Epilepsy
  Metabolic disorders (e.g., uremia, hypoglycemia, hypertensive encephalopathy, porphyria)
  Postconcussion (posttraumatic) amnesia
  Postoperative amnesia
Electroconvulsive therapy (or other strong electric shock)
Substance-induced (e.g., ethanol, sedative-hypnotics, anticholinergics, steroids, lithium, β-adrenergic receptor antagonists, pentazocine, phencyclidine, hypoglycemic agents, cannabis, hallucinogens, methyldopa)
Transient global amnesia
Wernicke-Korsakoff syndrome
Sleep-related amnesia (e.g., sleepwalking disorder)
Other dissociative disorders
Posttraumatic stress disorder
Acute stress disorder
Somatoform disorders (somatization disorder, conversion disorder)
Malingering (especially when associated with criminal activity)

TABLE 13–4
DSM-IV-TR DIAGNOSTIC CRITERIA FOR DISSOCIATIVE FUGUE

A. The predominant disturbance is sudden, unexpected travel away from home or one's customary place of work, with inability to recall one's past.
B. Confusion about personal identity or assumption of a new identity (partial or complete).
C. The disturbance does not occur exclusively during the course of dissociative identity disorder and is not due to the direct physiologic effects on a substance (e.g., a drug of abuse, a medication) or a general medical condition (e.g., temporal lobe epilepsy).
D. The symptoms cause clinically significant distress or impairment in social, occupational, or other important areas of functioning.

From American Psychiatric Association. *Diagnostic and Statistical Manual of Mental Disorders,* text revision, 4th ed. Washington, DC: American Psychiatric Association, Copyright 2000, with permission.

C. **Epidemiology.** See Table 13–2.

D. **Etiology.** See Table 13–2.

E. **Laboratory and psychological tests.** Drug-assisted interviews and hypnosis can help clarify the diagnosis. In some studies, positron emission tomography scans and cerebral blood flow studies have revealed metabolic differences between different personalities in the same person.

F. **Psychodynamics.** Severe psychological and physical abuse (most often sexual) in childhood leads to a profound need to distance the self from horror and pain. The need to distance oneself leads to an unconscious splitting off of different aspects of the original personality, with each personality expressing some necessary emotion or state (e.g., rage, sexuality, flamboyance, competence) that the original personality dares not express. During abuse, the child attempts to protect himself or herself from trauma by dissociating from the terrifying acts, becoming in essence another person or persons who are not experiencing abuse and who could not be subjected to abuse. The dissociated selves become a long-term, ingrained method of self-protection from perceived emotional threats.

G. **Differential diagnosis**

   1. **Schizophrenia.** Patients may be delusional in believing that they have different identities or are being controlled by others, but the formal thought disorder and social deterioration distinguish schizophrenia from dissociative identity disorder.

TABLE 13–5
DSM-IV-TR DIAGNOSTIC CRITERIA FOR DISSOCIATIVE IDENTITY DISORDER

A. The presence of two or more distinct identities or personality states (each with its own relatively enduring pattern of perceiving, relating to, and thinking about the environment and self).

B. At least two of these identities or personality states recurrently take control of the person's behavior.

C. Inability to recall important personal information that is too extensive to be explained by ordinary forgetfulness.

D. The disturbance is not due to the direct physiological effects of a substance (e.g., blackouts or chaotic behavior during alcohol intoxication) or a general medical conditions (e.g., complex partial seizures). **Note:** in children, the symptoms are not attributable to imaginary playmates or other fantasy play.

From American Psychiatric Association. *Diagnostic and Statistical Manual of Mental Disorders,* text revision, 4th ed. Washington, DC: American Psychiatric Association, Copyright 2000, with permission.

TABLE 13–6
SIGNS OF DISSOCIATIVE IDENTITY DISORDER

1. Reports of time distortions, lapses, and discontinuities.
2. Being told of behavioral episodes by others that are not remembered by the patient.
3. Being recognized by others or called by another name by people whom the patient does not recognize.
4. Notable changes in the patient's behavior reported by a reliable observer; the patient may call himself or herself by a different name or refer to himself or herself in the third person.
5. Other personalities are elicited under hypnosis or during amobarbital interviews.
6. Use of the word "we" in the course of an interview.
7. Discovery of writings, drawings, or other productions or objects (e.g., identification cards, clothing) among the patient's personal belongings that are not recognized or cannot be accounted for.
8. Headaches.
9. Hearing voices originating from within and not identified as separate.
10. History of severe emotional or physical trauma as a child (usually before the age of 5 years).

From Cummings JL. Dissociative states, depersonalization, multiple personality, episodic memory lapses. In: Cummings JL, ed. *Clinical Neuropsychiatry.* Orlando, FL: Grune & Stratton, 1985:122, with permission.

2. **Malingering.** The most difficult differential diagnosis; clear secondary gain must raise suspicion. Drug-assisted interview may help.

3. **Borderline personality disorder.** In many patients with coexisting borderline personality disorder, only the personality disorder is diagnosed because the different personalities are mistaken for the characteristic mood, behavior, and interpersonal instability of the patient with borderline personality disorder.

4. **Bipolar disorder with rapid cycling.** Symptoms appear to be similar to those of dissociative identity disorder, but discrete personalities are absent.

5. **Neurological disorders.** The symptoms of complex partial epilepsy are the most likely to mimic those of dissociative identity disorder.

H. **Course and prognosis.** See Table 13–2.

I. **Treatment.** Intensive insight-oriented psychotherapy, often with hypnotherapy or drug-assisted interviewing. Pharmacotherapy has not been very useful. Goals of therapy include reconciliation of disparate, split-off affects by helping the patient understand that the original reasons for the dissociation (overwhelming rage, fear, and confusion secondary to abuse) no longer exist, and that the affects can be expressed by one whole personality without the self being destroyed.

V. Depersonalization disorder

A. **Definition.** Persistent, recurrent episodes of feeling detached from one's self or body (e.g., feeling mechanical or as if in a dream).

B. **Diagnosis, signs, and symptoms.** See Table 13–7. Distortions in sense of time and space, a feeling that extremities are too large or too small, and derealization (sense of strangeness about external world) are common. Patients may feel robot-like. Dizziness, depressive and obsessive ruminations, anxiety, and somatic preoccupations are common.

C. **Epidemiology.** See Table 13–2.

D. **Etiology.** See Table 13–2.

E. **Differential diagnosis.** See Table 13–8. Depersonalization as a symptom can occur in many syndromes, both psychiatric and medical. Mood disorders, anxiety disorders, schizophrenia, dissociative identity disorder, substance use, adverse medication, brain tumors or injury, and seizure disorders

---

TABLE 13–7
DSM-IV-TR DIAGNOSTIC CRITERIA FOR DEPERSONALIZATION DISORDER

A. Persistant or recurrent experiences of feeling detached from, and as if one is an outside observer of, one's mental processes or body (e.g., feeling like one is in a dream).

B. During the depersonalization experience, reality testing remains intact.

C. The depersonalization causes clinically significant distress or impairment in social, occupational, or other important areas of functioning.

D. The depersonalization experience does not occur exclusively during the course of another mental disorder, such as schizophrenia, panic disorder, acute stress disorder, or another dissociative disorder, and is not due to the direct physiological effects of a substance (e.g., a drug of abuse, a medication) or a general medical condition (e.g., temporal lobe epilepsy).

From American Psychiatric Association. *Diagnostic and Statistical Manual of Mental Disorders,* text revision, 4th ed. Washington, DC: American Psychiatric Association, Copyright 2000, with permission.

TABLE 13–8
CAUSES OF DEPERSONALIZATION

Neurological disorders	*Idiopathic mental disorders*
Epilepsy	Schizophrenia
Migraine	Depressive disorders
Brain tumors	Manic episodes
Cerebrovascular disease	Conversion disorder
Cerebral trauma	Anxiety disorders
Encephalitis	Obsessive-compulsive disorder
General paresis	Personality disorders
Dementia of the Alzheimer's type	Phobic-anxiety depersonalization syndrome
Huntington's disease	*In normal persons*
Spinocerebellar degeneration	Exhaustion
Toxic and metabolic disorders	Boredom; sensory deprivation
Hypoglycemia	Emotional shock
Hypoparathyroidism	*In hemidepersonalization*
Carbon monoxide poisoning	Lateralized (usually right parietal) focal brain lesion
Mescaline intoxication	
Botulism	
Hyperventilation	
Hypothyroidism	

Adapted from Cummings JL. Dissociative states, depersonalization, multiple personality, episodic memory lapses. In: Cummings JL, ed. *Clinical Neuropsychiatry.* Orlando, FL: Grune & Stratton 1985:123, with permission.

(e.g., temporal lobe epilepsy) must be ruled out. Depersonalization disorder describes the condition in which depersonalization is predominant.

F. Course and prognosis. See Table 13–2.

G. Treatment. Anxiety usually responds to anxiolytics and to both supportive and insight-oriented therapy. As anxiety is reduced, episodes of depersonalization decrease.

IV. Dissociative disorder not otherwise specified

A. Definition. Dissociative symptoms are prominent, but the clinical picture does not fully meet the specific criteria for dissociative disorder. Disorders in which the predominant feature is a dissociative symptom (i.e., a disturbance or alteration in the normally integrative functions of identity, memory, or consciousness that does not meet the criteria for a specific dissociative disorder).

B. Examples

1. Ganse's syndrome—giving approximate answers to questions (e.g., 2 + 2 = 5) or talking past the point; commonly associated with other symptoms (e.g., amnesia, disorientation, perceptual disturbances, fugue, conversion symptoms).

2. Cases similar to dissociative identity disorder in which more than one personality state can assume executive control of the person, but not more than one personality state is sufficiently distinct to meet the full criteria for dissociative identity disorder; or cases in which a second personality never assumes complete executive control; or cases without amnesia for important information.

3. Derealization unaccompanied by depersonalization.

4. Dissociated states in persons who have been subjected to periods of prolonged and intense coercive persuasion (e.g., brainwashing or indoctrination while the captive of terrorists or cultists).

5. Dissociative trance disorder—disturbances in consciousness, identity, or memory that are indigenous to particular locations and cultures (e.g., amok [rage reaction], *pibloktoq* [self-injurious behavior]). Trance states are altered states of consciousness with markedly diminished or selectively focused responsiveness to environmental stimuli. In children, such states may follow physical abuse or trauma.

6. Coma, stupor, or loss of consciousness not resulting from a general medical condition. Cases in which sudden, unexpected travel and organized, purposeful behavior with inability to recall one's past are not accompanied by the assumption of a new identity, partial or complete.

For more detailed discussion of this topic, see Dissociative Disorders, Ch 18, p 1544, in CTP/VII.

14

Sexual Dysfunctions, Paraphilias, and Gender Identity Disorders

I. Sexual dysfunctions

A. Definition. Sexual function is affected by biological, psychological, and sociologic factors. Internal and external genitalia, hormones and neurohormones, intrapsychic dynamics, interpersonal relations, socioeconomic status, and the prevailing cultural mores all affect the expression of sexuality. A disturbance in one or more of these areas can result in sexual dysfunction. Several episodes of sexual dysfunction create anxiety about sexual performance, and anxiety aggravates and tends to perpetuate the dysfunction. The dysfunctions can be a **lifelong type** or **acquired type** (i.e., developing after a period of normal functioning); a **generalized type** or **situational type** (i.e., limited to a certain partner or a specific situation); and the consequence of **physiological factors, psychological factors,** or **combined factors.** The seven major categories of sexual dysfunction listed in DSM-IV-TR are (1) sexual desire disorders, (2) sexual arousal disorders, (3) orgasmic disorders, (4) sexual pain disorders, (5) sexual dysfunction resulting from a general medical condition, (6) substance-induced sexual dysfunction, and (7) sexual dysfunction not otherwise specified. Table 14–1 lists each DSM-IV-TR phase of the sexual response cycle and the sexual dysfunctions usually associated with it.

B. Sexual desire disorders. Sexual desire disorders are divided into two classes: hypoactive sexual desire disorder, characterized by a deficiency or absence of sexual fantasies and the desire for sexual activity, and sexual aversion disorder, characterized by an aversion to and avoidance of genital sexual contact with a sexual partner.

Patients with desire problems may use inhibition of desire defensively to protect against unconscious fears about sex. A lack of desire can also accompany chronic anxiety or depression, or the use of various psychotropic drugs and other drugs that depress the CNS. In sex therapy clinic populations, lack of desire is one of the most common complaints among married couples, with women more affected than men.

C. Sexual arousal disorders. These disorders include male erectile disorder and female arousal disorder. The diagnosis considers the focus, intensity, and duration of the patient's sexual activity. If sexual stimulation is inadequate in focus, intensity, or duration, the diagnosis should not be made.

1. Women. See Table 14–2. The prevalence of female sexual arousal disorder is generally underestimated. In one study of subjectively happily married couples, 33% of women described arousal problems. Difficulty in maintaining excitement can reflect psychologic conflicts (e.g., anxiety, guilt, and fear) or physiologic changes. Alterations in levels of testos-

TABLE 14-1
DSM-IV-TR PHASES OF THE SEXUAL RESPONSE CYCLE AND ASSOCIATED SEXUAL DYSFUNCTIONS^a

Phases	Characteristics	Dysfunction
1. Desire	Distinct from any identified solely through physiology and reflects the patient's motivations, drives, and personality; characterized by sexual fantasies and the desire to have sex.	Hypoactive sexual desire disorder; sexual aversion disorder; hypoactive sexual desire disorder due to a general medical condition (male or female); substance-induced sexual dysfunction with impaired desire.
2. Excitement	Subjective sense of sexual pleasure and accompanying physiological changes; all physiological responses noted in Masters and Johnson's excitement and plateau phases are combined in this phase.	Female sexual arousal disorder; male erectile disorder (may also occur in stages 3 and 4); male erectile disorder due to a general medical condition; dyspareunia due to a general medical condition (male or female); substance-induced sexual dysfunction with impaired arousal.
3. Orgasm	Peaking of sexual pleasure, with release of sexual tension and rhythmic contraction of the perineal muscles and pelvic reproductive organs.	Female orgasmic disorder; male orgasmic disorder; premature ejaculation; other sexual dysfunction due to a general medical condition (male or female); substance-induced sexual dysfunction with impaired orgasm.
4. Resolution	A sense of general relaxation, well-being, and muscle relaxation; men are refractory to orgasm for a period of time that increases with age, whereas women can have multiple orgasms without a refractory period.	Postcoital dysphoria; postcoital headache.

^{a} DSM-IV-TR consolidates the Masters and Johnson's excitement and plateau phases into a single excitement phase, which is preceded by the desire (appetitive) phase. The orgasm and resolution phases remain the same as originally described by Masters and Johnson.

TABLE 14-2
DSM-IV-TR DIAGNOSTIC CRITERIA FOR FEMALE SEXUAL AROUSAL DISORDER

A. Persistent or recurrent inability to attain, or to maintain until completion of the sexual activity, an adequate lubrication-swelling response of sexual excitement.
B. The disturbance causes marked distress or interpersonal difficulty.
C. The sexual dysfunction is not better accounted for by another Axis I disorder (except another sexual dysfunction) and is not due exclusively to the direct physiologic effects of a substance (e.g., a drug of abuse) or a general medical condition.

Specify type:
Lifelong type
Acquired type

Specify type:
Generalized type
Situational type

Specify:
Due to psychological factors
Due to combined factors

From American Psychiatric Association. *Diagnostic and Statistical Manual of Mental Disorders*, text revision, 4th ed. Washington, DC: American Psychiatric Association, Copyright 2000, with permission.

TABLE 14–3
DSM-IV-TR DIAGNOSTIC CRITERIA FOR MALE ERECTILE DISORDER

A. Persistent or recurrent inability to attain, or to maintain until completion of the sexual activity, an adequate erection.
B. The disturbance causes marked distress or interpersonal difficulty.
C. The erectile dysfunction is not better accounted for by another Axis I disorder (other than a sexual dysfunction) and is not due exclusively to the direct physiologic effects of a substance (e.g., a drug of abuse, a medication) or a general medical condition.

Specify type:
  Lifelong type
  Acquired type

Specify type:
  Generalized type
  Situational type

Specify:
  Due to psychological factors
  Due to combined factors

From American Psychiatric Association. *Diagnostic and Statistical Manual of Mental Disorders,* text revision, 4ᵗʰ ed. Washington, DC: American Psychiatric Association, Copyright 2000, with permission.

terone, estrogen, prolactin, serotonin, dopamine, and thyroxin have been implicated in arousal disorders, as have antihistamine medications.

   2. Men. See Table 14–3. The prevalence of erectile disorder, or impotence, in young men is estimated at 8%. However, this disorder may first appear later in life. A number of procedures, from benign to invasive, are used to differentiate organically (i.e., medically) caused impotence from functional (i.e., psychological) impotence. The most commonly used procedure is monitoring of nocturnal penile tumescence (erections that occur during sleep), normally associated with rapid eye movement (REM) sleep.

   A good history is invaluable in determining the cause. A history of spontaneous erections, morning erections, or good erections with masturbation or with partners other than the usual one indicates functional impotence. Psychological causes of erectile dysfunction include unresolved oedipal or pre-oedipal conflicts that result in a punitive superego, an inability to trust, or feelings of inadequacy. Erectile dysfunction also may reflect relationship difficulties between partners.

D. Orgasmic disorders

   1. Female. See Table 14–4. Female orgasmic disorder (anorgasmia) is a recurrent or persistent delay in or absence of orgasm following a normal sexual excitement phase. The estimated proportion of married women over age 35 who never have achieved orgasm is 5%. The proportion is higher in unmarried women and younger women. The overall prevalence of inhibited female orgasm is 30%. Psychological factors associated with inhibited orgasm include fears of impregnation or rejection by the sex partner, hostility toward men, feelings of guilt about sexual impulses, or marital conflicts.

   2. Male. In male orgasmic disorder (inhibited male orgasm), the man achieves ejaculation during coitus with great difficulty, if at all. Lifelong inhibited male orgasm usually indicates more severe psychopathology. Acquired ejaculatory inhibition frequently reflects interpersonal difficulties.

TABLE 14-4
DSM-IV-TR DIAGNOSTIC CRITERIA FOR FEMALE ORGASMIC DISORDER

A. Persistent or recurrent delay in, or absence of, orgasm following a normal sexual excitement phase. Women exhibit wide variability in the type or intensity of stimulation that triggers orgasm. The diagnosis of female orgasmic disorder should be based on the clinician's judgment that the woman's orgasmic capacity is less than would be reasonable for her age, sexual experience, and the adequacy of sexual stimulation she receives.
B. The disturbance causes marked distress or interpersonal difficulty.
C. The orgasmic dysfunction is not better accounted for by another Axis I disorder (except another sexual dysfunction) and is not due exclusively to the direct physiologic effects of a substance (e.g., a drug of abuse, a medication) or a general medical condition.

Specify type:
Lifelong type
Acquired type

Specify type:
Generalized type
Situational type

Specify:
Due to psychological factors
Due to combined factors

From American Psychiatric Association. *Diagnostic and Statistical Manual of Mental Disorders,* text revision, 4th ed. Washington, DC: American Psychiatric Association, Copyright 2000, with permission.

3. Premature ejaculation.

Premature ejaculation is the chief complaint of 35–40% of men treated for sexual disorders. The man persistently or recurrently achieves orgasm and ejaculates before he wishes to. It is more prevalent among young men, men with a new partner, and college-educated men than among men with less education; it is thought to be related to concern for partner satisfaction.

Premature ejaculation may be associated with unconscious fears about the vagina. It may also be the result of conditioning if the man's early sexual experiences occurred in situations in which discovery would have been embarrassing. A stressful marriage exacerbates the disorder.

This dysfunction is the one most amenable to cure when behavioral techniques are used in treatment. However, a subgroup of premature ejaculators may be biologically predisposed; they are more vulnerable to sympathetic stimulation or they have a shorter bulbocavernosus reflex nerve latency time, and they should be treated pharmacologically.

E. Sexual pain disorders

1. Vaginismus. Vaginismus is an involuntary muscle constriction of the outer third of the vagina that interferes with penile insertion and intercourse. This dysfunction most frequently afflicts women in higher socioeconomic groups. A sexual trauma, such as rape or childhood sexual abuse, can be the cause. Women with psychosexual conflicts may perceive the penis as a weapon. A strict religious upbringing that associates sex with sin or problems in the dyadic relationship are also noted in these cases.

2. Dyspareunia. Dyspareunia is recurrent or persistent genital pain occurring before, during, or after intercourse. Medical causes (endometriosis, vaginitis, cervicitis, and other pelvic disorders) must be ruled out in patients with this complaint.

Chronic pelvic pain is a common complaint in women with a history of rape or childhood sexual abuse. Painful coitus may result from tension and anxiety. Dyspareunia is uncommon in men and is usually associated with a medical condition.

F. Sexual dysfunction due to a general medical condition
   1. Male erectile disorder. Statistics indicate that erectile disorder is medically based in 50% of affected men. Medical causes of male erectile dysfunction are listed in Table 14–5.
   2. Dyspareunia. Pelvic disease is found in 30–40% of women with this complaint who are seen in sex therapy clinics. An estimated 30% of surgical procedures on the female pelvic or genital area also result in temporary dyspareunia. In most cases, however, dynamic factors are considered causative.

   Medical conditions leading to dyspareunia include irritated or infected hymenal remnants, episiotomy scars, infection of a Bartholin's gland, various forms of vaginitis and cervicitis, endometriosis, postmenopausal vaginal atrophy, and Peyronie's disease.

TABLE 14–5
MEDICAL CONDITIONS IMPLICATED IN ERECTILE DYSFUNCTION

Infectious and parasitic diseases
  Elephantiasis
  Mumps
Cardiovascular disease
  Atherosclerotic disease
  Aortic aneurysm
  Leriche's syndrome
  Cardiac failure
Renal and urological disorders
  Peyronie's disease
  Chronic renal failure
  Hydrocele and varicocele
Hepatic disorders
  Cirrhosis (usually associated with alcohol dependence)
Pulmonary disorders
  Respiratory failure
Genetic disorders
  Klinefelter's syndrome
  Congenital penile vascular and structural abnormalities
Nutritional disorders
  Malnutrition
  Vitamin deficiencies
Endocrine disorders
  Diabetes mellitus
  Dysfunction of the pituitary–adrenal–testis axis
  Acromegaly
  Addison's disease
  Chromophobe adenoma
  Adrenal neoplasia
  Myxedema
  Hyperthyroidism

Neurological disorders
  Multiple sclerosis
  Transverse myelitis
  Parkinson's disease
  Temporal lobe epilepsy
  Traumatic and neoplastic spinal cord diseases
  Central nervous system tumor
  Amyotrophic lateral sclerosis
  Peripheral neuropathy
  General paresis
  Tabes dorsalis
Pharmacological contributants
  Alcohol and other dependence-inducing substances (heroin, methadone, morphine, cocaine, amphetamines, and barbiturates)
  Prescribed drugs (psychotropic drugs, antihypertensive drugs, estrogens, and antiandrogens)
Poisoning
  Lead (plumbism)
  Herbicides
Surgical procedures
  Perineal prostatectomy
  Abdominal–perineal colon resection
  Sympathectomy (frequently interferes with ejaculation)
  Aortoiliac surgery
  Radical cystectomy
  Retroperitoneal lymphadenectomy
Miscellaneous
  Radiation therapy
  Pelvic fracture
  Any severe systemic disease or debilitating condition

TABLE 14–6
PHARMACOLOGICAL AGENTS IMPLICATED IN MALE SEXUAL DYSFUNCTIONS

Drug	Impairs Erection	Impairs Ejaculation
Psychiatric drugs		
Selective serotonin reuptake inhibitors[a]		
Citalopram (Celexa)	−	+
Fluoxetine (Prozac)	−	+
Paroxetine (Paxil)	−	+
Sertraline (Zoloft)	−	+
Cyclic drugs		
Imipramine (Tofranil)	+	+
Protriptyline (Vivactil)	+	+
Desipramine (Pertofrane)	+	+
Clomipramine (Anafranil)	+	+
Amitriptyline (Elavil)	+	+
Monoamine oxidase inhibitors		
Tranylcypromine (Parnate)	+	
Phenelizine (Nardil)	+	+
Pargyline (Eutonyl)	−	+
Isocarboxazid (Marplan)	−	+
Other mood-active drugs		
Lithium (Eskalith)	+	
Amphetamines	+	+
Trazodone (Desyrel)[b]	−	−
Venlafaxine (Effexor)	−	+
Antipsychotics[c]		
Fluphenazine (Prolixin)	+	
Thioridazine (Mellaril)	+	+
Chlorprothixene (Taractan)	−	+
Mesoridazine (Serentil)	−	+
Perphenazine (Trilafon)	−	+
Trifluoperazine (Stelazine)	−	+
Reserpine (Serpasil)	+	+
Haloperidol (Haldol)	−	+
Antianxiety agent[d]		
Chlordiazepoxide (Librium)	−	+
Antihypertensive drugs		
Clonidine (Catapres)	+	
Methyldopa (Aldomet)	+	+
Spironolactone (Aldactone)	+	−
Hydrochlorothiazide (Hydrodiuril)	+	−
Guanethidine (Ismelin)	+	+
Commonly abused substances		
Alcohol	+	+
Barbiturates	+	+
Cannabis	+	−
Cocaine	+	+
Heroin	+	+
Methadone	+	−
Morphine	+	+
Miscellaneous drugs		
Antiparkinsonian agents	+	+
Clofibrate (Atromid-S)	+	−
Digoxin (Lanoxin)	+	−
Glutethimide (Doriden)	+	+
Indomethacin (Indocin)	+	−
Phentolamine (Regitine)	−	+
Propranolol (Inderal)	+	−

[a] SSRIs also impair desire.
[b] Trazodone has been causative in some cases of priapism.
[c] Impairment of sexual function is less likely with atypical antipsychotics. Priapism has occasionally occurred in association with the use of antipsychotics.
[d] Benzodiazepines have been reported to decrease libido, but in some patients the diminution of anxiety caused by those drugs enhances sexual function.

3. **Hypoactive sexual desire disorder.** Desire commonly decreases after major illness or surgery. Drugs that depress the CNS, decrease testosterone or dopamine concentrations, or increase serotonin or prolactin concentrations can decrease desire.

4. **Other male sexual dysfunctions.** Male orgasmic dysfunction may have physiological causes and can occur after surgery on the genitourinary tract. It may also be associated with Parkinson's disease and other neurological disorders involving the lumbar or sacral sections of the spinal cord. Certain drugs (e.g., guanethidine monosulfate [Ismelin]) have been implicated in retarded ejaculation (Table 14–6).

5. **Other female sexual dysfunctions.** Some medical conditions—specifically, such endocrine diseases as hypothyroidism, diabetes mellitus, and primary hyperprolactinemia—can affect a woman's ability to have orgasms.

G. **Substance-induced sexual dysfunction.** In general, sexual function is negatively affected by serotonergic agents, dopamine antagonists, drugs that increase prolactin, and drugs that affect the autonomic nervous system. With commonly abused substances, dysfunction occurs within a month of significant substance intoxication or withdrawal. In small doses, many substances enhance sexual performance, but continued use impairs erectile, orgasmic, and ejaculatory capacities.

The interrelation between female sexual dysfunction and pharmacological agents has been less extensively evaluated than have male reactions. Oral contraceptives are reported to decrease libido in some women, and some drugs with anticholinergic side effects may impair arousal as well as orgasm. Benzodiazepines have been reported to decrease libido, but in some patients the diminution of anxiety caused by those drugs enhances sexual function. Both increase and decrease in libido have been reported with psychoactive agents. It is difficult to separate those effects from the

TABLE 14–7
SOME PSYCHIATRIC DRUGS IMPLEMENTED IN INHIBITED FEMALE ORGASM

Tricyclic antidepressants
  Imipramine (Tofranil)
  Clomipramine (Anafranil)
  Nortriptyline (Aventyl)
Monoamine oxidase inhibitors
  Tranylcypromine (Parnate)
  Phenelzine (Nardil)
  Isocarboxazid (Marplan)
Dopamine receptor antagonists
  Thioridazine (Mellaril)
  Trifluoperazine (Stelazine)
Selective serotonin reuptake inhibitors
  Fluoxetine (Prozac)
  Paroxetine (Paxil)
  Sertraline (Zoloft)
  Fluvoxamine (Luvox)
  Citalopram (Celexa)

underlying condition or from improvement of the condition. Sexual dysfunction associated with the use of a drug disappears when the drug is discontinued. Table 14–7 lists psychiatric medications that may inhibit female orgasm.

H. Sexual dysfunction not otherwise specified.   Includes sexual dysfunctions that do not meet the criteria for any specific dysfunction. Examples include orgasmic anhedonia and compulsive sexual behavior.

I. Treatment.   Methods that have proved effective singly or in combination include (1) training in behavioral-sexual skills, (2) systematic desensitization, (3) directive marital therapy, (4) psychodynamic approaches, (5) group therapy, (6) pharmacotherapy, (7) surgery, and (8) hypnotherapy. Evaluation and treatment must address the possibility of accompanying personality disorders and physical conditions.

  1. Analytically oriented sex therapy. One of the most effective treatment modalities is the integration of sex therapy (training in behavioral–sexual skills) with psychodynamic and psychoanalytically oriented psychotherapy. Psychodynamic conceptualizations are added to behavioral techniques for the treatment of patients with sexual disorders associated with other psychopathology.

  2. Behavioral techniques. The aim of these techniques is to establish or reestablish verbal and sexual communication between partners. Specific exercises are prescribed to help the person or couple with their particular problem. All exercises are carried out in privacy, never in the presence of the therapist.

  Beginning exercises focus on verbal interchange and then on heightening sensory awareness to sight, touch, and smell. Initially, intercourse is prohibited and partners caress each other, with stimulation of the genitalia excluded. Performance anxiety is reduced because responses of genital excitement and orgasm are unnecessary for the completion of the initial exercises.

  During these sensate focus exercises, patients receive encouragement and reinforcement to reduce their anxiety. They are urged to use fantasies to distract them from obsessive concerns about performance (spectatoring). The expression of mutual needs is encouraged. Resistances, such as claims of fatigue or not enough time to complete the exercises, are common and must be dealt with by the therapist. Genital stimulation is eventually added to general body stimulation. Finally, intromission and intercourse are permitted. Therapy sessions follow each new exercise period, and problems and satisfactions, both sexual and related to other areas of the patients' lives, are discussed.

    a. Dysfunction-specific techniques and exercises. Different techniques are used for specific dysfunctions.

      (1) Vaginismus—the woman is advised to dilate her vaginal opening with her fingers or with dilators.

      (2) Premature ejaculation—the squeeze technique is used to raise the threshold of penile excitability. The patient or his partner forcibly squeezes the coronal ridge of the glans at the first sensation of impending ejaculation. The erection is diminished and ejaculation inhibited. A variation is the stop–start technique. Stimulation is stopped as excitement increases, but no squeeze is used.

   (3) Male erectile disorder—the man is sometimes told to masturbate to demonstrate that full erection and ejaculation are possible.

   (4) Female orgasmic disorder (primary anorgasmia)—the woman is instructed to masturbate, sometimes with the use of a vibrator. The use of fantasy is encouraged.

   (5) Retarded ejaculation—managed by extravaginal ejaculation initially and gradual vaginal entry after stimulation to the point of near ejaculation.

   b. **Behavioral techniques.** Reported to be successful 40–85% of the time. Individual psychotherapy is required in 10% of refractory cases. Approximately one third of dysfunctional couples refractory to behavioral techniques alone require some combination of marital and sex therapy.

3. Biological

   a. **Pharmacotherapy.** Most pharmacological treatments involve male sexual dysfunctions. Studies are being conducted to test the use of drugs to treat women. Pharmacotherapy may be used to treat sexual disorders of physiological, psychological, or mixed causes. In the latter two cases, phamacological treatment is usually used in addition to a form of psychotherapy.

   (1) Treatment of erectile disorder and premature ejaculation. Sildenafil (Viagra), a nitric oxide enhancer, facilitates the inflow of blood to the penis necessary for an erection. The medication does not work in the absence of sexual stimulation. Its use is contraindicated for people taking organic nitrates.

   Other medications act as vasodilators in the penis. They include oral prostaglandin (Vasomax), alprostadil (Caverject), an injectable phentolamine, and a transurethral alprostadil suppository (MUSE).

   α-Adrenergic agents such as methylphenidate (Ritalin), dextroamphetamine (Dexedrine), and yohimbine (Yocon) are also used to treat erectile disorder.

   Selective serotonin reuptake inhibitors (SSRIs) and heterocyclic antidepressants alleviate premature ejaculation because of their side effect of inhibiting orgasm.

   (2) Treatment of sexual aversion disorder. Cyclic antidepressants and SSRIs are used if people with this dysfunction are considered phobic of the genitalia.

   b. **Surgery.** Penile implants, revascularization.

II. Gender identity disorders

   A. Definition. A group of disorders that have as their main symptom a persistent preference for the role of the opposite sex and the feeling that one was born into the wrong sex. The feeling of discontent with one's biological sex is labeled *gender dysphoria*.

People with disordered gender identity try to live as or pass as members of the opposite sex. *Transsexuals* want biological treatment (surgery, hormones) to change their biological sex and acquire the anatomic characteristics of the opposite sex. The disorders may coexist with other pathology or be circumscribed, with patients functioning ably in many areas of their lives.

B. Diagnosis, signs, and symptoms.   See Table 14–8.

C. Epidemiology

1. Unknown, but rare.

2. Male-to-female ratio is 4:1.

   a. Almost all gender-disordered females have a homosexual orientation.

   b. Fifty percent of gender-disordered males have a homosexual orien-

---

TABLE 14–8
DSM-IV-TR DIAGNOSTIC CRITERIA FOR GENDER IDENTITY DISORDER

A. A strong and persistent cross-gender identification (not merely a desire for any perceived cultural advantages of being the other sex).

   In children, the disturbance is manifested by four (or more) of the following:
   (1) repeatedly stated desire to be, or insistence that he or she is, the other sex
   (2) in boys, preference for cross-dressing or simulating female attire; in girls, insistence on wearing only stereotypical masculine clothing
   (3) strong and persistent preferences for cross-sex roles in make-believe play or persistent fantasies of being the other sex
   (4) intense desire to participate in the stereotypical games and pastimes of the other sex
   (5) strong preference for playmates of the other sex

   In adolescents and adults, the disturbance is manifested by symptoms such as a stated desire to be the other sex, frequent passing as the other sex, desire to live or be treated as the other sex, or the conviction that he or she has the typical feelings and reactions of the other sex.

B. Persistent discomfort with his or her sex or sense of inappropriateness in the gender role of that sex.

   In children, the disturbance is manifested by any of the following: in boys, assertion that his penis or testes are disgusting or will disappear or assertion that it would be better not to have a penis, or aversion toward rough-and-tumble play and rejection of male stereotypical toys, games, and activities: in girls, rejection of urinating in a sitting position, assertion that she has or will grow a penis, or assertion that she does not want to grow breasts or menstruate, or marked aversion toward normative feminine clothing.

   In adolescents and adults, the disturbance is manifested by symptoms such as preoccupation with getting rid of primary and secondary sex characteristics (e.g., request for hormones, surgery, or other procedures to physically alter sexual characteristics to stimulate the other sex) or belief that he or she was born the wrong sex.

C. The disturbance is not concurrent with a physical intersex condition.

D. The disturbance causes clinically significant distress or impairment in social, occupational, or other important areas of functioning.

Code based on current age:
   Gender identity disorder in children
   Gender identity disorder in adolescents or adults

Specify if (for sexually mature individuals):
   Sexually attracted to males
   Sexually attracted to females
   Sexually attracted to both
   Sexually attracted to neither

From American Psychiatric Association. *Diagnostic and Statistical Manual of Mental Disorders*, text revision, 4th ed. Washington, DC: American Psychiatric Association, Copyright 2000, with permission.

tation, and 50% have a heterosexual, bisexual, or asexual orientation.

3. The prevalence rate for transsexualism is 1/10,000 males and 1/30,000 females.

D. Etiology

1. Biological. Testosterone affects brain neurons that contribute to masculinization of the brain in such areas as the hypothalamus. Whether testosterone contributes to so-called masculine or feminine behavioral patterns in gender identity disorders remains controversial. Sex steroids influence the expression of sexual behavior in mature men and women (i.e., testosterone can increase libido and aggressiveness in women, and estrogen or progesterone can decrease libido and aggressiveness in men).

2. Psychosocial. The absence of same-sex role models and explicit or implicit encouragement from caregivers to behave like the other sex contributes to gender identity disorder in childhood. Mothers may be depressed or withdrawn. Inborn temperamental traits sometimes result in sensitive, delicate boys and energetic, aggressive girls. Physical and sexual abuse may predispose.

E. Differential diagnosis

1. Transvestic fetishism. Cross-dressing for purpose of sexual excitement; can coexist (dual diagnosis).

2. Intersex conditions. See Table 14–9.

3. Schizophrenia. Rarely, true delusions of being other sex.

F. Course and prognosis

1. Children. Course varies. Symptoms may diminish spontaneously or with treatment. Prognosis depends on age of onset and intensity of symptoms. The disorder begins in boys before the age of 4 years, and peer conflict develops at about the age of 7 or 8 years. Tomboyism is generally better tolerated. The age of onset is also early for girls, but most give up masculine behavior by adolescence. Fewer than 10% of children go on to transsexualism.

2. Adults. Course tends to be chronic.

Transsexualism—after puberty, distress with one's biological sex and a desire to eliminate one's primary and secondary sex characteristics and acquire those of the other sex. Most transsexuals have had gender identity disorder in childhood; cross-dressing is common; associated mental disorder is common, especially borderline personality disorder or depressive disorder; suicide is a risk, but persons may mutilate their sex organs to coerce surgeons to perform sex reassignment surgery.

G. Treatment

1. Children. Improve existing role models or, in their absence, provide one from the family or elsewhere (e.g., big brother or sister). Caregivers are helped to encourage sex-appropriate behavior and attitudes. Any associated mental disorder is addressed.

TABLE 14-9
CLASSIFICATION OF INTERSEXUAL DISORDERS^a

Syndrome	Description
Virilizing adrenal hyperplasia (andrenogenital syndrome)	Results from excess androgens in fetus with XX genotype; most common female intersex disorder; associated with enlarged clitoris, fused labia, hirsutism in adolescence.
Turner's syndrome	Results from absence of second female sex chromosome (XO); associated with web neck, dwarfism, cubitus valgus; no sex hormones produced; infertile; usually assigned as females because of female-looking genitals.
Klinefelter's syndrome	Genotype is XXY; male habitus present with small penis and rudimentary testes because of low androgen production; weak libido; usually assigned as male.
Androgen insensitivity syndrome (testicular-feminizing syndrome)	Congenital X-linked recessive disorder that results in inability of tissues to respond to androgens; external genitals look female and cryptorchid testes present; assigned as females, even though they have XY genotype; in extreme form patient has breasts, normal external genitals, short blind vagina, and absence of pubic and axillary hair.
Enzymatic defects in XY genotype (e.g., 5-α-reductase deficiency, 17-hydroxysteroid deficiency)	Congenital interruption in production of testosterone that produces ambiguous genitals and female habitus; usually assigned as female because of female-looking genitalia.
Hermaphroditism	True hermaphrodite is rare and characterized by both testes and ovaries in same person (may be 46 XX or 46 XY).
Pseudohermaphroditism	Usually the result of endocrine or enzymatic defect (e.g., adrenal hyperplasia) in persons with normal chromosomes; female pseudohermaphrodites have masculine-looking genitals but are XX; male pseudohermaphrodites have rudimentary testes and external genitals and are XY; assigned as males or females, depending on morphology of genitals.

^{a} Intersexual disorders include a variety of syndromes that produce persons with gross anatomical or physiological aspects of the opposite sex.

2. **Adolescents.** Difficult to treat because of the coexistence of normal identity crises and gender identity confusion. Acting out is common, and adolescents rarely have a strong motivation to alter their stereotypic cross-gender roles.

3. **Adults**

   a. **Psychotherapy**—set the goal of helping patients become comfortable with the gender identity they desire; the goal is not to create a person with a conventional sexual identity. Therapy also explores sex-reassignment surgery and the indications and contraindications for such procedures, which severely distressed and anxious patients often decide to undergo impulsively.

   b. **Sex-reassignment surgery**—definitive and irreversible. Patients must go through a 3- to 12-month trial of cross-dressing and receive hormone treatment. Seventy percent to eighty percent of patients are satisfied by the results. Dissatisfaction correlates with severity of preexisting psychopathology. A reported 2% commit suicide.

   c. **Hormonal treatments**—many patients are treated with hormones in lieu of surgery.

TABLE 14-10
PARAPHILIAS

Disorder	Definition	General Considerations	Treatment
Exhibitionism	Exposing genitals in public; rare in females.	Person wants to shock female—her reaction is affirmation to patient that penis is intact.	Insight-oriented psychotherapy, aversive conditioning. Female should try to ignore exhibitionistic male, who is offensive but not dangerous, or call police.
Fetishism	Sexual arousal with inanimate objects (e.g., shoes, hair, clothing).	Almost always in men. Behavior often followed by guilt.	Insight-oriented psychotherapy; aversive conditioning; implosion, i.e., patient (masturbates with fetish until it loses its arousal effect (masturbatory satiation)).
Frotteurism	Rubbing genitals against female to achieve arousal and orgasm.	Occurs in crowded places, such as subways usually by passive, nonassertive men.	Insight-oriented psychotherapy; aversive conditioning; group therapy; antiandrogenic medication.
Pedophilia	Sexual activity with children under age 13; most common paraphilia.	95% heterosexual, 5% homosexual. High risk of repeated behavior. Fear of adult sexuality in patient; low self-esteem. 10–20% of children have been molested by age 18.	Place patient in treatment unit; group therapy; insight-oriented psychotherapy; antiandrogen medication to diminish sexual urge.
Sexual masochism	Sexual pleasure derived from being abused physically or mentally or from being humiliated (moral masochism).	Defense against guilt feelings related to sex—punishment turned inwards.	Insight-oriented psychotherapy; group therapy.
Sexual sadism	Sexual arousal resulting from causing mental or physical suffering to another person.	Mostly seen in men. Named after Marquis de Sade. Can progress to rape in some cases.	Insight-oriented psychotherapy; aversive conditioning.
Transvestic fetishism	Cross-dressing.	Most often used in heterosexual arousal. Most common is male-to-female cross-dressing. Do not confuse with transsexualism-wanting to be opposite sex.	Insight-oriented psychotherapy.
Voyeurism	Sexual arousal by watching sexual acts (e.g., coitus or naked person). Can occur in women but more common in men. Variant is listening to erotic conversations (e.g., telephone sex).	Masturbation usually occurs during voyeuristic activity. Usually arrested for loitering or peeping-tomism.	Insight-oriented psychotherapy; aversive conditioning.
Other paraphilias Excretory paraphilias	Defecating (corprophilia) or urinating (urophilia) on a partner or vice versa.	Fixation at anal stage of development; klismaphilia (enemas).	Insight-oriented psychotherapy.
Zoophilia	Sex with animals.	More common in rural areas; may be opportunistic.	Behavior modification, insight-oriented psychotherapy.

III. Paraphilias

These are disorders characterized by sexual impulses, fantasies, or practices that are unusual, deviant, or bizarre. More common in men than in women. Cause is unknown. A biological predisposition (abnormal electroencephalogram, hormone levels) may be reinforced by psychological factors, such as childhood abuse. Psychoanalytic theory holds that paraphilia results from fixation at one of the psychosexual phases of development or is an effort to ward off castration anxiety. Learning theory holds that association of the act with sexual arousal during childhood leads to conditioned learning.

Paraphiliac activity often is compulsive. Patients repeatedly engage in deviant behavior and are unable to control the impulse. When stressed, anxious, or depressed, the patient is more likely to engage in the deviant behavior. The patient may make numerous resolutions to stop the behavior but is generally unable to abstain for long, and acting out is followed by strong feelings of guilt. Treatment techniques, which result in only moderate success rates, include insight-oriented psychotherapy, behavior therapy, and pharmacotherapy alone or in combination. Table 14–10 lists the common paraphilias.

For more detailed discussion of this topic, see Normal Human Sexuality and Sexual and Gender Identity Disorder, Ch 19, p 1577, in CTP/VII.

15
Eating Disorders and Obesity

I. General introduction

Disorders characterized by a marked disturbance in eating behavior. The two major eating disorders are anorexia nervosa and bulimia nervosa. Obesity is also covered in this chapter. However, it is not a DSM-IV-TR diagnostic category.

II. Anorexia nervosa

A. Definition. A serious and potentially fatal condition characterized by a disturbed body image and self-imposed severe dietary limitations that usually result in serious malnutrition. The range of mortality is 5–18% of patients.

B. Diagnosis, signs, and symptoms. Two types: restricting type (no binge eating) and binge-eating/purging type (Table 15–1).

C. Epidemiology

1. Lifetime prevalence among women is 0.5–3.7%.
2. Onset is usually between the ages of 10 and 30 years; often associated with stressful life event.
3. Male-to-female ratio is 1:10 to 1:20.
4. Most common in professions that require thinness (e.g., modeling, ballet) and in developed countries.

D. Etiology

1. **Biological.** Higher concordance rates in monozygotic twins than in dizygotic twins. An increase in familial depression, alcohol dependence, or eating disorders has been noted. Some evidence of increased anorexia nervosa in sisters and a higher concordance in monozygotic than in dizygotic twins. Neurobiologically, a reduction in 3-methoxy-4-hydroxyphenylglycol (MHPG) in urine and CSF suggests lessened norepinephrine turnover and activity. Endogenous opioid activity appears lessened as a consequence of starvation. In one positron emission tomography (PET) study, caudate nucleus metabolism was higher during the anorectic state than after weight gain. Magnetic resonance imaging (MRI) may show volume deficits of gray matter during illness, which may persist during recovery. A genetic predisposition may be a factor.
2. **Psychological.** Appears to be a reaction to demands for independence and social or sexual functioning in adolescence.
3. **Social.** Society's emphasis on thinness and exercise. Patient may have close but troubled relationship with parents.

E. Psychodynamics

1. Patients are unable to separate psychologically from their mothers.
2. Fear of pregnancy.
3. Repressed sexual or aggressive drives.

TABLE 15-1
DSM-IV-TR DIAGNOSTIC CRITERIA FOR ANOREXIA NERVOSA

A. Refusal to maintain body weight at or above a minimally normal weight for age and height (e.g., weight loss leading to maintenance of body weight less than 85% of that expected; or failure to make expected weight gain during period of growth, leading to body weight less than 85% of that expected).
B. Intense fear of gaining weight or becoming fat, even though underweight.
C. Disturbance in the way in which one's body weight or shape is experienced, undue influence of body weight or shape on self-evaluation, or denial of the seriousness of the current low body weight.
D. In postmenarcheal females, amenorrhea, i.e., the absence of at least three consecutive menstrual cycles. A woman is considered to have amenorrhea if her periods occur only following hormone, e.g., estrogen, administration.

Specify type:
  Restricting type: during the current episode of anorexia nervosa, the person has not regularly engaged in binge-eating or purging behavior (i.e., self-induced vomiting or the misuse of laxatives, diuretics, or enemas)
  Binge-eating/purging type: during the current episode of anorexia nervosa, the person has regularly engaged in binge-eating or purging behavior (i.e., self-induced vomiting or the misuse of laxatives, diuretics, or enemas)

From American Psychiatric Association. *Diagnostic and Statistical Manual of Mental Disorders*, text revision, 4th ed. Washington, DC: American Psychiatric Association, Copyright 2000, with permission.

F. Differential diagnosis

1. **Medical conditions and substance use disorders.** Medical illness, (e.g., cancer, brain tumor, gastrointestinal disorders, drug abuse) that can account for weight loss.

2. **Depressive disorder.** Patient has a decreased appetite; patient with anorexia nervosa claims to have a normal appetite and feel hungry (loss of appetite occurs only late in illness). No preoccupation with caloric content of food. No intense fear of obesity or disturbance of body image. Comorbid major depression or dysthymia has been found in 50% of patients with anorexia.

3. **Somatization disorder.** Weight loss not as severe; no morbid fear of becoming overweight; amenorrhea unusual.

4. **Bulimia nervosa.** Patient's weight loss is seldom more than 15%. Bulimia nervosa develops in 30–50% of patients with anorexia nervosa within 2 years of the onset of anorexia.

G. Course and prognosis. Of these patients, 40% recover, 30% improve, and 30% are chronic cases.

H. Treatment. May be outpatient or inpatient pediatric, medical, or psychiatric unit, depending on degree of weight loss and physical condition. Psychiatry unit is indicated, if physical condition permits, in cases with depression, a high risk for suicide, or a family crisis. Inpatient treatment of starvation provides for (1) ensured weight gain and (2) monitoring and treatment of the potentially life-threatening effects of starvation (and metabolic complications of bulimia nervosa, if present). A desired weight is set and a strategy devised, which may include supervised meals, food supplements, and nasogastric feedings for uncooperative patients.

1. **Pharmacological.** Patients with anorexia nervosa often resist medication, and no drugs are of proven efficacy. Antidepressants are tried if major depressive disorder coexists. Serotoninergic agents (e.g., 40 mg of fluoxetine [Prozac] daily) may be useful. Additionally, weight gain is a side effect of cyproheptadine (Periactin).

2. **Psychological.** Psychosocial treatment and group therapy are educational, supportive, and inspirational. Individual psychodynamic psychotherapy is generally ineffective. Cognitive behavior therapy aimed at changing attitudes and habits concerning food, eating, and body image is of value. Family therapy is useful to deal with relational problems and may help reduce symptoms.

III. Bulimia nervosa

A. Definition.
Episodic, uncontrolled, compulsive, and rapid ingestion of large amounts of food within a short period of time (binge eating) followed by self-induced vomiting, use of laxatives or diuretics, fasting, or vigorous exercise to prevent weight gain (binge and purge).

B. Diagnosis, signs, and symptoms.
See Table 15–2.

C. Epidemiology
1. Lifetime prevalence in women is 1–4%.
2. Age at onset is usually 16 to 18 years.
3. Male-to-female ratio is 1:10.

D. Etiology
1. **Biological.** Metabolic studies indicate decreased norepinephrine and serotonin activity and turnover. Plasma levels of endorphins are raised in some patients with bulimia nervosa after vomiting, which may reinforce behavior. Many are depressed; increased family history of depression and obesity.
2. **Social.** Reflects society's premium on thinness. Patients tend to be perfectionists and achievement-oriented. Family strife, rejection, and neglect are more common than in anorexia nervosa.
3. **Psychological.** Patients have difficulties with adolescent demands, but patients with bulimia nervosa are more outgoing, angry, and impul-

---

TABLE 15–2
DSM-IV-TR DIAGNOSTIC CRITERIA FOR BULIMIA NERVOSA

A. Recurrent episodes of binge eating. An episode of binge eating is characterized by both of the following:
  (1) eating, in a discrete period of time (e.g., within any 2-hour period), an amount of food that is definitely larger than most people would eat during a similar period of time and under similar circumstances
  (2) a sense of lack of control over eating during the episode (e.g., a feeling that one cannot stop eating or control what or how much one is eating)
B. Recurrent inappropriate compensatory behavior in order to prevent weight gain, such as self-induced vomiting; misuse of laxatives, diuretics, enemas, or other medications; fasting; or excessive exercise.
C. The binge eating and inappropriate compensatory behaviors both occur, on average, at least twice a week for 3 months.
D. Self-evaluation is unduly influenced by body shape and weight.
E. The disturbance does not occur exclusively during episodes of anorexia nervosa.

Specify type:
  Purging type: during the current episode of bulimia nervosa, the person has regularly engaged in self-induced vomiting or the misuse of laxatives, diuretics, or enemas
  Nonpurging type: during the current episode of bulimia nervosa, the person has used other inappropriate compensatory behaviors, such as fasting or excessive exercise, but has not regularly engaged in self-induced vomiting or the misuse of laxatives, diuretics, or enemas

From American Psychiatric Association. *Diagnostic and Statistical Manual of Mental Disorders*, text revision, 4th ed. Washington, DC: American Psychiatric Association, Copyright 2000, with permission.

sive than those with anorexia nervosa. They may fear leaving the family to go to school. Anxiety and depressive symptoms are common; suicide is a risk. Alcohol abuse occurs, and approximately one third engage in shoplifting (food).

E. Psychodynamics
1. Struggle for separation from the maternal figure is played out in ambivalence toward food.
2. Sexual and aggressive fantasies are unacceptable and disgorged symbolically.

F. Differential diagnosis
1. **Neurological disease.** Epileptic-equivalent seizures, CNS tumors, Klüver-Bucy syndrome, Kleine-Levin syndrome.
2. **Borderline personality disorder.** Patients sometimes binge eat, but the eating is associated with other signs of the disorder.
3. **Major depressive disorder.** Patients rarely have peculiar attitudes or idiosyncratic practices regarding food.

G. Course and prognosis.
Course is usually chronic but not debilitating when not complicated by electrolyte imbalance and metabolic alkalosis. Sixty percent may recover with treatment; however, relapse rate can approach 50% during a 5-year period.

H. Treatment
1. **Hospitalization.** Electrolyte imbalance, metabolic alkalosis, and suicidality may necessitate hospitalization. Careful attention must be given to the physical complications of bulimia, which can be life-threatening.
2. **Pharmacological.** Antidepressants appear to be more beneficial than in anorexia nervosa. Imipramine (Tofranil), desipramine (Norpramin), trazodone (Desyrel), and the monoamine oxidase inhibitors (e.g., phenelzine [Nardil]) have reduced symptoms in studies. Fluoxetine (Prozac) is also of reported benefit in reducing binge eating and subsequent purging episodes.
3. **Psychological.** Lack of control over eating usually motivates desire for therapy, which may include individual psychotherapy, cognitive behavioral therapy, and group psychotherapy. Normalization of eating habits, attitudes about food, and pursuit of the ideal body must be addressed.

IV. Obesity
A. Definition.
Obesity is a condition characterized by excessive accumulation of fat in the body.

B. Diagnosis.
By convention, obesity is said to be present when body weight exceeds by 20% the standard weight listed in the usual height–weight tables.

Another and more precise measurement of obesity is the amount of fat in the body, or the body mass index (BMI). In general, a healthful BMI is in the range of 20 to 25.

C. **Epidemiology**
  1. More than half of people in the United States are obese.
  2. Obesity is six times more common among women of lower socioeconomic status than among women of higher socioeconomic status.
  3. More common in women than in men.

D. **Etiology**
  1. **Biological.** One theory is that the metabolic signal to the receptors in the hypothalamus after eating may be impaired, so that the sense of hunger remains and the person continues to eat.

    Another theory is that leptin, a hormone made by fat cells, acts as a fat thermostat. When the blood level of leptin is low, more fat is consumed; when the level is high, less fat is consumed. Further research is needed. Evidence suggests that the CNS, particularly the lateral and ventromedial hypothalamic areas, adjusts to food intake in response to changing energy requirements so as to maintain fat stores at a baseline determined by a specific set point. This set point varies from one person to another and depends on height and body build.

  2. **Genetics.** About 80% of patients who are obese have a family history of obesity. Identical twins raised apart can both be obese, an observation that suggests a hereditary role. To date, no specific genetic marker of obesity has been identified.

  3. **Psychological.** No specific mental illness is associated with obesity. Generally, stress produces hyperphagia. Obese persons have to deal with prejudice against them in a society that overvalues youth and slimness.

E. **Psychodynamic.**   Strong dependency needs produce overeating as compensation. For some persons who were not nurtured as children, food equals love and gratifies overall needs. Some persons ward off outside sexual stimuli by becoming obese and less sexually attractive to others.

F. **Differential diagnosis.**   A variety of clinical disorders are associated with obesity. Cushing's disease is associated with a characteristic fat distribution (buffalo adiposity). Myxedema is associated with weight gain, although not invariably. Other neuroendocrine disorders include adiposogenital dystrophy (Fröhlich's syndrome), which is characterized by obesity and sexual and skeletal abnormalities. The prolonged use of serotonergic agonists in the treatment of depression may be associated with weight gain. Certain antipsychotics (especially atypical drugs) are known to cause obesity.

G. **Course and prognosis.**   Obesity has adverse effects on health and is associated with a broad range of illnesses (Table 15–3). Obese men, regardless of smoking habits, have higher rates of mortality from colon, rectal, and prostate cancer than do men of normal weight. Obese women have higher rates of mortality from cancer of the gallbladder, biliary passages, breast (postmenopause), uterus (including cervix and endometrium), and ovaries than do women of normal weight.

   Obesity is associated with earlier mortality overall.

   The prognosis for weight reduction is poor, and the course of obesity tends toward inexorable progression. Of the patients who lose significant amounts of weight, 90% regain it eventually.

TABLE 15–3
HEALTH DISORDERS THOUGHT TO BE CAUSED OR EXACERBATED BY OBESITY

Heart
 Premature coronary heart disease
 Left ventricular hypertrophy
 Angina pectoris
 Sudden death (ventricular arrhythmia)
 Congestive heart failure
Vascular system
 Hypertension
 Cerebrovascular disorder (cerebral infarction or hemorrhage)
 Venous stasis (with lower-extremity edema, varicose veins)
Respiratory system
 Obstructive sleep apnea
 Pickwickian syndrome (alveolar hypoventilation)
 Secondary polycythemia
 Right ventricular hypertrophy (sometimes leading to failure)
Hepatobiliary system
 Cholelithiasis and cholecystitis
 Hepatic steatosis
Hormonal and metabolic functions
 Diabetes mellitus (insulin-independent)
 Gout (hyperuricemia)
 Hyperlipidemias (hypertriglyceridemia and hypercholesterolemia)
Kidney
 Proteinuria and, in very severe obesity, nephrosis
 Renal vein thrombosis
Joints, muscles, and connective tissue
 Osteoarthritis of knees
 Bone spurs of the heel
 Osteoarthrosis of spine (in women)
 Aggravation of preexisting postural faults
Neoplasia
 In woman: increased risk of cancer of endometrium, breast, cervix, ovary, gallbladder, and biliary passages
 In men: increased risk of cancer of colon, rectum, and prostate

From Van Itallie TB. Obesity: adverse effects on health and longevity. *Am J Clin Nutr* 1979;32:2723, with permission.

H. Treatment

1. **Diet.** In general, the best method of weight loss is a balanced diet of 1,100 to 1,200 calories. Such a diet can be followed for long periods but should be supplemented with vitamins, particularly iron, folic acid, zinc, and vitamin B_6. Unmodified fasts are used for short-term weight loss, but associated morbidity includes orthostatic hypotension, sodium diuresis, and impaired nitrogen balance.

2. **Exercise.** Increased physical activity may actually cause a decrease in food intake for formerly sedentary people. The combination of increased caloric expenditure and decreased food intake makes an increase in physical activity a highly desirable feature of any weight-reduction program. Exercise also helps maintain weight loss.

3. **Pharmacotherapy.** Various drugs, some more effective than others, are used to treat obesity. Table 15–4 lists the drugs currently available. An initial trial period of 4 weeks with a specific drug can be used; then, if the patient responds with weight loss, the drug can be continued to determine whether tolerance develops. If a drug remains effective, it can be dispensed until the desired weight is achieved. Some drugs (e.g., sibu-

TABLE 15–4
DRUGS FOR THE TREATMENT OF OBESITY

Generic Name	Trade Name	Usual Dosage (mg/d)
Orlistat[a]	Xenical	260
Sibutramine[b]	Meridia	10–20
Phentermine	Adipex-P, Fastin, Ionamin	15–37.5
Phendimetrazine	Bontril SR, Prelu-2, Plegine	70–105
Benzphetamine	Didrex	75–150
Diethylpropion	Tenuate	75
Mazindol	Anorex, Mazanor	3–9
Phenylpropanolamine	Dexatrim, Acutrim	75

[a] Lipase inhibitor that decreases fat absorption by 30%.
[b] Serotonin–norepinephrine reuptake inhibitor.

tramine [Meridia], orlistat [Xenical]) are also used to maintain a healthful weight.

4. **Surgery.** *Gastric bypass* is a procedure in which the stomach is made smaller by transecting or stapling one of its curvatures. In *gastroplasty,* the size of the stomach stoma is reduced so that the passage of food slows. Results are successful, although vomiting, electrolyte imbalance, and obstruction may occur.

5. **Psychotherapy.** Behavior modification has been the most successful of the psychotherapies. Patients are taught to recognize eating cues and develop patterns of eating behavior.

Group therapy helps to maintain motivation, promote identification among members who have lost weight, and provide education about nutrition. Insight-oriented psychotherapy generally has not proved useful.

For more detailed discussion of this topic, see Eating Disorders and Obesity, Ch 15, p 1663, in CTP/VII.

16

Sleep Disorders

I. General introduction

About one third of all adults in the United States experience a sleep disorder during their lifetime. More than half of persons do not seek treatment for sleep problems. Insomnia is the most common of many types of sleep disorders. Disturbed sleep can be a component of another medical or psychiatric disorder (Table 16–1) or can be a primary diagnosis itself. Careful diagnosis and specific treatment are essential. Sleep disorders can have serious consequences, including fatal accidents related to sleepiness. Female sex, advanced age, medical and mental disorders, and substance abuse are associated with an increased prevalence of sleep disorders.

In DSM-IV-TR, sleep disorders are classified on the basis of clinical diagnostic criteria and presumed etiology. The three major categories are (1) primary sleep disorders, (2) sleep disorders related to another mental disorder, and (3) other sleep disorders (due to a general medical condition and substance-induced).

A. Sleep stages. Sleep is measured with a polysomnograph, which simultaneously measures brain activity (EEG), eye movement (electrooculogram), and muscle tone (electromyogram). Other physiological tests can be applied during sleep and measured along with the above. EEG findings are used to describe sleep stages (Table 16–2).

It takes the average person 15 to 20 minutes to fall asleep. During the next 45 minutes, one descends to stages III and IV (deepest sleep, largest stimulus needed to arouse). Approximately 45 minutes after stage IV, the first rapid eye movement (REM) period is reached (average REM latency is 90 minutes). As the night progresses, each REM period becomes longer, and stages III and IV disappear. Further into the night, persons sleep more lightly and dream (REM sleep).

B. Characteristics of REM sleep
   1. Tonic inhibition of skeletal muscle tone.
   2. Reduced hypercapnic respiratory drive.
   3. Relative poikilothermia (cold-bloodedness).
   4. Penile tumescence or vaginal lubrication.

C. Sleep and aging
   1. Subjective reports of elderly.
      a. Time in bed increases.
      b. Number of nocturnal awakenings increases.
      c. Total sleep time at night decreases.
      d. Time to fall asleep increases.
      e. Dissatisfaction with sleep.

      f. Tired and sleepy in the daytime.

      g. More frequent napping.

  2. Objective evidence of age-related changes in sleep cycle.

      a. Reduced total REM sleep.

      b. Reduced stages III and IV.

      c. Frequent awakenings.

      d. Reduced duration of nocturnal sleep.

      e. Need for daytime naps.

      f. Propensity for phase advance.

  3. Certain sleep disorders are more common in the elderly.

      a. Nocturnal myoclonus.

      b. Restless legs syndrome.

      c. REM sleep behavior disturbance.

      d. Sleep apnea.

      e. Sundowning (confusion from sedation).

  4. Medications and medical disorders also contribute to the problem.

TABLE 16–1
COMMON CAUSES OF INSOMNIA

Symptom	Insomnias Secondary to Medical Conditions	Insomnias Secondary to Psychiatric or Environmental Conditions
Difficulty in falling asleep	Any painful or uncomfortable condition CNS lesions Conditions listed below, at times	Anxiety Tension anxiety, muscular Environmental changes Circadian rhythm sleep disorder
Difficulty in remaining asleep	Sleep apnea syndromes Nocturnal myoclonus and restless legs syndrome Dietary factors (probably) Episodic events (parasomnias) Direct substance effects (including alcohol) Substance withdrawal effects (including alcohol) Substance interactions Endocrine or metabolic diseases Infectious, neoplastic, or other diseases Painful or uncomfortable conditions Brainstem or hypothalamic lesions or diseases Aging	Depression, especially primary depression Environmental changes Circadian rhythm sleep disorder Posttraumatic stress disorder Schizophrenia

Courtesy of Ernest L. Hartmann, M.D.

TABLE 16–2
SLEEP STAGES

Awake	Low voltage, random, very fast
Drowsiness	Alpha waves random and fast (8 to 12 CPS)
Stage I	Slight slowing, 3 to 7 CPS, theta waves
Stage II	Further slowing, K complex (triphasic complexes), 12 to 14 CPS (sleep spindles); this stage marks the onset of true sleep
Stage III	High-amplitude slow waves (delta waves) at 0.5 to 2.5 CPS
Stage IV	At least 50% delta waves on EEG (stages III and IV constitute delta sleep)
REM sleep	Sawtooth waves, similar to drowsy sleep on EEG

CPS, cycles per second.

II. Primary sleep disorders

Sleep disorders caused by an abnormal sleep–wake mechanism and often by conditioning. Primary sleep disorders are not caused by another mental disorder, a physical condition, or a substance. Primary sleep disorders are categorized as dyssomnias and parasomnias.

A. Dyssomnias.   Characterized by abnormalities in the quality, amount, or timing of sleep.

   1. Primary insomnia. Diagnosed when the chief complaint is nonrestorative sleep or difficulty in initiating or maintaining sleep for at least 1 month.

   a. Treatment can include deconditioning techniques, transcendental meditation, relaxation tapes, or sedative-hypnotic drugs.

   b. Nonspecific measures (sleep hygiene) are described in Table 16–3.

   2. Primary hypersomnia. Diagnosed when no other cause for excessive somnolence occurring for at least 1 month can be found. Treatment consists of stimulant drugs (e.g., amphetamines) taken in the morning or early evening.

   3. Narcolepsy

   a. Characterized by symptom tetrad—(1) excessive daytime somnolence, (2) cataplexy, (3) sleep paralysis, and (4) hypnagogic hallucinations. Narcolepsy is an abnormality of REM-inhibiting mechanisms (sleep attacks).

   (1) Excessive daytime somnolence.

   (a) Considered to be the primary symptom of narcolepsy; others are auxiliary.

   (b) Distinguished from fatigue by irresistible sleep attacks of short duration—less than 15 minutes.

   (c) Sleep attacks may be precipitated by monotonous or sedentary activity.

   (d) Naps are highly refreshing—effects last 30 to 120 minutes.

   (2) Cataplexy.

   (a) Reported by 70–80% of narcoleptic patients.

   (b) Brief (seconds to minutes) episodes of muscle weakness or paralysis.

   (c) No loss of consciousness if episode is brief.

TABLE 16–3
NONSPECIFIC MEASURES TO INDUCE SLEEP (SLEEP HYGIENE)

1. Arise at the same time daily.
2. Limit daily in-bed time to the usual amount before the sleep disturbance.
3. Discontinue CNS-acting drugs (caffeine, nicotine, alcohol, stimulants).
4. Avoid daytime naps (except when sleep chart shows they induce better night sleep).
5. Establish physical fitness by means of a graded program of vigorous exercise early in the day.
6. Avoid evening stimulation; substitute radio or relaxed reading for television.
7. Try very hot, 20-minute, body temperature-raising bath soaks near bedtime.
8. Eat at regular times daily; avoid large meals near bedtime.
9. Practice evening relaxation routines, such as progressive muscle relaxation or meditation.
10. Maintain comfortable sleeping conditions.

From Regestein QR. Sleep disorders. In: Stoudemire A, ed. *Clinical Psychiatry for Medical Students.* Philadelphia: Lippincott, 1990:578.

(d) When attack is over, the patient is completely normal.
(e) Often triggered by the following:
- (i) Laughter (common).
- (ii) Anger (common).
- (iii) Athletic activity.
- (iv) Excitement or elation.
- (v) Sexual intercourse.
- (vi) Fear.
- (vii) Embarrassment.

(f) Flat affect or lack of expressiveness develops in some patients as an attempt to control emotions.
(g) May manifest as partial loss of muscle tone (weakness, slurred speech, buckled knees, dropped jaw).

(3) Sleep paralysis.
- (a) Reported by 25–50% of general population.
- (b) Temporary partial or complete paralysis in sleep–wake transitions.
- (c) Most commonly occurs on awakening.
- (d) Conscious but unable to move.
- (e) Generally lasts less than 1 minute.

(4) Hypnagogic hallucinations.
- (a) Dreamlike experience during transition from wakefulness to sleep.
- (b) Patient is aware of surroundings.
- (c) Vivid auditory or visual hallucinations or illusions.
- (d) Appear several years after onset of sleep attacks.

b. Sleep-onset REM periods (SOREMPs).
(1) Narcolepsy can be distinguished from other disorders of excessive daytime sleepiness by SOREMPs.
(2) Defined as appearance of REM within 10 to 15 minutes of onset of sleep.
(3) Multiple sleep latency test (MSLT) measures excessive sleepiness—several recorded naps at 2-hour intervals. More than one SOREMP is considered diagnostic of narcolepsy (seen in 70% of patients with narcolepsy, in fewer than 10% of patients with other hypersomnias).

c. Increased incidence of other clinical findings in narcolepsy.
(1) Periodic leg movement.
(2) Sleep apnea—predominantly central.
(3) Short sleep latency.
(4) Memory problems.
(5) Ocular symptoms—blurring, diplopia, flickering.
(6) Depression.

d. Onset and clinical course.
(1) Insidious onset before age 15. Once established, condition is chronic without major remissions.
(2) Typically, full syndrome emerges in late adolescence or early 20s.

(3) A long delay may occur between the earliest symptoms (excessive somnolence) and the late appearance of cataplexy.

e. Human leukocyte antigen (HLA)-DR2 and narcolepsy.

(1) Strong association between narcolepsy and HLA-DR2, a type of human lymphocyte antigen.

(2) Some experts maintain that the presence of HLA-DR2 is necessary for the diagnosis of idiopathic narcolepsy.

f. Treatment.

(1) Regular bedtime.

(2) Daytime naps.

(3) Safety considerations, such as caution in driving or avoiding furniture with sharp edges.

(4) Stimulants (e.g., modafinil [Provigil]) for daytime sleepiness. High-dose propranolol (Inderal) may be effective.

(5) Tricyclics and monoamine oxidase inhibitors for REM-related symptoms, especially cataplexy (Table 16–4).

3. **Breathing-related sleep disorder.** Characterized by sleep disruption leading to excessive sleepiness or insomnia that is caused by a sleep-related breathing disturbance. The three types of sleep apnea are (1) obstructive, (2) central, and (3) mixed.

   a. **Obstructive sleep apnea**

      (1) Typically occurs in older, middle-aged, overweight men.

      (2) Main symptoms are loud snoring with intervals of apnea.

      (3) Extreme daytime sleepiness with long and unrefreshing daytime sleep attacks.

      (4) Patients unaware of episodes of apnea.

      (5) Other symptoms include severe morning headaches, morning confusion, depression, and anxiety.

TABLE 16–4
NARCOLEPSY DRUGS CURRENTLY AVAILABLE

Drug	Maximal Daily Dosage (mg) (All Drugs Administered Orally)
Treatment of excessive daytime somnolence (EDS)	
Stimulants	
Methylphenidate	≤60
Pemoline	≤150
Modafinil	≤400
Amphetamine–dextroamphetamine	≤60
Dextroamphetamine	≤60
Adjunct-effect drugs (i.e., improve EDS if associated with stimulant)	
Protriptyline	≤10
Treatment of cataplexy, sleep paralysis, and hypnogogic hallucinations	
Tricyclic antidepressants (with atropine-like side effects)	
Protriptyline	≤20
Imipramine	≤200
Clomipramine	≤200
Desipramine	≤200
Antidepressants (without major atropine-like side effects)	
Bupropion	≤300

Adapted from Guilleminault C. Narcolepsy syndrome. In: Kryger MH, Roth T, Dement WC, eds. *Principles and Practice of Sleep Medicine*. Philadelphia: Saunders, 1989:344, with permission.

(6) Findings include hypertension, arrhythmias, right-sided heart failure, and peripheral edema; progressively worsens without treatment.

(7) Sleep laboratory evaluation reveals cessation of air flow in the presence of continued thoracic breathing movements.

(8) In severe cases, patients have more than 500 episodes of apnea a night.

(9) Each lasts 10 to 20 seconds.

(10) Treatment consists of nasal continuous positive airway pressure (CPAP), uvulopharyngopalatoplasty, weight loss, or tricyclic drugs, which reduce REM periods, the stage during which obstructive apnea is usually more frequent. If a specific abnormality of the upper airway is found, surgical intervention is indicated.

b. Central sleep apnea

(1) Rare.

(2) Cessation of air flow secondary to lack of respiratory effort.

(3) Treatment consists of mechanical ventilation or nasal CPAP.

c. Mixed type. Elements of both obstructive and central sleep apnea.

d. Central alveolar hypoventilation. Central apnea followed by an obstructive phase.

(1) Impaired ventilation in which the respiratory abnormality appears or greatly worsens only during sleep and in which significant apneic episodes are absent.

(2) The ventilatory dysfunction is characterized by inadequate tidal volume or respiratory rate during sleep.

(3) Death may occur during sleep (Ondine's curse).

(4) Central alveolar hypoventilation is treated with some form of mechanical ventilation (e.g., nasal ventilation).

4. Circadian rhythm sleep disorder. Includes a wide range of conditions involving a misalignment between desired and actual sleep periods.

a. Transient disturbances associated with jet lag and changes in work shifts.

(1) Self-limited. Resolves as body readjusts to new sleep–wake schedule.

(2) Adjusting to an advance of sleep time is more difficult than adjusting to a delay.

b. Disturbances include (1) delayed sleep phase type, (2) jet lag type, (3) shift work type, and (4) unspecified type (e.g., advanced sleep phase, non–24-hour, and irregular or disorganized sleep–wake pattern).

(1) Quality of sleep basically is normal, but timing is off.

(2) Patient can adjust through gradual delay of sleep time until new schedule is achieved.

c. Most effective treatment of sleep–wake schedule disorders is a regular schedule of bright light therapy to entrain the sleep cycle. More useful in transient than in persistent disturbances. Melatonin, a natural hormone produced by the pineal gland that induces sleep, has been used orally to alter sleep–wake cycles, but its effect is uncertain.

5. Dyssomnia not otherwise specified

a. Periodic leg movement disorder (formerly called *nocturnal myoclonus*).

  (1) Stereotypic, periodic leg movements (every 30 seconds).
  (2) No seizure activity.
  (3) Most prevalent in patients over age 55.
  (4) Frequent awakenings.
  (5) Unrefreshing sleep.
  (6) Daytime sleepiness a major symptom.
  (7) Patient unaware of the myoclonic events.
  (8) Various drugs have been reported to help. These include clonazepam (Klonopin), opioids, and levodopa (Larodopa).

b. Restless legs syndrome

  (1) Uncomfortable sensations in legs at rest.
  (2) Not limited to sleep, but can interfere wtih falling asleep.
  (3) Relieved by movement.
  (4) Patient may have associated sleep-related myoclonus.
  (5) Benzodiazepines (e.g., clonazepam) are the treatment of choice. In severe cases, levodopa or opioids may be used.

c. Kleine-Levin syndrome

  (1) Periodic disorder of hypersomnolence.
  (2) Usually affects young men, who sleep excessively for several weeks.
  (3) Patient awakens only to eat (voraciously).
  (4) Associated with hypersexuality and extreme hostility.
  (5) Amnesia follows attacks.
  (6) May resolve spontaneously after several years.
  (7) Patients are normal between episodes.
  (8) Treatment consists of stimulants (amphetamines, methylphenidate [Ritalin], and pemoline [Cylert]) for hypersomnia and preventive measures for other symptoms. Lithium also has been used successfully.

d. Menstruation-associated syndrome. Some women experience intermittent marked hypersomnia, altered behavior patterns, and voracious eating at or shortly before the onset of menses.

e. Insufficient sleep. Characterized by complaints of daytime sleepiness, irritability, inability to concentrate, and impaired judgment by a person who persistently fails to sleep enough to support alert wakefulness.

f. Sleep drunkenness

  (1) Inability to become fully alert for sustained period after awakening.
  (2) Most commonly seen in persons with sleep apnea or after sustained sleep deprivation.
  (3) Can occur as an isolated disorder.
  (4) No specific treatment. Stimulants may be of limited value.

g. **Altitude insomnia**
   (1) Insomnia secondary to change in sleep onset ventilatory set point and resulting breathing problems.
   (2) More severe at higher altitudes as oxygen level declines.
   (3) Patients may awaken with apnea.
   (4) Acetazolamide (Diamox) can increase ventilatory drive and decrease hypoxemia.

B. Parasomnias

1. Nightmare disorder
   a. Nightmares almost always occur during REM sleep.
   b. Can occur at any time of night.
   c. Good recall (quite detailed).
   d. Long, frightening dream in which one awakens frightened.
   e. Less anxiety, vocalization, motility, and autonomic discharge than in sleep terrors.
   f. No specific treatment; benzodiazepines may be of help.

2. Sleep terror disorder
   a. Especially common in children.
   b. Sudden awakening with intense anxiety.
   c. Autonomic overstimulation.
   d. Movement.
   e. Crying out.
   f. Patient does not remember the event.
   g. Occurs during deep, non-REM sleep.
   h. Often occurs within the first hour or two of sleep.
   i. Treatment rarely needed in childhood.
   j. Awakening child before regular night terror for several days may eliminate terrors for extended periods.

3. Sleepwalking disorder
   a. Also known as *somnambulism*.
   b. Most common in children; generally disappears spontaneously with age.
   c. Patients often have familial history of other parasomnias.
   d. Complex activity—leaving bed and walking about without full consciousness.
   e. Episodes brief.
   f. Amnesia for the event—patient does not remember the episode.
   g. Occurs during deep non-REM sleep.
   h. Initiated during first third of the night.
   i. In adults and elderly persons, may reflect psychopathology—rule out CNS pathology.
   j. Can sometimes be initiated by placing a child who is in stage IV sleep in the standing position.
   k. Potentially dangerous.
   l. Drugs that suppress stage IV sleep, such as benzodiazepines, can be used to treat somnambulism.
   m. Precautions include window guards and other measures to prevent injury.

4. Parasomnia not otherwise specified

a. Sleep bruxism

(1) Primarily occurs in stages I and II or during partial arousals or transitions.

(2) No EEG abnormality (no seizure activity).

(3) Treatment consists of bite plates to prevent dental damage.

b. REM sleep behavior disorder

(1) Chronic and progressive, chiefly in elderly men.

(2) Loss of atonia during REM sleep, with emergence of complex and violent behaviors.

(3) Potential for serious injury.

(4) Neurological cause in many cases.

(5) May occur as rebound to sleep deprivation.

(6) Treat with 0.5 to 2.0 mg of clonazepam daily, or 100 mg of carbamazepine (Tegretol) three times daily.

c. Sleep talking (somniloquy)

(1) Sometimes accompanies night terrors and sleepwalking.

(2) Requires no treatment.

d. Rhythmic movement disorder (*jactatio capitis nocturna*)

(1) Rhythmic head or body rocking just before or during sleep; may extend into light sleep.

(2) Usually limited to childhood.

(3) Usually observed in period immediately before sleep; sustained into light sleep.

(4) No treatment required in most infants and young children. Crib padding or helmets may be used. Behavior modification, benzodiazepines, and tricyclic drugs may be effective.

e. Sleep paralysis

(1) Isolated symptom.

(2) Not associated with narcolepsy.

(3) Episode terminates with touch, noise (some external stimulus), or voluntary repetitive eye movements.

e. Other. Confusional arousals, sleep starts, nocturnal leg cramps, impaired or painful sleep-related penile erections, REM sleep-related sinus arrest, sleep enuresis, nocturnal paroxysmal dystonia, sleep-related abnormal swallowing syndrome, and primary snoring.

III. Sleep disorders related to another mental disorder

A. Insomnia that is related to a mental disorder (e.g., major depressive disorder, panic disorder, schizophrenia) and that lasts for at least 1 month. In 35% of patients who present to sleep disorder centers with a complaint of insomnia, the underlying cause is a psychiatric disorder. Half of these patients have major depression.

B. Hypersomnia related to a mental disorder is usually found in a variety of conditions (e.g., the early stages of mild depressive disorder, grief, personality disorders, dissociative disorders, and somatoform disorders).

IV. Other sleep disorders

A. Sleep disorder resulting from a general medical condition

1. Insomnia, hypersomnia, parasomnia, or combination can be caused by a general medical condition.

    a. Sleep-related epileptic seizures—seizures occur almost exclusively during sleep.

    b. Sleep-related cluster headaches and chronic paroxysmal hemicrania.

    (1) Sleep-related cluster headaches are severe and unilateral, appear often during sleep, and are marked by an on–off pattern of attacks.

    (2) Chronic paroxysmal hemicrania is a unilateral headache that occurs frequently and has a sudden onset.

    c. Sleep-related asthma—asthma that is exacerbated by sleep; in some people, may result in significant sleep disturbances.

    d. Sleep-related cardiovascular symptoms—associated with disorders of cardiac rhythm, myocardial incompetence, coronary artery insufficiency, and blood pressure variability that may be induced or exacerbated by alterations in cardiovascular physiology during sleep.

    e. Sleep-related gastroesophageal reflux—patient awakes from sleep with burning substernal pain, a feeling of tightness or pain in the chest, or a sour taste in the mouth. Often associated with hiatal hernia.

    f. Sleep-related hemolysis (paroxysmal nocturnal hemoglobinuria)—rare, acquired, chronic hemolytic anemia. The hemolysis and consequent hemoglobinuria are accelerated during sleep, so that the morning urine appears brownish red.

2. Treatment, whenever possible, should be of the underlying medical condition.

B. Substance-induced sleep disorder.
Insomnia, hypersomnia, parasomnia, or combination caused by the use a medication or by intoxication or withdrawal from a drug of abuse.

1. Somnolence can be related to tolerance or withdrawal from a CNS stimulant or to sustained use of CNS depressants.

2. Insomnia is associated with tolerance to or withdrawal from sedative-hypnotic drugs and CNS stimulants, and with long-term alcohol consumption.

3. Sleep problems may occur as a side effect of many drugs (e.g., antimetabolites, thyroid preparations, anticonvulsant agents, antidepressants).

For a more detailed discussion of this topic, see Sleep Disorders, Ch 21, p 1677, in CTP/VII.

17

Impulse-Control and Adjustment Disorders

I. Impulse-control disorders not elsewhere classified

A. Definition. Patients with disorders of impulse control do not resist impulses, drives, or enticements to do something harmful to themselves or others. Patients may or may not consciously try to resist the impulses, and they may or may not plan their behaviors. Patients sense increasing tension or arousal before they act; afterward, they experience feelings of pleasure, satisfaction, or freedom and may or may not feel sincere remorse, guilt, or self-reproach. The six DSM-IV-TR categories are the following:

1. **Intermittent explosive disorder**—episodes of aggression resulting in harm to others.
2. **Kleptomania**—repeated shoplifting or stealing.
3. **Pathologicalal gambling**—repeated episodes of gambling that result in socioeconomic disruption, indebtedness, and illegal activities.
4. **Pyromania**—deliberately setting fires.
5. **Trichotillomania**—compulsive hair pulling that produces bald spots (alopecia areata).
6. **Impulse-control disorder not otherwise specified**—residual category. Examples: compulsive buying, internet addiction, compulsive sexual behavior.

B. Diagnosis, signs, and symptoms. See Tables 17–1 through 17–5.

C. Epidemiology

1. Intermittent explosive disorder, pathological gambling, pyromania—affected men outnumber affected women.
2. Kleptomania, trichotillomania—women are affected more often than men.
3. Pathological gambling—affects 1–3% of adult population in the United States.

D. Etiology. Usually unknown. Some disorders (e.g., intermittent explosive disorder) may be associated with abnormal electroencephalogram (EEG) results, mixed cerebral dominance, or soft neurological signs. Alcohol reduces the patient's ability to control impulses (disinhibition).

E. Psychodynamics. Acting out of impulses related to the need to express sexual or aggressive drive. Gambling often is associated with underlying depression and represents an unconscious need to lose and experience punishment.

F. Differential diagnosis. See Table 17–6.

1. **Temporal lobe epilepsy.** Characteristic foci of EEG abnormalities in the temporal lobe account for aggressive outbursts, kleptomania, or pyromania.

TABLE 17–1
DSM-IV-TR DIAGNOSTIC CRITERIA FOR INTERMITTENT EXPLOSIVE DISORDER

A. Several discrete episodes of failure to resist aggressive impulses that result in serious assaultive acts or destruction of property.
B. The degree of aggressiveness expressed during the episodes is grossly out of proportion to any precipitating psychosocial stressors.
C. The aggressive episodes are not better accounted for by another mental disorder (e.g., antisocial personality disorder, borderline personality disorder, a psychotic disorder, a manic episode, conduct disorder, or attention-deficit/hyperactivity disorder) and are not due to the direct physiological effects of a substance (e.g., a drug of abuse, a medication) or a general medical condition (e.g., head trauma, Alzheimer's disease).

From American Psychiatric Association. *Diagnostic and Statistical Manual of Mental Disorders*, text revision, 4th ed. Washington, DC: American Psychiatric Association, Copyright 2000, with permission.

TABLE 17–2
DSM-IV-TR DIAGNOSTIC CRITERIA FOR KLEPTOMANIA

A. Recurrent failure to resist impulses to steal objects that are not needed for personal use or for their monetary value.
B. Increasing sense of tension immediately before committing the theft.
C. Pleasure, gratification, or relief at the time of committing the theft.
D. The stealing is not committed to express anger or vengeance and is not in response to a delusion or a hallucination.
E. The stealing is not better accounted for by conduct disorder, a manic episode, or antisocial personality disorder.

From American Psychiatric Association. *Diagnostic and Statistical Manual of Mental Disorders*, text revision, 4th ed. Washington, DC: American Psychiatric Association, Copyright 2000, with permission.

TABLE 17–3
DSM-IV-TR DIAGNOSTIC CRITERIA FOR PYROMANIA

A. Deliberate and purposeful fire setting on more than one occasion.
B. Tension or affective arousal before the act.
C. Fascination with, interest in, curiosity about, or attraction to fire and its situational contexts (e.g., paraphernalia, uses, consequences).
D. Pleasure, gratification, or relief when setting fires, or when witnessing or participating in their aftermath.
E. The fire setting is not done for monetary gain, as an expression of sociopolitical ideology, to conceal criminal activity, to express anger or vengeance, to improve one's living circumstances, in response to a delusion or hallucination, or as a result of impaired judgment (e.g., in dementia, mental retardation, substance intoxication).
F. The fire setting is not better accounted for by conduct disorder, a manic episode, or antisocial personality disorder.

From American Psychiatric Association. *Diagnostic and Statistical Manual of Mental Disorders*, text revision, 4th ed. Washington, DC: American Psychiatric Association, Copyright 2000, with permission.

TABLE 17–4
DSM-IV-TR DIAGNOSTIC CRITERIA FOR PATHOLOGICAL GAMBLING

A. Persistent and recurrent maladaptive gambling behavior as indicated by five (or more) of the following:
    (1) is preoccupied with gambling (e.g., preoccupied with reliving past gambling experiences, handicapping or planning the next venture, or thinking of ways to get money with which to gamble)
    (2) needs to gamble with increasing amounts of money in order to achieve the desired excitement
    (3) has repeated unsuccessful efforts to control, cut back, or stop gambling
    (4) is restless or irritable when attempting to cut down or stop gambling
    (5) gambles as a way of escaping from problems or of relieving a dysphoric mood (e.g., feelings of helplessness, guilt, anxiety, depression)
    (6) after losing money gambling, often returns another day to get even ("chasing" one's losses)
    (7) lies to family members, therapist, or others to conceal the extent of involvement with gambling
    (8) has committed illegal acts such as forgery, fraud, theft, or embezzlement to finance gambling
    (9) has jeopardized or lost a significant relationship, job, or educational or career opportunity because of gambling
    (10) relies on others to provide money to relieve a desperate financial situation caused by gambling
B. The gambling behavior is not better accounted for by a manic episode.

From American Psychiatric Association. *Diagnostic and Statistical Manual of Mental Disorders*, text revision, 4th ed. Washington, DC: American Psychiatric Association, Copyright 2000, with permission.

TABLE 17–5
DSM-IV-TR DIAGNOSTIC CRITERIA FOR TRICHOTILLOMANIA

A. Recurrent pulling out of one's hair resulting in noticeable hair loss.
B. An increasing sense of tension immediately before pulling out the hair or when attempting to resist the behavior.
C. Pleasure, gratification, or relief when pulling out the hair.
D. The disturbance is not better accounted for by another mental disorder and is not due to a general medical condition (e.g., a dermatological condition).
E. The disturbance causes clinically significant distress or impairment in social, occupational, or other important areas of functioning.

From American Psychiatric Association. *Diagnostic and Statistical Manual of Mental Disorders,* text revision, 4th ed. Washington, DC: American Psychiatric Association, Copyright 2000, with permission.

TABLE 17–6
DIFFERENTIAL DIAGNOSIS, COURSE, AND PROGNOSIS FOR IMPULSE-CONTROL DISORDERS

Disorder	Differential Diagnosis	Course and Prognosis
Intermittent explosive disorder	Delirium, dementia Personality change due to a general medical condition, aggressive type Substance intoxication or withdrawal Oppositional defiant disorder, conduct disorder, antisocial disorder, manic episode, schizophrenia Purposeful behavior, malingering Temporal lobe epilepsy	May increase in severity with time
Kleptomania	Ordinary theft Malingering Antisocial personality disorder, conduct disorder Manic episode Delusions, hallucinations, (e.g., schizophrenia) Dementia Temporal lobe epilepsy	Frequently arrested for shoplifting
Pyromania	Arson: profit, sabotage, revenge, political statement Childhood experimentation Conduct disorder Manic episode Antisocial personality disorder Delusions, hallucinations (e.g., schizophrenia) Dementia Mental retardation Substance intoxication Temporal lobe epilepsy	Often produces increasingly larger fires over time
Pathological gambling	Social or professional gambling Manic episode Antisocial personality disorder	Progressive, with increasing financial losses, writing bad checks, total deterioration
Trichotillomania	Alopecia areata, male pattern baldness, chronic discoid lupus erythematosus, lichen planopilaris, or other cause of alopecia Obsessive-compulsive disorder Stereotypic movement disorder Delusion, hallucination Factitious disorder	Remissions and exacerbations

2. **Head trauma.** Brain imaging techniques show residual signs of trauma.

3. **Bipolar I disorder.** Gambling may be an associated feature of manic episodes.

4. **Substance-related disorder.** History of drug or alcohol use or a positive test result on drug screen may suggest that the behavior is drug- or alcohol-related.

5. **Medical condition.** Rule out organic disorder, brain tumor, degenerative disease, and endocrine disorder on the basis of characteristic findings for each.

6. **Schizophrenia.** Shows delusions or hallucinations to account for acting out of impulse.

G. **Course and prognosis.**   See Table 17–6. Course usually is chronic for all impulse-control disorders.

H. **Treatment**

1. **Intermittent explosive disorder.** Combined pharmacotherapy and psychotherapy. May have to try different medications (e.g., β-adrenergic receptor antagonists, anticonvulsants [carbamazepine (Tegretol)], lithium [Eskalith]) before result is achieved. Serotonergic drugs such as buspirone (BuSpar), trazodone (Desyrel), and SSRIs (e.g., fluoxetine [Prozac]) may be helpful. Benzodiazepines can aggravate the condition through disinhibition. Other measures include supportive psychotherapy, setting limits, and family therapy if the patient is a child or adolescent. Group therapy must be used cautiously if the patient is liable to attack fellow group members.

2. **Kleptomania.** Insight-oriented psychotherapy to understand motivation (e.g., guilt, need for punishment) and control impulse. Behavior therapy to learn new patterns of behavior. SSRIs, tricyclics, trazodone, lithium, and valproate (Depacon) may be effective in some patients.

3. **Pathological gambling.** Insight-oriented psychotherapy coupled with peer support groups, especially Gamblers Anonymous. Total abstinence is the goal. Treat associated depression, mania, substance abuse, or sexual dysfunction. Family therapy may be helpful.

4. **Pyromania.** Insight-oriented therapy, behavior therapy. Patients require close supervision because of repeated fire-setting behavior and consequent danger to others. May require inpatient facility, night hospital, or other structured setting.

5. **Trichotillomania.** Supportive and insight-oriented psychotherapies are of value, but medications may also be required: benzodiazepines for patients with high level of anxiety; antidepressant drugs, especially serotoninergic agents (e.g., SSRIs, clomipramine [Anafranil]), for patients with or without depressed mood. Consider hypnosis and biofeedback in some cases.

II. Adjustment disorders

A. **Definition.**   Defined in DSM-IV-TR as "clinically significant emotional or behavioral symptoms" that develop "in response to an identifiable psychosocial stressor or stressors." The reaction should be disproportionate to

TABLE 17–7
DSM-IV DIAGNOSTIC CRITERIA FOR ADJUSTMENT DISORDERS

A. The development of emotional or behavioral symptoms in response to an identifiable stressor(s) occurring within 3 months of the onset of the stressor(s).
B. These symptoms or behaviors are clinically significant as evidenced by either of the following:
  (1) marked distress that is in excess of what would be expected from exposure to the stressor
  (2) significant impairment in social or occupational (academic) functioning
C. The stress-related disturbance does not meet the criteria for another specific Axis I disorder and is not merely an exacerbation of a preexisting Axis I or Axis II disorder.
D. The symptoms do not represent bereavement.
E. Once the stressor (or its consequences) has terminated, the symptoms do not persist for more than an additional 6 months.

Specify if:
  Acute: If the disturbance lasts less than 6 months
  Chronic: If the disturbance lasts for 6 months or longer

Adjustment disorders are coded based on the subtype, which is selected to the predominant symptoms. The specific stressor(s) can be specified on Axis IV.
  With depressed mood
  With anxiety
  With mixed anxiety and depressed mood
  With disturbance of conduct
  With mixed disturbance of emotions and conduct
  Unspecified

From American Psychiatric Association. *Diagnostic and Statistical Manual of Mental Disorders*, text revision, 4th ed. Washington, DC: American Psychiatric Association, Copyright 2000, with permission.

the nature of the stressor, or social or occupational functioning should be significantly impaired. Stressors are within the range of normal experience (e.g., birth of a baby, going away to school, marriage, loss of job, divorce, illness).

B. Diagnosis, signs, and symptoms.   See Table 17–7.

C. Epidemiology.   Most frequent in adolescence, but can occur at any age.

D. Etiology

1. **Genetic.** High-anxiety temperament more prone to overreacting to a stressful event and experiencing subsequent adjustment disorder.

2. **Biological.** Greater vulnerability with history of serious medical illness or disability.

3. **Psychosocial.** Greater vulnerability in persons who lost a parent during infancy or who had poor mothering experiences. Ability to tolerate frustration in adult life correlates with gratification of basic needs in infant life.

E. Differential diagnosis

1. **Posttraumatic stress disorder and acute stress disorder.** Psychosocial stressor determines diagnosis. Stressor is outside the range of normal human experience (e.g., war, rape, mass catastrophe, floods, being taken hostage).

2. **Brief psychotic disorder.** Characterized by hallucinations and delusions.

3. **Uncomplicated bereavement.** Occurs before, immediately, or shortly after death of a loved one; occupational or social functioning is impaired within expected bounds and remits spontaneously.

4. **Anxiety and mood disorders.** Symptoms not directly related to stressor and occur frequently.

F. **Course and prognosis.** Most symptoms diminish over time without treatment, especially after stressor is removed; subgroup maintains chronic course, with risk for secondary depression, anxiety, and substance use disorder.

G. **Treatment**
1. **Psychological**
   a. **Psychotherapy**—the treatment of choice. Explore meaning of stressor to the patient, provide support, encourage alternative ways of coping, offer empathy. Biofeedback, relaxation techniques, and hypnosis for anxious mood.
   b. **Crisis intervention**—aimed at helping the person resolve the situation quickly through supportive techniques, suggestion, reassurance, environmental modifications, and hospitalization, if necessary.
2. **Pharmacological.** Patients can be treated with anxiolytic or antidepressant agents depending on the type of adjustment disorder (e.g., with anxiety, with depressed mood, but be careful to avoid drug dependency, especially if benzodiazepines are used).

For a more detailed discussion of this topic, see Impulse-Control Disorders Not Elsewhere Classified, Ch 22, p 1701, and Adjustment Disorders, Ch 23, p 1714, in CTP/VII.

18

Psychosomatic Medicine

I. Psychosomatic disorders

A. Definition. Psychosomatic medicine deals with the relation between psychological and physiological factors in the causation or maintenance of disease states. Although most physical disorders are influenced by stress, conflict, or generalized anxiety, some disorders are more affected than others. In DSM-IV-TR, psychosomatic disorders are subsumed under the classification of psychological factors affecting medical condition (Table 18–1).

B. Etiology

1. **Specific stress factors.** This theory postulates specific stresses or personality types for each psychosomatic disease and is typified by the work of the following investigators:

   a. **Flanders Dunbar**—described personality traits that are specific for a psychosomatic disorder (e.g., coronary personality). Type A personality is hard-driving, aggressive, irritable, and susceptible to heart disease.

   b. **Franz Alexander**—described unconscious conflicts that produce anxiety, are mediated through the autonomic nervous system, and result in a specific disorder (e.g., repressed dependency needs contribute to peptic ulcer).

2. **Nonspecific stress factors.** This theory states that any prolonged stress can cause physiological changes that result in a physical disorder. Each person has a shock organ that is genetically vulnerable to stress: some patients are cardiac reactors, others are gastric reactors, and others are skin reactors. Persons who are chronically anxious or depressed are more vulnerable to physical or psychosomatic disease. Table 18–2 lists life stressors that may herald a psychosomatic disorder.

3. **Physiological factors.** Hans Selye described the general adaption syndrome, which is the sum of all the nonspecific systemic reactions of the body that follow prolonged stress. The hypothalamic–pituitary–adrenal axis is affected, with excess secretion of cortisol producing structural damage to various organ systems. George Engel postulated that in the stressed state, all neuroregulatory mechanisms undergo functional changes that depress the body's homeostatic mechanisms, so that the body is left vulnerable to infection and other disorders.

   Neurophysiological pathways thought to mediate stress reactions include the cerebral cortex, limbic system, hypothalamus, adrenal medulla, and sympathetic and parasympathetic nervous systems. Neuromessengers include such hormones as cortisol and thyroxine (Table 18–3).

TABLE 18-1
DSM-IV-TR DIAGNOSTIC CRITERIA FOR PSYCHOLOGICAL FACTORS AFFECTING MEDICAL CONDITION

A. A general medical condition (coded on Axis III) is present.
B. Psychological factors adversely affect the general medical condition in one of the following ways:
   (1) the factors have influenced the course of the general medical condition as shown by a close temporal association between the psychological factors and the development or exacerbation of, or delayed recovery from, the general medical condition
   (2) the factors interfere with the treatment of the general medical condition
   (3) the factors constitute additional health risks for the individual
   (4) stress-related physiological responses precipitate or exacerbate symptoms of a general medical condition

Choose name based on the nature of the psychological factors of more than one factor is present indicate the most prominent

Mental disorder affecting medical condition (e.g., an Axis I disorder such as major depressive disorder delaying recovery from a myocardial infarction).

Psychological symptoms affecting medical condition (e.g., depressive symptoms delaying recovery from surgery, anxiety, exacerbating asthma).

Personality traits or coping style affecting medical condition (e.g., pathological denial of the need for surgery in a patient with cancer hostile, pressured behavior contributing to cardiovascular disease).

Maladaptive health behaviors affecting medical condition (e.g., lack of exercise, unsafe sex, over eating).

Stress-related physiological response affecting general medical condition (e.g., stress-related exacerbation of ulcer hypertension, arrhythmia or tension headache).

Other or unspecified psychological factors affecting medical condition (e.g., interpersonal, cultural or religious factors).

From American Psychiatric Association. *Diagnostic and Statistical Manual of Mental Disorders,* text revision, 4th ed. Washington, DC: American Psychiatric Association; Copyright 2000, with permission.

TABLE 18-2
1994 RANKING OF 10 LIFE-CHANGE STRESSORS

1. Death of spouse
2. Divorce
3. Death of close family member
4. Marital separation
5. Serious personal injury or illness
6. Fired from work
7. Jail term
8. Death of a close friend
9. Pregnancy
10. Business readjustment

Adapted from Richard H. Rahe, M.D., and Thomas Holmes.

TABLE 18-3
FUNCTIONAL RESPONSES TO STRESS

Neurotransmitter response
   Increased synthesis of brain norepinephrine.
   Increased serotonin turnover may result in eventual depletion of serotonin.
   Increased dopaminergic transmission.
Endocrine response
   Increased adrenocortotropic hormone (ACTH) stimulates adrenal cortisol.
   Testosterone decrease with prolonged stress.
   Decrease in thyroid hormone.
Immune response
   Immune activation occurs with release of hormonal immune factors (cytokines) in acute stress.
   Number and activity of natural killer cells decreased in chronic stress.

TABLE 18-4
PHYSICAL CONDITIONS AFFECTED BY PSYCHOLOGICAL FACTORS

Disorder	Observations/Comments/Theory/Approach
Angina, arrhythmias, coronary spasms	Type A person is aggressive, irritable, easily frustrated, and prone to coronary artery disease. Arrhythmias common in anxiety states. Sudden death from ventricular arrhythmia in some patients who experience massive psychological shock or catastrophe. Lifestyle changes: cease smoking, curb alcohol intake, lose weight, lower cholesterol to limit risk factors. Propranolol (Inderal) prescribed for patients who develop tachycardia as part of social phobia—protects against arrhythmia and decreased coronary blood flow.
Asthma	Attacks precipitated by stress, respiratory infection, allergy. Examine family dynamics, especially when child is the patient. Look for overprotectiveness and try to encourage appropriate independent activities. Propranolol and beta blockers contraindicated in asthma patients for anxiety. Psychological theories: strong dependency and separation anxiety; asthma wheeze is suppressed cry for love and protection.
Connective tissue diseases: systemic lupus erythematosus, rheumatoid arthritis	Disease can be heralded by major life stress, especially death of loved one. Worsens with chronic stress, anger, or depression. Important to keep patient as active as possible to minimize joint deformities. Treat depression with antidepressant medications or psychostimulants, and treat muscle spasm and tension with benzodiazepines.
Headaches	Tension headache results from contraction of strap muscles in neck, constricting blood flow. Associated with anxiety, situational stress. Relaxation therapy, antianxiety medication useful. Migraine headaches are unilateral and can be triggered by stress, exercise, foods high in tyramine. Manage with ergotamine (Cafergot). Propranolol prophylaxis can produce associated depression. Sumatriptan (Imitrex) can be used to treat nonhemiplegic and nonbasilar migraine attacks.
Hypertension	Acute stress produces catecholamines (epinephrine), which raise systolic blood pressure. Chronic stress associated with essential hypertension. Look at lifestyle. Prescribe exercise, relaxation therapy, biofeedback. Benzodiazepines of use in acute stress if blood pressure rises as shock organ. Psychological theories: inhibited rage, guilt over hostile impulses, need to gain approval from authority.
Hyperventilation syndrome	Accompanies panic disorder, generalized anxiety disorder with associated hyperventilation, tachycardia, vasoconstriction. May be hazardous in patients with coronary insufficiency. Antianxiety agents of use: some patients respond to monoamine oxidase inhibitors, tricyclic antidepressants, or serotonergic agents.
Inflammatory bowel diseases: Crohn's disease, irritable bowel syndrome, ulcerative colitis	Depressed mood associated with illness; stress exacerbates symptoms. Onset after major life stress. Patients respond to stable doctor-patient relationship and supportive psychotherapy in addition to bowel medication. Psychological theories: passive personality, childhood intimidation, obsessive traits, fear of punishment, masked hostility.
Metabolic and endocrine disorders	Thyrotoxicosis following sudden severe stress. Glycosuria in chronic fear and anxiety. Depression alters hormone metabolism: especially adrenocorticotropic hormone (ACTH).
Neurodermatitis	Eczema in patients with multiple psychosocial stressors—especially death of loved one, conflicts over sexuality, repressed anger. Some respond to hypnosis in symptom management.
Obesity	Hyperphagia reduces anxiety. Night-eating syndrome associated with insomnia. Failure to perceive appetite, hunger, and satiation. Psychological theories: conflicts about orality and pathologic dependency. Behavioral techniques, support groups, nutritional counseling, and supportive psychotherapy useful. Treat underlying depression.
Osteoarthritis	Lifestyle management includes weight reduction, isometric exercises to strengthen joint musculature, maintenance of physical activity, pain control. Treat associated anxiety or depression with supportive psychotherapy.
Peptic ulcer disease	Idiopathic type not related to specific bacterium or physical stimulus. Increased gastric acid and pepsin relative to mucosal resistance: both sensitive to anxiety, stress, coffee, alcohol. Lifestyle changes. Relaxation therapy. Psychological theories: strong frustrated dependency needs, cannot express anger, superficial self-sufficiency.

TABLE 18–4—*continued*

Disorder	Observations/Comments/Theory/Approach
Raynaud's disease	Peripheral vasoconstriction associated with smoking, stress. Lifestyle changes: cessation of smoking, moderate exercise. Biofeedback can raise hand temperature by increased vasodilation.
Syncope, hypotension	Vasovagal reflex with acute anxiety or fear produces hypotension and fainting. More common in patients with hyperreactive autonomic nervous system. Aggravated by anemia, antidepressant medications (produce hypotension as side effect).
Urticaria, angioedema	Idiopathic type not related to specific allergens or physical stimulus. May be associated with stress, chronic anxiety, depression. Pruritis worse with anxiety; self-excoriation associated with repressed hostility. Some phenothiazines have antipruritic effect. Psychological theories: conflict between dependence–independence, unconscious guilt feelings, itching as sexual displacement.

C. Diagnosis. To meet the diagnostic criteria for psychological factors affecting a medical condition, the following two criteria must be met: (1) a medical condition is present, and (2) psychological factors affect it adversely (e.g., the psychologically meaningful environmental stimulus is temporally related to the initiation or exacerbation of the specific physical condition or disorder). The physical condition must demonstrate either organic disease (e.g., rheumatoid arthritis) or a known pathophysiologic process (e.g., migraine headache). A number of physical disorders meet these criteria and are listed in Table 18–4.

D. Medical, surgical, and neurological conditions that present with psychiatric symptoms. A host of medical and neurological disorders, summarized in Table 18–5, may present with psychiatric symptoms, which must be differentiated from primary psychiatric disorders.

E. Differential diagnosis. As outlined in Table 18–6, various psychiatric syndromes and disorders can be confused with psychosomatic disorders. Each lacks a demonstrable organic pathological lesion or known pathophysiological process.

F. Treatment

1. **Collaborative approach.** Collaborate with internist or surgeon who manages the physical disorder, with psychiatrist attending to psychiatric aspects.

2. **Psychotherapy**

   a. **Supportive psychotherapy.** When patients have a therapeutic alliance, they are able to ventilate fears of illness, especially death fantasies, with the psychiatrist. Many patients have strong dependency needs, which are partially gratified in treatment.

   b. **Dynamic insight-oriented psychotherapy.** Explore unconscious conflicts regarding sex and aggression. Anxiety associated with life stresses is examined and mature defenses are established. More patients will benefit from supportive psychotherapy than insight-oriented therapy when they have psychosomatic disorders.

   c. **Group therapy.** Group therapy is of use for patients who have similar physical conditions (e.g., patients with colitis, those undergoing hemodialysis). They share experiences and learn from one another.

TABLE 18–5
MEDICAL PROBLEMS THAT PRESENT WITH PSYCHIATRIC SYMPTOMS

Disease	Sex and Age Prevalence	Common Medical Symptoms	Psychiatric Symptoms and Complaints	Impaired Performance and Behavior	Diagnostic Problems
AIDS	Males > females; IV drug abusers, homosexuals, female sex partners of bisexual men	Lymphadenopathy, fatigue, opportunistic infections, Kaposi's sarcoma	Depression, anxiety, disorientation	Dementia with global impairment	Seropositive HIV virus is diagnostic when clinical signs present
Hyperthyroidism (thyrotoxicosis)	Females 3:1; 20 to 50 years	Tremor, sweating, loss of weight and strength, heat intolerance	Anxiety, depression	Occasional hyperactive or grandiose behavior	Long lead time; rapid onset resembles anxiety attack
Hypothyroidism (myxedema)	Females 5:1; 30 to 50 years	Puffy face, dry skin, cold intolerance	Lethargy, anxiety with irritability, thought disorder, somatic delusions, hallucinations	Myxedema madness; delusional, paranoid, belligerent behavior	Madness may mimic schizophrenia; mental status is clear, even during most disturbed behavior
Hyperparathyroidism	Females 3:1; 40 to 60 years	Weakness, anorexia, fractures, calculi, peptic ulcers			Anorexia and fatigue of slow-growing adenoma resembles involutional depression
Hypoparathyroidism	Females, 40 to 60 years	Hyperreflexia, spasms, tetany	Either state may cause anxiety, hyperactivity, and irritability or depression, apathy, and withdrawal	Either state may proceed to a toxic psychosis: confusion, disorientation, and clouded sensorium	None; rare condition except after surgery
Hyperadrenalism (Cushing's disease)	Adults, both sexes	Weight gain, fat alteration, easy fatigability	Varied; depression, anxiety, thought disorder with somatic delusions	Rarely produces aberrant behavior	Bizarre somatic delusions caused by bodily changes; resemble those of schizophrenia
Adrenal cortical insufficiency (Addison's disease)	Adults, both sexes	Weight loss, hypotension, skin pigmentation	Depression—negativism, apathy; thought disorder—suspiciousness	Toxic psychosis with confusion and agitation	Long lead time; weight loss, apathy, despondency resemble involutional depression

Porphyria—acute intermittent type	Females, 20 to 40 years	Abdominal crises, paresthesias, weakness	Anxiety—sudden onset, severe; mood swings	Extremes of excitement or withdrawal; emotional or angry outbursts	Patients often have truly neurotic lifestyles; crises resemble conversion reactions or anxiety attacks
Pernicious anemia	Females, 40 to 60 years	Weight loss, weakness, glossitis, extremity neuritis	Depression—feelings of guilt and worthlessness	Eventual brain damage with confusion and memory loss	Long lead time, sometimes many months; easily mistaken for involutional depression; normal early blood studies may give false reassurance
Hepatolenticular degeneration (Wilson's disease)	Males 2:1; adolescence	Liver and extrapyramidal symptoms	Mood swings—sudden and changeable; anger—explosive	Eventual brain damage with memory and I.Q. loss; combativeness	In late teens, may resemble adolescent storm, incorrigibility, or schizophrenia
Hypoglycemia (islet cell adenoma)	Adults, both sexes	Tremor, sweating, hunger, fatigue, dizziness	Anxiety—fear and dread, depression with fatigue	Agitation, confusion; eventual brain damage	Can mimic anxiety attack or acute alcoholism; bizarre behavior may draw attention away from somatic symptoms
Intracranial tumors	Adults, both sexes	None early; headache, vomiting, papilledema later	Varied; depression, anxiety, personality changes	Loss of memory, judgment; self-criticism; clouding of consciousness	Tumor location may not determine early symptoms
Pancreatic carcinoma	Males 3:1; 50 to 70 years	Weight loss, abdominal pain, weakness, jaundice	Depression, sense of imminent doom but without severe guilt	Loss of drive and motivation	Long lead time; exact age and symptoms of involutional depression
Pheochromocytoma	Adults, both sexes	Headache, sweating during elevated blood pressure	Anxiety, panic, fear, apprehension, trembling	Inability to function during an attack	Classic symptoms of anxiety attack; intermittently normal blood pressures may discourage further studies

continued

TABLE 18-5—*continued*

Disease	Sex and Age Prevalence	Common Medical Symptoms	Psychiatric Symptoms and Complaints	Impaired Performance and Behavior	Diagnostic Problems
Multiple sclerosis	Females, 20 to 40 years	Motor and sensory losses, scanning speech, nystagmus	Varied; personality changes, mood swings, depression; bland euphoria uncommon	Inappropriate behavior resulting from personality changes	Long lead time; early neurological symptoms mimic hysteria or conversion disorders
Systemic lupus erythematosus	Females 8:1; 20 to 40 years	Multiple symptoms of cardiovascular, genitourinary, gastrointestinal, other systems	Varied; thought disorder, depression, confusion	Toxic psychosis unrelated to steroid treatment	Long lead time, perhaps many years; psychiatric picture variable over time; thought disorder resembles schizophrenia, steroid psychosis

Adapted from Maurice J. Martin, M.D.

TABLE 18–6
CONDITIONS MIMICKING PSYCHOSOMATIC DISORDERS

Diagnosis	Definition and Example
Conversion disorder	There is an alteration of physical function that suggests a physical disorder but is an expression of psychological conflict (e.g., psychogenic aphonia). The symptoms are falsely neuroanatomic in distribution, are symbolic in nature, and allow much secondary gain.
Body dysmorphic disorder	Preoccupation with an imagined physical defect in appearance in a normal-appearing person (e.g., preoccupation with facial hair).
Hypochondriasis	Imaged overconcern about physical disease when objective examination reveals none to exist (e.g., angina pectoris with normal heart functioning).
Somatization disorder	Recurrent somatic and physical complaints with no demonstrable physical disorder despite repeated physical examinations and no organic basis.
Pain disorder	Preoccupation with pain with no physical disease to account for intensity. It does not follow a neuroanatomical distribution. There may be a close correlation between stress and conflict and the initiation or exacerbation of pain.
Physical complaints associated with classic psychological disorders	Somatic accompaniment of depression (e.g., weakness, asthenia).
Physical complaints with substance abuse disorder	Bronchitis and cough associated with nicotine and tobacco dependence.

   d. Family therapy. Family relationships and processes are explored, with emphasis placed on how the patient's illness affects other family members.
   e. Cognitive–behavioral therapy
      (1) Cognitive. Patients learn how stress and conflict translate into somatic illness. Negative thoughts about disease are examined and altered.
      (2) Behavioral. Relaxation and biofeedback techniques affect the autonomic nervous system positively. Of use in asthma, allergies, hypertension, and headache.
3. Pharmacotherapy
   a. Always take nonpsychiatric symptoms seriously and use appropriate medication (e.g., laxatives for simple constipation). Consult with referring physician.
   b. Use antipsychotic drugs when associated psychosis is present. Be aware of side effects and their impact on the disorder.
   c. Antianxiety drugs diminish harmful anxiety during period of acute stress. Limit use so as to avoid dependency, but do not hesitate to prescribe in a timely manner.
   d. Antidepressants can be used with depression resulting from a medical condition. Selective serotonin reuptake inhibitors can help when the patient obsesses or ruminates about his or her illness.

II. Consultation–liaison psychiatry
   Psychiatrists serve as consultants to medical colleagues (either another psychiatrist or, more commonly, a nonpsychiatric physician) or to other mental health professionals (psychologist, social worker, or psychiatric nurse). In

TABLE 18–7
COMMON CONSULTATION-LIAISON PROBLEMS

Reason for Consultation	Comments
Suicide attempt or threat	High-risk factors are men over 45, no social support, alcohol dependence, previous attempt, incapacitating medical illness with pain, and suicidal ideation. If risk is present, transfer to psychiatric unit or start 24-hour nursing care.
Depression	Suicidal risks must be assessed in every depressed patient (see above); presence of cognitive defects in depression may cause diagnostic dilemma with dementia; check for history of substance abuse or depressant drugs (e.g., reserpine, propranolol); use antidepressants cautiously in cardiac patients because of conduction side effects, orthostatic hypotension.
Agitation	Often related to cognitive disorder, withdrawal from drugs, (e.g., opioids, alcohol, sedative-hypnotics); haloperidol most useful drug for excessive agitation; use physical restraints with great caution; examine for command hallucinations or paranoid ideation to which patient is responding in agitated manner; rule out toxic reaction to medication.
Hallucinations	Most common cause in hospital is delirium tremens; onset 3 to 4 days after hospitalization. In intensive care units, check for sensory isolation; rule out brief psychotic disorder, schizophrenia, cognitive disorder. Treat with antipsychotic medication.
Sleep disorder	Common cause is pain; early morning awakening associated with depression; difficulty in falling asleep associated with anxiety. Use antianxiety or antidepressant agent, depending on cause. Those drugs have no analgesic effect, so prescribe adequate painkillers. Rule out early substance withdrawal.
No organic basis for symptoms	Rule out conversion disorder, somatization disorder, factitious disorder, and malingering; glove and stocking anesthesia with autonomic nervous system symptoms seen in conversion disorder; multiple body complaints seen in somatization disorder; wish to be hospitalized seen in factitious disorder; obvious secondary gain in malingering (e.g., compensation case).
Disorientation	Delirium versus dementia; review metabolic status, neurological findings, substance history. Prescribe small dose of antipsychotics for major agitation; benzodiazepines may worsen condition and cause sundown syndrome (ataxia, confusion); modify environment so patient does not experience sensory deprivation.
Noncompliance or refusal to consent to procedure	Explore relationship of patient and treating doctor; negative transference is most common cause of noncompliance; fears of medication or of procedure require education and reassurance. Refusal to give consent is issue of judgment; if impaired, patient can be declared incompetent, but only by a judge; cognitive disorder is main cause of impaired judgment in hospitalized patients.

addition, consultation–liaison psychiatrists provide consultation regarding patients in medical or surgical settings and provide follow-up psychiatric treatment as needed. Consultation–liaison psychiatry is associated with all the diagnostic, therapeutic, research, and teaching services that psychiatrists perform in the general hospital and serves as a bridge between psychiatry and other specialties.

Because more than 50% of medical inpatients have psychiatric problems that may require treatment, the consultation–liaison psychiatrist is important in the hospital setting. Table 18–7 lists the most common consultation–liaison problems encountered in general hospitals.

III. Special medical settings

Besides the usual medical wards in a hospital, special settings produce uncommon, distinctive forms of stress.

A. **ICU.** ICUs contain seriously ill patients who have life-threatening ill-nesses (e.g., coronary care units). Among the defensive reactions encoun-tered are fear, anxiety, acting out, signing out against medical advice, hos-tility, dependency, depression, grief, and delirium.

B. **Hemodialysis.** Patients on hemodialysis have a lifelong dependency on machines and health care providers. They have problems with prolonged

TABLE 18–8
TRANSPLANTATION AND SURGICAL PROBLEMS

Organ	Biological Factors	Psychological Factors
Kidney	50–90% success rate; may not be done if patient is over age 55; increasing use of cadaver kidneys rather than those from living donors	Living donors must be emotionally stable; parents are best donors, siblings may be ambivalent; donors are subject to depression. Patients who panic before surgery may have poor prognoses; altered body image with fear of organ rejection is common. Group therapy for patients is helpful.
Bone marrow	Used in aplastic anemias and immune system disease	Patients are usually ill and must deal with death and dying; compliance is important. The pro-cedure is commonly done in children who pre-sent problems of prolonged dependence; siblings are often donors and may be angry or ambivalent about procedure.
Heart	End-stage coronary artery disease and cardiomyopathy	Donor is legally dead; relatives of the deceased may refuse permission or be ambivalent. No fallback is available if the organ is rejected; kidney rejection patient can go on hemodialysis. Some patients seek transplantation hoping to die. Postcardiotomy delirium is seen in 25% of patients.
Breast	Radical mastectomy versus lumpectomy	Reconstruction of breast at time of surgery leads to postoperative adaptation; veteran patients are used to counsel new patients; lumpectomy patients are more open about surgery and sex than are mastectomy patients; group support is helpful.
Uterus	Hysterectomy performed on 10% of women over 20	Fear of loss of sexual attractiveness with sexual dysfunction may occur in a small percentage of women; loss of childbearing capacity is upsetting.
Brain	Anatomical location of lesion determines behavioral change	Environmental dependence syndrome in frontal lobe tumors is characterized by inability to show initiative; memory disturbances are involved in periventricular surgery; hallucinations are involved in parieto-occipital area.
Prostate	Cancer surgery has more negative psychobiological effects and is more tech-nically difficult than surgery for benign hypertrophy	Sexual dysfunction is common except in trans-urethral prostatectomy. Perineal prostatectomy produces the absence of emission, ejaculation, and erection; penile implant may be of use.
Colon and rectum	Colostomy and ostomy are common outcomes, especially for cancer	One third of patients with colostomies feel worse about themselves than before bowel surgery; shame and self-consciousness about the stoma can be alleviated by self-help groups that deal with those issues.
Limbs	Amputation performed for massive injury, diabetes, or cancer	Phantom-limb phenomenon occurs in 98% of cases; the experience may last for years; some-times the sensation is painful, and neuroma at the stump should be ruled out; the condition has no known cause or treatment; it may stop spontaneously.

TABLE 18–9
PHYSIOLOGICAL CLASSIFICATION OF PAIN

Type	Subtypes	Example	Comment
Nociceptive	Somatic	Bone metastasis	Caused by activation of
	Visceral	Intestinal obstruction	pain-sensitive fibers; usually aching or pressure.
Neuropathic	Peripheral	Causalgia	Caused by interruption of
	Central	Thalamic pain	afferent pathways.
	Somatic	Causalgia	Pathophysiology poorly
	Visceral	Visceral pain in paraplegics	understood, with most syndromes probably
	Sympathetic-dependent	Post-herpetic pain	involving both peripheral
	Non-sympathetic-dependent	Phantom pain	and central nervous system changes. Usually dysesthetic, often burning and lancinating.
Psychogenic	Somatization disorder	Failed low back	Does not include factitious
	Psychogenic pain	Atypical facial pain	disorders (i.e., malingering,
	Hypochondriasis	Chronic headache	Munchausen's syndrome).
	Specific pain diagnoses with organic contribution		

Adapted from Berkow R, ed. *Merck Manual,* 15th ed. Rahway, NJ: Merck, Sharp & Dohme Research Laboratories. 1987:1341, with permission.

dependency, regression to childhood states, hostility, and negativism in following doctors' directions. It is advisable that all patients for whom dialysis is being considered undergo a psychological evaluation.

Dialysis dementia is a disorder characterized by a loss of cognitive functions, dystonias, and seizures. It usually ends in death. It tends to occur in patients who have been on dialysis for long periods of time.

C. Surgery.   Patients who have undergone severe surgical procedures have a variety of psychological reactions, depending on their premorbid personality and the nature of the surgery. These reactions are summarized in Table 18–8.

IV. Pain

Pain is a complex symptom consisting of a sensation underlying potential disease and an associated emotional state. Acute pain is a reflex biological response to injury. By definition, chronic pain is pain that lasts at least 6 months. A physiological classification of pain is listed in Table 18–9, and characteristics of pain are listed in Table 18–10.

TABLE 18–10
CHARACTERISTICS OF SOMATIC AND NEUROPATHIC PAIN

Somatic Pain	Neuropathic Pain
Nociceptive stimulus usually evident	No obvious nociceptive stimulus
Usually well localized; visceral pain may be referred	Often poorly localized
Similar to other somatic pains in patient's experience	Unusual, dissimilar from somatic pain
Relieved by anti-inflammatory or narcotic analgesics	Only partially relieved by narcotic analgesics

Adapted from Braunwald E, Isselbacher K, Petersdorf RG, Wilson JD, Martin JB, Fauci AS. *Harrison's Principles of Internal Medicine,* 11th ed., *Companion Handbook.* New York, McGraw-Hill, 1988:1.

V. Analgesia

Analgesia is the loss or absence of pain. The most effective analgesics are the narcotics (drugs derived from opium or an opium-like substance), which relieve pain, alter mood and behavior, and have the potential to cause dependence and tolerance. *Opioids* is a generic term that includes drugs that bind to opioid

TABLE 18–11
OPIOID ANALGESICS FOR MANAGEMENT OF CANCER PAIN

Drug and Equianalgesic Dose Relative Potency	Dose (mg IM or oral)	Plasma Half-Life (h)	Starting Oral Dose[a] (mg)	Available Commercial Preparations
Opioid agonists				
Morphine	10 IM 60 oral	3–4	30–60	Oral: tablet, liquid, slow-release tablet Rectal: 5–30 mg Injectable: SC, IM, IV, epidural, intrathecal
Hydromophone	1.5 IM 7.5 oral	2–3	2–48	Oral: tablets—1, 2, 4 mg Injectable: SC, IM, IV 2, 3 and 10 mg/mL
Methadone	10 IM 20 oral	12–24	5–10	Oral: tablets, liquid Injectable: SC, IM, IV
Levorphanol	2 IM 4 oral	12–16	2–4	Oral: tablets Injectable: SC, IM, IV
Oxymorphone	1 IM	2–3	NA	Rectal: 10 mg Injectable: SC, IM, IV
Heroin	5 IM 60 oral	3–4	NA	NA
Meperidine	75 IM 300 oral	3–4 (norme-peridine 12–16)	75	Oral: tablets Injectable: SC IM, IV
Codeine	30 IM 200 oral	3–4	60	Oral: tablets and combination with acetyl-salicylic acid, acetaminophen, liquid
Oxycodone	15 oral 30 oral	—	5	Oral: tablets, liquid, oral formulation in combination with aceta-minophen (tablet and liquid) and aspirin (tablet)

The times of peak analgesia in nontolerant patients ranges from ½ to 1 h, and the duration from 4 to 6 h. The peak analgesic effect is delayed, and the duration is prolonged after oral administrations.

[a] Recommended starting IM doses; the optimal dose for each patient is determined by titration, and the maximal dose is limited by adverse effects.
Adapted from Foley K. Management of cancer pain. In: DeVita VT, Hellman S, Rosenberg SA, eds. *Cancer: Principles and Practice of Oncology*, 4th ed. Philadelphia: Lippincott, 1993:22, with permission.

TABLE 18–12
PHYTOMEDICINALS WITH PSYCHOACTIVE EFFECTS

Name	Ingredients	Use	Adverse Effects	Interactions	Dosage[a]	Comments
Echinacea L. *Echinacea purpurea*	Flavonoids,[b] polysaccharides, caffeic acid derivatives, alkamides	Stimulates immune system; for lethargy, malaise, respiratory and lower urinary tract infections	Allergic reaction, fever, nausea, vomiting	Undetermined.	1–3 g/d	Use in HIV and AIDS, patients is controversial.
Ephedra, ma-huang L. *Ephedra sinica*	Ephedrine, pseudoephedrine	Stimulant: for lethargy, malaise, diseases of respiratory tract	Sympathomimetic overload: arrhythmias, increased blood pressure, headache, irritability, nausea, vomiting	Synergistic with sympathomimetics, serotoninergic agents. Avoid with MAOIs.	1–2 g/d	Administer for short periods as tachyphylaxis and dependence can occur.
Ginkgo L. *Ginkgo biloba*	Flavonoids,[b] ginkgolide A, B	Symptomatic relief of delirium, dementia; improves concentration and memory deficits; possible antidote to SSRI induced sexual dysfunction	Allergic skin reactions, gastro-intestinal upset, muscle spasms, headache	Anticoagulant: use with caution because of its inhibitory effect on platelet-activating factor; increased bleeding possible.	120–240 mg/d	Studies indicate improved cognition in Alzheimer's patients after 4 to 5 weeks of use, possibly because of increased blood flow.
Ginseng L. *Panax ginseng*	Triterpenes, ginsenosides	Stimulant: for fatigue, elevation of mood immune system	Insomnia, hypertonia, and edema (called *ginseng abuse syndrome*)	Not to be used with sedatives, hypnotic agents, MAOIs, antidiabetic agents, or steroids.	1–2 g/d	Several varieties exist: Korean (most highly valued), Chinese, Japanese, American (*Panax quinquefolius*).
Kava kava L. *Piperis methysticum rhizoma*	Kava lactones, kava pyrone	Sedative-hypnotic, antispasmodic	Lethargy, impaired cognition, dermatitis with long-term unreported use	Synergistic with anxiolytics, alcohol; avoid with levodopa and dopaminergic agents.	600–800 mg/d	May be GABAergic. Contraindicated in patients with endogenous depression; may increase the danger of suicide.

St. John's wort L. *Hypericum perforatum*	Hypericin, flavonoids, xanthones	Antidepressant, sedative, anxiolytic	Headaches, photosensitivity (may be severe), constipation	Report of manic reaction when used with sertraline (Zoloft). Do not combine with SSRIs or MAOIs; possible serotonin syndrome. Do not use with alcohol, opioids.	100–950 mg/d	Under investigation by National Institutes of Health. May act as MAOI or SSRI. Allow 4- to 6-week trial for mild depressive moods; if no apparent improvement, another therapy should be tried. May be chemically unstable.
Valerian L. *Valeriana officinalis*	Valepotriates, valerenic acid, caffeic acid	Sedative, muscle relaxant, hypnotic	Cognitive and motor impairment, gastrointestinal upset, hepatotoxicity; with long-term use: contact allergy; headache, restlessness, insomnia, mydriasis, cardiac dysfunction	Avoid concomitant use with alcohol or CNS depressants.	1–2 g/d	

[a] No reliable, consistent, or valid data on dosages or adverse affects are available for most phytomedicinals.
[b] Flavonoids are common to many herbs. They are plant by-products that act as antioxidants (i.e. agents that prevent the deterioration of material such as DNA via oxidation).
MAOI, monoamine oxidase inhibitor; GABA, γ–aminobutyric acid; SSRI, selective serotonin reuptake inhibitor.

receptors and produce a narcotic effect. They are most useful in the short-term management of severe, acute, serious pain. A goal should be to lower the pain level so that the patient can eat and sleep with minimal upset. A guideline should be to give the drug at the request of the patient. The self-administration by patients with pain of measured amounts of narcotics through an intravenous pump, when carried out in a hospital, is a new approach to pain control that is proving effective. The major opioid analgesics are listed in Table 18–11.

A. Nonnarcotic analgesics. Typical of this group is aspirin. Unlike narcotic analgesics, which act on the CNS, salicylates act at the peripheral or local level—the site of origin of the pain. Usually taken every 3 hours.

With most analgesics, peak plasma concentrations occur in 45 minutes, and analgesic effects last 3 to 4 hours. Other nonsteroidal anti-inflammatory drugs (NSAIDs) can also be used for analgesia (200 to 400 mg of ibuprofen every 4 hours). Drug equivalents: 650 mg of aspirin = 32 mg of codeine = 65 mg of propoxyphene (Darvon) = 50 mg of oral pentazocine (Talwin).

B. Placebos. Substances with no known pharmacological activity that act through suggestion rather than biological action. It has recently been demonstrated, however, that naloxone (Narcan), an opioid antagonist, can block the analgesic effects of a placebo, which suggests that a release of endogenous opioids may explain some placebo effects.

Long-term treatment with placebos should never be undertaken when patients have clearly stated an objection to such treatment. Furthermore, deceptive treatment with placebos seriously undermines patients' confidence in their physicians. Finally, placebos should not be used when an effective therapy is available.

VI. Alternative (or complementary) medicine

In increasing use at present. One in three persons use such therapies at some point for such common ailments as depression, anxiety, chronic pain, low back pain, headaches, and digestive problems. Some commonly taken herbal preparations with psychoactive properties are listed in Table 18–12.

For more detailed discussion of this topic, see Psychological Factors Affecting Medical Conditions, Ch 25, p 1765, in CTP/VII.

19
Personality Disorders

I. General introduction

A. Definition.
Personality may be described as a person's characteristic configuration of behavioral response patterns apparent in ordinary life, a totality that is usually stable and predictable. When this totality appears to differ in a way that exceeds the range of variation found in most people, and when personality traits are rigid and maladaptive and produce functional impairment and subjective distress, a personality disorder may be diagnosed.

B. Features and diagnosis

1. The traits are pervasive and persistent. The diagnosis requires a history of long-term difficulties in various spheres of life (i.e., love and work).

2. The traits are ego-syntonic (i.e., acceptable to the ego), not ego-dystonic or ego-alien.

3. The traits are alloplastic (i.e., the patient seeks to alter the environment rather than the self), not autoplastic.

4. The traits are held rigidly.

5. The armoring against internal impulses and external stress involves idiosyncratic patterns of defenses. Underneath the protective armor is anxiety. The defenses may or may not effectively bind anxiety. Common defense mechanisms include the following:

   a. **Fantasy.** Schizoid patients with a fear of intimacy may seem aloof and create imaginary lives and friends.

   b. **Dissociation.** Unpleasant affects are repressed or replaced with pleasant ones. Histrionic patients may seem dramatic and emotionally shallow.

   c. **Isolation.** Facts are recalled without affect. This is characteristic of obsessive-compulsive patients.

   d. **Projection.** Unacknowledged feelings are attributed to others. This is common in paranoid patients.

   e. **Splitting.** Others are seen as all good or all bad. This is seen in borderline patients.

   f. **Turning against the self.** This involves deliberate failure and self-destructive acts. It often involves passive-aggressive behavior against others.

   g. **Acting out.** Wishes or conflicts are expressed in action, without reflective awareness of the idea or affect. This is seen most commonly in antisocial personality disorder.

   h. **Projective identification.** Others are coerced to identify with a projected aspect of the self, so that the other person experiences feelings similar to those of the patient. This is common in borderline patients.

6. The patient shows developmental fixation and immaturity.

7. Internal object relations are disturbed. The patient shows interpersonal difficulties in love and work and characteristically does not appreciate his or her impact on others.

8. The patient lacks insight and does not tend to seek help.

9. Frequently, problems develop in medical situations, and the patients may elicit strong negative responses from health care personnel.

10. Stress tolerance tends to be poor.

C. Epidemiology

1. The prevalence is 6–9%, possibly as high as 15%.

2. An early analogue is a disorder of temperament. Usually, a personality disorder is first evident in late adolescence or early adulthood, but it can be evident in childhood.

3. Overall, women and men are affected equally.

4. The patient's family often has a nonspecific history of psychiatric disorders. With most personality disorders, a partially genetic transmission is established.

D. Etiology

1. The etiology of personality disorders is multifactorial.

2. Biological determinants are sometimes evident (genetics, perinatal injury, encephalitis, head trauma). The concordance rates in monozygotic twins are high for most personality disorders. Some show biological features of other disorders. (Patients with obsessive-compulsive disorders have a shortened rapid eye movement [REM] latency and abnormal dexamethasone suppression test results.)

   a. Impulsive traits are associated with increased levels of testosterone, 17-estradiol, and estrone. Low levels of platelet monoamine oxidase may be associated with sociability or with schizotypal personality disorder.

   b. Saccadic eye movements are associated with introversion, low self-esteem, social withdrawal, and schizotypal personality disorder.

   c. High levels of endorphins may be associated with phlegmatic features.

   d. Low levels of hydroxyindoleacetic acid (5-HIAA) are associated with suicide attempts, impulsiveness, and aggression. Raising serotonin levels pharmacologically may be associated with diminished sensitivity to rejection and increased assertiveness, self-esteem, and stress tolerance.

   e. Electroencephalogram (EEG) slow-wave activity may be associated with some personality disorders. Early neurological soft signs are associated with antisocial and borderline personality disorders.

   f. The brain dysfunction associated with personality disorders, especially antisocial disorders, is minimal.

3. Developmental histories frequently reveal individual difficulties and family problems, sometimes severe (abuse, incest, neglect, parental illness and death). Parent–child goodness of fit is also important.

E. Psychological tests

1. Neuropsychological tests may reveal organicity. EEG, computed tomography (CT), and electrophysiological mapping may also be useful.

2. Projective tests can reveal preferred personality patterns and styles (Minnesota Multiphasic Personality Inventory-2 [MMPI-2], thematic apperception test [TAT], Rorschach test, Draw-a-Person).

F. Pathophysiology of personality syndromes resulting from medical factors

1. Frontal lobe dysfunction is associated with impulsivity, poor judgment, abulia.

2. Temporal lobe lesions or dysfunction can be associated with Klüver-Bucy traits, hypersexuality, religiosity, possible violence.

3. Parietal lobe lesions are associated with denial or euphoric features.

G. Psychodynamics. These vary with different disorders. Most personality disorders tend to involve the problems listed below.

1. Ego function impairment.

2. Superego impairment.

3. Self-image, self-esteem problems.

4. Enactments of inner psychological conflicts based on past experiences, with impairments in judgment.

H. Course and prognosis. Variable. Patients are usually stable or deteriorate, but some patients improve. A tendency to the development of Axis I disorders has been noted.

I. Treatment. Usually, patients are not motivated. Otherwise, differing and sometimes mixed modalities are employed: psychoanalysis, psychoanalytic psychotherapy, supportive psychotherapy, cognitive therapy, group therapy, family therapy, milieu therapy, hospitalization (short- and long-term), pharmacotherapy.

J. Classification. DSM-IV-TR groups the personality disorders into three clusters.

1. Cluster A is the odd, eccentric cluster and consists of the paranoid, schizoid, and schizotypal personality disorders. These disorders involve the use of fantasy and projection and are associated with a tendency toward psychotic thinking. Patients may have a biological vulnerability toward cognitive disorganization when stressed.

2. Cluster B is the dramatic, emotional, and erratic cluster and includes the histrionic, narcissistic, antisocial, and borderline personality disorders. These disorders involve the use of dissociation, denial, splitting, and acting out. Mood disorders may be common.

3. Cluster C is the anxious or fearful cluster and includes the avoidant, dependent, and obsessive-compulsive personality disorders. These disorders involve the use of isolation, passive aggression, and hypochondriasis.

4. Some personality disorders are included in an appendix to DSM-IV-TR (depressive and passive-aggressive personality disorders). Personality disorder not otherwise specified is also listed. When a patient meets the criteria for more than one personality disorder, clinicians should diagnose each; this circumstance is not uncommon.

5. Clinicians should be aware of the following additional Axis I disorders: personality change secondary to a general medical condition; substance-related disorder not otherwise specified, gender identity disorder, impulse control disorders, psychological factors affecting medical condition, relational problems, problems related to abuse or neglect, noncompliance with treatment, malingering, adult antisocial behavior, child or adolescent antisocial behavior, identity problem, acculturation problem, phase-of-life problem.

II. Odd and eccentric cluster

A. Paranoid personality disorder

1. **Definition.** Patients with paranoid personality disorder have a tendency to attribute malevolent motives to others. They are suspicious and mistrustful; often hostile, irritable, or angry; and often bigots, injustice collectors, pathologically jealous spouses, or litigious cranks.

2. **Diagnosis, signs, and symptoms.** See Table 19–1. These patients tend to be reluctant to confide. They see hidden meanings, tend to bear grudges, and are quick to counterattack. They have a formal manner and can exhibit considerable muscle tension, with an inability to relax. They may scan the environment. They are often humorless and serious. Projection is employed, and they can be quite prejudiced. They show ideas of reference, seeing others as demeaning or threatening. They dispute others' loyalty or trustworthiness and may be quite restricted, lacking warmth. At times, they are proud of being rational and objective. They often attend excessively to power and rank and express disdain for the weak, sickly, or impaired. They may appear business-like and efficient but often generate fear or conflict in others. Some are involved in extremist groups.

TABLE 19–1
DSM-IV-TR DIAGNOSTIC CRITERIA FOR PARANOID PERSONALITY DISORDER

A. A pervasive distrust and suspiciousness of others such that their motives are interpreted as malevolent, beginning by early adulthood and present in a variety of contexts, as indicated by four (or more) of the following:
  (1) suspects, without sufficient basis. that others are exploiting, harming, or deceiving him or her
  (2) is preoccupied ith unjustified doubts about the loyalty or trustworthiness of friends or associates
  (3) is reluctant to confide in others because of unwarranted fear that the information will be used maliciously against him or her
  (4) reads hidden demeaning or threatening meanings into benign remarks or events
  (5) persistently bears grudges, i.e., is unforgiving of insults, injuries, or slights
  (6) perceives attacks on his or her character or reputation that are not apparent to others and is quick to react angrily or to counterattack
  (7) has recurrent suspicions, without justification, regarding fidelity of spouse or sexual partner
B. Does not occur exclusively during the course of schizophrenia, a mood disorder with psychotic features, or another psychotic disorder and is not due to the direct physiological effects of a general medical condition.

Note: If criteria are met prior to the onset of schizophrenia odd "premorbid," e.g., "paranoid personality disorder (premorbid)"

From American Psychiatric Association. *Diagnostic and Statistical Manual of Mental Disorders*, text revision, 4th ed. Washington, DC: American Psychiatric Association, Copyright 2000, with permission.

3. Epidemiology
   a. The prevalence is 0.5–2.5%.
   b. The incidence is increased in families of probands with schizophrenia and delusional disorders.
   c. The disorder is more common in men than in women.
   d. The prevalence is higher among minorities, immigrants, and the deaf.

4. Etiology
   a. A genetic component is established.
   b. Nonspecific early family difficulties are often present. Histories of childhood abuse are common.

5. Psychodynamics
   a. The classic defenses are projection, denial, and rationalization.
   b. Shame is a prominent feature.
   c. The superego is projected onto authority.
   d. Unresolved separation and autonomy issues are a factor.

6. Differential diagnosis
   a. Delusional disorder—the patient has fixed delusions.
   b. Paranoid schizophrenia—the patient has hallucinations and a formal thought disorder.
   c. Schizoid, borderline, and antisocial personality disorders—the patient does not show similar active involvement with others, is less stable, and has superego deficits.
   d. Substance abuse (e.g., stimulants) can produce paranoid features.

7. Course and prognosis.
These vary, depending on individual ego strengths and life circumstances; possible complications are delusional disorders, schizophrenia, depression, anxiety disorders, and substance-related disorders. Patients rarely seek treatment.

8. Treatment.
Paranoid patients tend to become more paranoid. Health practitioners should expect this and remain honest, courteous, and professional.
   a. Rarely, low-dose antipsychotics (e.g., 2.5 mg of olanzapine [Zyprexa] a day) can be used; an antianxiety agent (e.g., 0.5 mg of clonazepam [Klonopin] as needed) can be prescribed to deal with agitation and anxiety.
   b. Usually, supportive psychotherapy is employed, with attention to openness, consistency, and avoidance of humor. Healthy portions of the ego should be supported. Alternative explanations can be presented, but without confrontation.

B. Schizoid personality disorder

1. Definition.
The patient leads an isolated lifestyle without overt longing for others.

2. Diagnosis, signs, and symptoms.
See Table 19–2. Solitary jobs are held. The patients are ill at ease with others and may show poor eye contact. Their affect is often constricted or aloof. They may be inappropriately serious and are often fearful or indifferent in the presence of others. Humor may be off the mark. They may give short answers, avoid spontaneous speech, and use occasional odd metaphors. They may be fascinated with inanimate objects or metaphysical constructs, or inter-

TABLE 19–2
DSM-IV-TR DIAGNOSTIC CRITERIA FOR SCHIZOID PERSONALITY DISORDER

A. A pervasive pattern of detachment from social relationships and a restricted range of supression of emotions in interpersonal settings, beginning by early adulthood and present in a variety of contexts, as indicated by four (or more) of the following:
   (1) neither desires nor enjoys close relationships, including being part of a family
   (2) almost always chooses solitary activities
   (3) has little, if any, interest in having sexual experiences with another person
   (4) takes pleasure in few, if any, activities
   (5) lacks close friends or confidants other than first-degree relatives
   (6) appears indifferent to the praise or criticism of others
   (7) shows emotional coldness, detachment, or flattened affectivity
B. Does not occur exclusively during the course of schizophrenia, a mood disorder with psychotic features, another psychotic disorder, or a pervasive developmental disorder and is not due to the direct physiological effects of a general medical condition.

Note: If criteria are met prior to the onset of schizophrenia, add "premorbid," e.g., "schizoid personality disorder (premorbid)"

From American Psychiatric Association. *Diagnostic and Statistical Manual of Mental Disorders*, text revision, 4th ed. Washington, DC: American Psychiatric Association, Copyright 2000, with permission.

ested in mathematics, astronomy, or philosophical movements. They are often reserved and uninvolved in the everyday events and concerns of others or may have an unwarranted sense of intimacy with others. They lack any apparent need or longing for ties to others but may be very attached to animals. These patients may be very passive and noncompetitive, with solitary interests. Their sexuality may involve fantasy only. Men often remain single, but women may passively agree to marriage. They may have an inability to express anger. Threats from others may be dealt with by fantasized omnipotence or resignation.

3. **Epidemiology**
   a. This disorder may affect 7.5% of the general population.
   b. The incidence is increased among family members of schizophrenic probands.
   c. The incidence is greater among men than among women, with a possible ratio of 2:1.

4. **Etiology**
   a. Genetic factors are likely.
   b. A history of disturbed early family relationships often is elicited.

5. **Psychodynamics**
   a. Social inhibition is pervasive.
   b. Social needs are repressed to ward off aggression.

6. **Differential diagnosis**
   a. Paranoid personality disorder—the patient is involved with others.
   b. Schizotypal personality disorder—the patient exhibits oddities and eccentricities of manners.
   c. Avoidant personality disorder—the patient is isolated but wants to be involved with others.

7. **Course and prognosis**
   a. These are variable.
   b. Complications of delusional disorder, schizophrenia, other psychoses, or depression may develop.

8. Treatment
   a. Supportive psychotherapy with a focus on relatedness, fears of closeness, and identification of emotions may be helpful.
   b. Group psychotherapy may be helpful.
   c. Milieu therapy may be helpful for some patients.
   d. Pharmacotherapy—some patients respond to antidepressants, psychostimulants, or low-dose antipsychotics.
   e. Because closeness is threatening, patients with this disorder may flee.

C. Schizotypal personality disorder
   1. Definition. Patients with schizotypal personality disorder have multiple oddities and eccentricities of behavior, thought, affect, speech, appearance. They appear strange to others. They engage in magical thinking; have peculiar ideas, ideas of reference, and illusions; and exhibit derealization.

   2. Diagnosis, signs, and symptoms. See Table 19–3. These patients seem "strange" or "odd." Their speech may be distinctive, idiosyncratic, or peculiar. They may not know their own feelings and be very sensitive to a negative affect in others. Many are superstitious or believe in extrasensory perception. They have an active fantasy life. They tend to be isolated and may exhibit transient psychotic symptoms under stress. They may be involved in cults, strange religious practices, or the occult. Few have close friends, and social anxiety is excessive in most.

   ### 3. Epidemiology
   a. The prevalence of this disorder is 3%.
   b. The prevalence is increased in families of schizophrenic probands. A higher concordance in monozygotic twins has been shown.
   c. This disorder is seen more commonly in men than in women.

TABLE 19–3
DSM-IV-TR DIAGNOSTIC CRITERIA FOR SCHIZOTYPAL PERSONALITY DISORDER

A. A pervasive pattern of social and interpersonal deficits marked by acute discomfort with and reduced capacity for close relationships as well as by cognitive or perceptual distortions and eccentricities of behavior, beginning by early adulthood and present in a variety of contexts, as indicated by five (or more) of the following:
   (1) ideas of reference (excluding delusions of reference)
   (2) odd beliefs or magical thinking that influences behavior and is inconsistent with subcultural norms (e.g., superstitiousness, belief in clairvoyance, telepathy, or "sixth sense"; in children and adolescents, bizarre fantasies or preoccupations)
   (3) unusual perceptual experiences, including bodily illusions
   (4) odd thinking and speech (e.g., vague, circumstantial, metaphorical, overelaborate, or stereotyped)
   (5) suspiciousness or paranoid ideation
   (6) inappropriate or constricted affect
   (7) behavior of appearance that is odd, eccentric, or peculiar
   (8) lack of close friends or confidants other than first-degree relatives
   (9) excessive social anxiety that does not diminish with familiarity and tends to be associated with paranoid fears rather than negative judgments about self
B. Does not occur exclusively during the course of schizophrenia, a mood disorder with psychotic features, another psychotic disorder, or a pervasive developmental disorder.

Note: If criteria are met prior to the onset of schizophrenia, add "premorbid," e.g., "schizotypal personality disorder (premorbid)"

4. **Etiology.** Etiological models of schizophrenia may apply. See Chapter 8.
5. **Psychological tests.** Thought disorder is common on the Rorschach test.
6. **Pathophysiology**
   a. Diminished monoamine oxidase.
   b. Impairments in smooth-pursuit eye tracking.
   c. Diminished brain mass, especially in the temporal lobe.
7. **Psychodynamics.** Dynamics of magical thinking, splitting, isolation of affect.
8. **Differential diagnosis**
   a. **Paranoid personality disorder**—the patient is suspicious and guarded.
   b. **Schizoid personality disorder**—the patient has no particular eccentricities.
   c. **Borderline personality disorder**—the patient shows emotional instability, intensity, and impulsiveness.
   d. **Schizophrenia**—the patient's reality testing is lost.
9. **Course and prognosis**
   a. The prognosis is guarded.
   b. Schizophrenia develops in some patients.
   c. Up to 10% of patients may commit suicide.
10. **Treatment.** Patients may need the auxiliary ego of the therapist to help with reality testing.
    a. Pharmacological—low-dose antipsychotics (e.g., 2.5 mg of olanzapine a day) or antidepressants may be helpful.
    b. Supportive psychotherapy is often helpful.
    c. Group psychotherapy may be useful.
    d. Milieu therapy may be indicated for some.

III. Dramatic, emotional, and erratic cluster

A. Antisocial personality disorder

1. **Definition.** This disorder involves maladaptive behavior in which the patient does not recognize the rights of others. It is not strictly synonymous with criminality.
2. **Diagnosis, signs, and symptoms.** See Table 19–4.
   a. Patients may show "psychopathic features": a "mask of sanity" (term originated by H. Cleckley). They may be manipulative and appear trustworthy.
   b. Criminal or dishonest activities are common, including lying, truancy, and running away from home. The patient may have a history of violence or be at risk for violent behavior. Promiscuity and spouse and child abuse are common. These patients lack remorse.
   c. Impulse dyscontrol and a failure to plan are present.
   d. Patients characteristically show a lack of sensitivity to others.
   e. Irritability and aggression are common.
   f. Deceit and irresponsibility are a way of life.
   g. They show a disregard for the safety of others and themselves.

TABLE 19-4
DSM-IV-TR DIAGNOSTIC CRITERIA FOR ANTISOCIAL PERSONALITY DISORDER

A. There is a pervasive pattern of disregard for and violation of the right of others occurring since age 15 years as indicated by three (or more) of the following:
   (1) failure to conform to social norms with respect to lawful behaviors as indicated by repeatedly performing acts that are grounds for arrest
   (2) deceitfulness, as indicated by repeated lying, use of all cases, or conning others for personal profit or pleasure
   (3) impulsivity or failure to plan ahead
   (4) irritability and aggressiveness, as indicated by repeated physical fights or assaults
   (5) reckless disregard for safety of self or others
   (6) consistent irresponsibility as indicated by repeated failure to sustain consistent work behavior or honor financial obligations
   (7) lack of remorse, as indicated by being indifferent to or rationalizing having hurt, mistreated, or stolen from another
B. The individual is at least age 18 years.
C. There is evidence of conduct disorder with onset before age 15 years.
D. The occurrence of antisocial behavior is not exclusively during the course of schizophrenia or a manic episode.

From American Psychiatric Association. *Diagnostic and Statistical Manual of Mental Disorders*, text revision, 4th ed. Washington, DC: American Psychiatric Association, Copyright 2000, with permission.

3. Epidemiology
   a. The prevalence is 3% in men (it may be as high as 7%) and 1% in women. In prison populations, it may be as high as 75%.
   b. Antisocial personality disorder, somatization disorder, and alcoholism cluster in some families. The disorder is five times more common among first-degree relatives of men than among controls.
   c. The disorder is more common in lower socioeconomic groups.
   d. Predisposing conditions include attention-deficit/hyperactivity disorder (ADHD) and conduct disorder.

4. Etiology
   a. Adoptive studies demonstrate that genetic factors are involved in this disorder.
   b. Brain damage or dysfunction is a feature of this disorder, which can be secondary to such conditions as perinatal brain injury, head trauma, and encephalitis.
   c. Histories of parental abandonment or abuse are very common. Repeated, arbitrary, or harsh punishment by parents is thought to be a factor.

5. Pathophysiology
   a. If brain damage is present, impulsivity usually is a consequence of frontal lobe injury or dysfunction, as shown by positron emission tomography.
   b. Other brain lesions (e.g., lesions of the amygdala or possibly other temporal lesions) can predispose to violence.
   c. Abnormal EEG findings may be present.
   d. Soft neurological signs may be present.

6. Psychodynamics
   a. Patients with this disorder are impulse-ridden, with associated ego deficits in planning and judgment.
   b. Superego deficits or lacunae are present; conscience is primitive or poorly developed.

c. Object relational difficulties are significant, with a failure in empathy, love, and basic trust.
d. Aggressive features are prominent.
e. Associated features are sadomasochism, narcissism, and depression.

7. Differential diagnosis
a. Adult antisocial behavior—the patient does not meet all the criteria in Table 19–4.
b. Substance use disorders—the patient may exhibit antisocial behavior as a consequence of substance abuse and dependence; the problems may coexist.
c. Mental retardation—the patient may demonstrate antisocial behavior as a consequence of impaired intellect and judgment; the problems may coexist.
d. Psychoses—the patient may engage in antisocial behavior as a consequence of psychotic delusions; the problems may coexist.
e. Borderline personality disorder—the patient often attempts suicide and exhibits self-loathing and intense, ambivalent attachments.
f. Narcissistic personality disorder—the patient is law-abiding.
g. Personality change secondary to a general medical condition—the patient has had a different premorbid personality or shows features of an organic disorder.
h. ADHD—cognitive difficulties and impulse dyscontrol are present.

8. Course and prognosis
a. The prognosis varies. The condition often significantly improves after early or middle adulthood.
b. Complications include death by violence, substance abuse, suicide, physical injury, legal and financial difficulties, depressive disorders. Many medical disorders are associated with this personality disorder.

9. Treatment
a. Treatment is often difficult, if not impossible.
b. The patient may be superficially charming but manipulative in a medical setting or may be defiant and refuse medical care.
c. The treatment of substance abuse may effectively treat antisocial traits.
d. Long-term hospitalization or a residence in a therapeutic community sometimes is effective.
e. Usually, effective treatment is behavioral (e.g., behavior may be modified by the threat of legal sanctions or the fear of punishment). Among healthier patients with this disorder, treatment tends to include overt setting of limits.
f. Some success has been reported with group psychotherapy, including self-help groups.
g. Pharmacotherapy.
  (1) Stimulants (e.g., 5 to 20 mg of methylphenidate [Ritalin] three times daily) may be given for ADHD.
  (2) Anticonvulsants (e.g., 500 to 1,000 mg of divalproex [Depakote] twice daily), mood stabilizers (e.g., 300 to 600 mg of lithium carbonate three times daily), or beta-blockers (e.g., 40 to 180 mg of nadolol [Corgard] daily) may be given for impulse dyscontrol.

B. Borderline personality disorder
1. Definition
   a. Defining this disorder entails multiple complexities and controversies. Conceptualizations often involve overlap with psychosis, mood disorders, other personality disorders, and cognitive disorders. It was formerly considered to be on the border between neurosis and psychosis.
   b. Separation–individuation problems, affective control problems, and intense, personal attachments appear central, in addition to self-image problems.
2. Diagnosis, signs, and symptoms. See Table 19–5.
   a. Patients are "always in crisis."
   b. They tend to have micropsychotic episodes, often with paranoia or transient dissociative symptoms.
   c. Self-destructive, self-mutilating, or suicidal gestures, threats, or acts are frequent.
   d. Relationships with others are often tumultuous.
   e. They are intolerant of being alone and driven by object hunger. They engage in frantic efforts to avoid real or imagined abandonment.
   f. They may be easily enraged.
   g. They are often manipulative, sometimes transparently so.
   h. Their self-image and identity are unstable.
   i. They are impulsive in regard to money and sex, and engage in substance abuse, reckless driving, or binge eating.
   j. Mood reactivity is usually present. They can have "affect storms."
   k. Pananxiety and chaotic sexuality are common features.
3. Epidemiology
   a. The prevalence of borderline personality disorder is about 2% of the general population.
   b. It is more common in women than in men.

TABLE 19–5
DSM-IV-TR DIAGNOSTIC CRITERIA FOR BORDERLINE PERSONALITY DISORDER

A pervasive pattern of instability of interpersonal relationships, self-image, and affects, and marked impulsivity beginning by early adulthood and present in a variety of contexts, as indicated by five (or more) of the following:
   (1) frantic efforts to avoid real or imagined abandonment. **Note:** Do not include suicidal or self-mutilating behavior, covered in Criterion 5
   (2) a pattern of unstable and intense interpersonal relationships characterized by alternating between extremes of idealization and devaluation
   (3) identity disturbance: markedly and persistently unstable self-image or sense of self
   (4) impulsivity in at least two areas that are potentially self-damaging (e.g., spending, sex, substance abuse, reckless driving, binge eating). **Note:** Do not include suicidal or self-mutilating behavior covered in Criterion 5
   (5) recurrent suicidal behavior, gestures, or threats, or self-mutilating behavior
   (6) affective instability due to a marked reactivity of mood (e.g., intense episodic dysphoria, irritability, or anxiety usually lasting a few hours and only rarely more than a few days)
   (7) chronic feelings of emptiness
   (8) inappropriate, intense anger or difficulty controlling anger (e.g., frequent displays of temper, constant anger, recurrent physical fights)
   (9) transient, stress-related paranoid ideation or severe dissociative symptoms

From American Psychiatric Association. *Diagnostic and Statistical Manual of Mental Disorders*, text revision, 4th ed. Washington, DC: American Psychiatric Association, Copyright 2000, with permission.

c. Of these patients, 90% have one other psychiatric diagnosis, and 40% have two.

d. The prevalence of mood and substance-related disorders in families is increased.

e. The prevalence of borderline personality disorder is increased in the mothers of borderline patients.

4. Etiology

a. Brain damage may be present and represent perinatal brain injury, encephalitis, head injury, and other brain disorders.

b. Histories of physical and sexual abuse, abandonment, or overinvolvement are the rule.

5. Psychological tests. Projective tests reveal impaired reality testing.

6. Pathophysiology

a. Frontal lesions can impair judgment and affective control.

b. Temporal lesions can produce Klüver-Bucy traits.

c. Serotonin deficiency may be present.

7. Psychodynamics

a. Splitting—the patient manifests rage without a consciousness of ambivalent or positive emotions toward someone. It is usually transient. An associated feature is an ability to divide persons into those who like and those who hate the patient, and into those who are all "good" and all "bad." This can become a problem for a treatment team managing a patient.

b. Primitive idealization.

c. Projective identification—the patient attributes idealized positive or negative features to another, then seeks to engage the other in various interactions that confirm the patient's belief. The patient tries, unconsciously, to induce the therapist to play the projected role.

d. The patient has both intense aggressive needs and intense object hunger, often alternating.

e. The patient has a marked fear of abandonment.

f. The rapprochement subphase of separation–individuation (theory of M. Mahler) is unresolved; object constancy is impaired. This results in a failure of internal structuralization and control.

g. Turning against the self—self-hate, self-loathing—is prominent.

h. Generalized ego dysfunction results in identity disturbance.

8. Differential diagnosis

a. **Psychotic disorder**—impaired reality testing persists.

b. **Mood disorders**—the mood disturbance is usually nonreactive. Major depressive disorder with atypical features is often a difficult differential diagnosis. At times, only a treatment trial will tell. Atypical patients often have sustained episodes of depression, however.

c. **Personality change secondary to a general medical condition**—results of testing for medical illness are positive.

d. **Schizotypal personality disorder**—the affective features are less severe.

e. **Antisocial personality disorder**—the defects in conscience and attachment ability are more severe.

f. **Histrionic personality disorder**—suicide and self-mutilation are less common. The patient tends to have more stable interpersonal relationships.

g. **Narcissistic personality disorder**—identity formation is more stable.

h. **Dependent personality disorder**—attachments are stable.

i. **Paranoid personality disorder**—suspiciousness is more extreme and consistent.

9. Course and prognosis

a. These are variable; some improvement may occur in later years.

b. Suicide, self-injury, mood disorders, somatoform disorders, psychoses, substance abuse, and sexual disorders are possible complications.

10. Treatment.
Patients with borderline personality disorder can be problematic. The patient may have "affect storms" and require considerable attention.

a. Treatment usually involves mixed supportive and exploratory psychotherapy. Management of transference psychosis, countertransference, acting out, and suicide threats and wishes is problematic. The therapist functions as an auxiliary ego, sets limits, and offers structure.

b. Behavior therapy may be useful to control impulses and angry outbursts and to reduce sensitivity to criticism and rejection; social skills training is used. Dialectical behavior therapy is a recent innovation.

c. Psychopharmacology—some medications may be useful for mood stabilization and impulse control. These include antidepressants (e.g., 50 to 200 mg of sertraline [Zoloft] per day, 300 to 600 mg of lithium carbonate two or three times a day, 200 to 400 mg of carbamazepine [Tegretol] three times a day, divalproex at therapeutic levels). Low-dose antipsychotics (e.g., 2.5 mg of olanzapine a day) may be useful for limited periods.

e. Hospitalizations for crises are usually brief, but some patients require long-term hospitalization for structural change.

f. The therapist must monitor countertransference and often seek consultation.

g. The patient can unconsciously split the staff. The patient engages the staff in such a way that they take sides against each other. This can be managed by educating the staff and must be anticipated.

C. Histrionic personality disorder

1. Definition.
Patients with histrionic personality disorder have a dramatic, emotional, impressionistic style.

2. Diagnosis, signs, and symptoms.
See Table 19–6.

a. Often cooperative and eager to be helped.

b. Tend to be colorful, possibly flamboyant, attention-seeking, and seductive.

TABLE 19–6
DSM-IV-TR DIAGNOSTIC CRITERIA FOR HISTRIONIC PERSONALITY DISORDER

A pervasive pattern of excessive emotionality and attention seeking, beginning by early adulthood and present in a variety of contexts, as indicated by five (or more) of the following:
(1) is uncomfortable in situations in which he or she is not the center of attention
(2) interaction with others is often characterized by inappropriate sexually seductive or provocative behavior
(3) displays rapidly shifting and shallow expression of emotions
(4) consistently uses physical appearance to draw attention to self
(5) has a style of speech that is excessively impressionistic and lacking in detail
(6) shows self-dramatization, theatricality, and exaggerated expression of emotion
(7) is suggestible, i.e., easily influenced by others or circumtances
(8) considers relationships to be more intimate than they actually are

From American Psychiatric Association. *Diagnostic and Statistical Manual of Mental Disorders*, text revision, 4th ed. Washington, DC: American Psychiatric Association, Copyright 2000, with permission.

    c. Show dependent behavior.
    d. Emotionality may be shallow or insincere.
    e. Speech may be dramatic.
    f. Often suggestible.
    g. Superficially likable, even gregarious.

3. Epidemiology
    a. The prevalence of histrionic personality disorder is 2–3%. Of the patients in treatment, 10–15% are reported to have this disorder.
    b. The prevalence is greater in women than in men, but the disorder is probably underdiagnosed in men.
    c. This disorder is associated with somatization disorder, mood disorders, and alcohol use.

4. Etiology
    a. Early interpersonal difficulties may have been resolved by dramatic behavior.
    b. Distant or stern father with a seductive mother may be a pattern.

5. Psychodynamics
    a. Fantasy in "playing a role," with emotionality and a dramatic style, is typical.
    b. Common defenses include repression, regression, identification, somatization, conversion, dissociation, denial, and externalization.
    c. A faulty identification with the same-sex parent and an ambivalent and seductive relationship with the opposite-sex parent are often noted.
    d. Fixation at the early genital level.
    e. Prominent oral traits.
    f. Fear of sexuality, despite overt seductiveness.

6. Differential diagnosis
    a. Borderline personality disorder—more overt despair and suicidal and self-mutilating features; the disorders can coexist.
    b. Somatization disorder—physical complaints predominate.
    c. Conversion disorder—physical deficits are apparent.
    d. Dependent personality disorder—the emotional style is lacking.

7. Course and prognosis

a. The course is variable.

b. Possible complications of somatization disorders, conversion disorders, dissociative disorders, sexual disorders, mood disorders, and substance abuse.

8. Treatment. The patient is often very emotional and may seek attention excessively.

a. Treatment is usually individual psychotherapy, insight-oriented or supportive, depending on ego strength. The focus is on the patient's deeper feeling and use of superficial drama as a defense against them.

b. Psychoanalysis is appropriate for some patients.

c. Group therapy can be useful.

d. Adjunctive use of medications, usually an anxiolytic (e.g., 0.5 to 1.0 mg of clonazepam daily), for transient emotional states can be helpful.

D. Narcissistic personality disorder

1. Definition. Pervasive pattern of grandiosity and overconcern with issues of self-esteem.

2. Diagnosis, signs, and symptoms. See Table 19–7.

a. Patients with narcissistic personality disorder have a grandiose sense of self-importance.

b. A sense of specialness and entitlement is associated.

c. The patient handles criticism or defeat with rage or depression; a fragile self-esteem is evident.

d. Can be exploitative, lacking empathy.

e. An excessive concern about appearance, rather than substance, is present, and the patient often requires excessive admiration.

3. Epidemiology

a. The established prevalence is less than 1% in the general population, but the disorder is thought to be significantly more common than this

---

TABLE 19–7
DSM-IV-TR DIAGNOSTIC CRITERIA FOR NARCISSISTIC PERSONALITY DISORDER

A pervasive pattern of grandiosity (in fantasy or behavior), need for admiration, and lack of empathy, beginning by early adulthood and present in a variety of contexts, as indicated by five (or more) of the following:

(1) has a grandiose sense of self-importance (e.g., exaggerates achievements and talents, expects to be recognized as superior without commensurate achievements)

(2) is preoccupied with fantasies of unlimited success, power, brilliance, beauty, or ideal love

(3) believes that he or she is "special" and unique and can only be understood by, or should associate with other special or high-status people (or institutions)

(4) requires excessive admiration

(5) has a sense of entitlement, i.e., unreasonable expectations of especially favorable treatment or automatic compliance with his or her expectations

(6) is interpersonality exploitative, i.e., takes advantage of others to achieve his or her own ends

(7) lacks empathy: is unwilling to recognize or identify with the feelings and needs of others

(8) is often envious of others or believes that others are envious of him or her

(9) shows arrogant, naughty behavior or attitudes

---

figure would indicate, and the number of affected persons may be increasing.

   b. The prevalence is 2–16% in the clinical population.

   c. A familial transmission is suspected.

4. **Etiology.** A commonly cited factor is a failure in maternal empathy, with early rejection or loss.

5. **Psychodynamics.** Are narcissistic traits developmental arrests or defenses? This is a matter of controversy. One view stresses that grandiosity and empathic failure defend against primitive aggression. The grandiosity is commonly viewed as a compensation for a sense of inferiority.

6. **Differential diagnosis**

   a. **Antisocial personality disorder**—the patient overtly disregards the law and the rights of others.

   b. **Paranoid schizophrenia**—the patient has overt delusions.

   c. **Borderline personality disorder**—the patient shows greater emotionality, greater instability.

   d. **Histrionic personality disorder**—the patient displays more emotion.

7. **Course and prognosis.** The disorder can be chronic and difficult to treat.

   a. Aging is handled poorly because it is a narcissistic injury.

   b. Possible complications include mood disorders, transient psychoses, somatoform disorders, and substance use disorders.

   c. The overall prognosis is guarded, although the narcissistic preoccupation of some patients may be much greater in early adulthood.

8. **Treatment**

   a. Individual psychotherapy, supportive or insight-oriented, depending on ego strength.

   b. Milieu therapy is helpful for patients with severe disorders.

   c. The treatment challenge is often the preservation of the patient's self-esteem, which is threatened by psychiatric interventions that are experienced as criticisms.

   d. Group psychotherapy can be helpful.

   e. Medical setting.

      (1) Illness may be a threat to a grandiose self-image.

      (2) Physicians may be idealized or devalued as patients measure themselves by the company they keep.

      (3) Such patients may expect special treatment.

IV. Anxious or fearful cluster

A. Obsessive-compulsive personality disorder

1. **Definition.** Perfectionism, orderliness, and inflexibility tend to predominate.

2. **Diagnosis, signs, and symptoms.** See Table 19–8.

   a. Excessively concerned with orderliness, including rules, regulations, and neatness.

   b. Perseverance is a common feature and often reaches a level of stubbornness.

TABLE 19–8
DSM-IV-TR DIAGNOSTIC CRITERIA FOR OBSESSIVE-COMPULSIVE PERSONALITY DISORDER

A pervasive pattern of preoccupation with orderliness, perfectionism, and mental and interpersonal control, of the expense of flexibility openness, and efficiency, beginning by early adulthood and present in a variety of contexts, as indicated by four (or more) of the following:

(1) is preoccupied with details, rules, lists, order, organization, or schedules to the extent that the major point of the activity is lost

(2) shows perfectionism that interferes with task completion (e.g., is unable to complete a project because his or her own overly strict standards are not met)

(3) is excessively devoted to work and productivity to the exclusion of leisure activities and friendships (not accounted for by obvious economic necessity)

(4) is overconscientious, scrupulous, and inflexible about matters of morality, ethics, or values (not accounted for by cultural or religious identification)

(5) is unable to discard worn-out or worthless objects even when they have no sentimental value

(6) is reluctant to delegate tasks or work with others unless they submit to exactly his or her way of doing things

(7) adopts a miserly spending style toward both self and others; money is viewed as something to be hoarded for future catastrophies

(8) shows rigidly and stubborness

From American Psychiatric Association. *Diagnostic and Statistical Manual of Mental Disorders*, text revision, 4th ed. Washington, DC: American Psychiatric Association, Copyright 2000, with permission.

c. Indecisiveness is a problem when decisions must be made intuitively.

d. Emotional constriction is common.

e. Perfectionism is frequent.

f. Patients seek control of themselves and their situations.

g. They may have a stiff, formal demeanor and tend to be serious, lacking spontaneity.

h. They may be circumstantial and detail-bound, preferring routine or ritual over novelty.

i. They may lack interpersonal skills, humor, warmth, or an ability to compromise.

j. They may have an authoritarian manner, with an excessive devotion to work and productivity.

k. Patients may hoard objects and are often miserly.

3. **Epidemiology**

a. The prevalence is greater in men than in women.

b. Familial transmission is likely.

c. The concordance is increased in monozygotic twins.

d. The disorder is diagnosed most often in oldest children.

4. **Etiology.** Patients may have backgrounds characterized by harsh discipline.

5. **Psychodynamics**

a. Isolation, reaction formation, undoing, intellectualization, and rationalization are the classic defenses.

b. Emotions are distrusted.

c. Issues of defiance and submission are psychologically important.

d. Fixation at the anal period.

6. **Differential diagnosis.** The patient with obsessive-compulsive disorder has true obsessions or compulsions, whereas the patient with obsessive-compulsive personality disorder does not.

7. Course and prognosis

a. The patient may flourish in arrangements in which methodical or detailed work is required.

b. The patient's personal life is likely to remain barren.

c. Complications of anxiety disorders, depressive disorders, and somatoform disorders may develop.

8. Treatment

a. Individual psychotherapy, supportive or insight-oriented, depending on ego strengths.

b. Group therapy can be beneficial.

c. Therapeutic issues include control, submission, and intellectualization.

d. Pharmacotherapy may be useful (e.g., 0.5 mg of clonazepam twice daily for anxiety; 75 to 225 mg of clomipramine [Anafranil] at bedtime or 20 to 200 mg daily of a selective serotonin reuptake inhibitor [SSRI] such as sertraline for obsessional or depressive features).

e. Medical setting—illness and treatment may be experienced as a threat to control or as punishment. Patients often react with intensified efforts to regain control (e.g., charting, calculating, monitoring).

B. Avoidant personality disorder

1. Definition. The patient has a shy or timid personality, also called *phobic*.

2. Diagnosis, signs, and symptoms. See Table 19–9.

a. Easily hurt and sensitive to rejection.

b. Socially withdrawn, requiring uncritical acceptance by others.

c. Desirous of social involvement.

d. "Inferiority complex" is often present: the patient lacks self-confidence and is self-effacing. The patient may misinterpret others' comments as derogatory and sees himself or herself as inept and unappealing.

3. Epidemiology

a. The prevalence is 0.05–1% of the general population. Figures as high as 10% have been reported.

b. Possible predisposing factors include avoidant disorder of childhood or adolescence or a deforming physical illness.

TABLE 19–9
DSM-IV-TR DIAGNOSTIC CRITERIA FOR AVOIDANT PERSONALITY DISORDER

A pervasive pattern of social inhibition, feeling of inadequacy, and hypersensitivity to negative evaluation, beginning by early adulthood and present in a variety of contexts, as indicated by four (or more) of the following:

(1) avoids occupational activities that involve significant interpersonal contact, because of fears of criticism, disapproval, or rejection

(2) is unwilling to get involved with people unless certain of being liked

(3) shows restraint within intimate relationships because of the fear of being shamed or ridiculed

(4) is preoccupied with being criticized or rejected in social situations

(5) is inhibited in new interpersonal situation because of feelings of inadequacy

(6) views self as socially inept, personally unappealing, or inferior to others

(7) is unusually reluctant to take personal risks or to engage in any new activities because they may prove embarrassing

From American Psychiatric Association. *Diagnostic and Statistical Manual of Mental Disorders,* text revision, 4th ed. Washington, DC: American Psychiatric Association, 2000, with permission.

4. Etiology. Overt parental deprecation, overprotection, or phobic features in the parents themselves are possible etiological factors.

5. Psychodynamics

a. The avoidance and inhibition are defensive.

b. The overt fears of rejection cover underlying aggression, either oedipal or preoedipal.

6. Differential diagnosis

a. **Schizoid personality disorder**—the patient has no overt desire for involvement with others.

b. **Social phobia**—specific social situations, rather than personal relationships, are avoided. The disorders may coexist. However, generalized social phobia is phenomenologically the same as avoidant personality disorder.

c. **Dependent personality disorder**—the patient does not avoid attachments and has a greater fear of abandonment.

7. Course and prognosis

a. The patient functions best in a protected environment, although he or she longs for more.

b. Possible complications are social phobia and mood disorders.

8. Treatment. The patient may be undemanding and cooperative but is sensitive to ambiguous statements as possibly demeaning.

a. Individual psychotherapy, supportive or insight-oriented, depending on ego strength.

b. Group therapy is often helpful.

c. Social skills and assertiveness training may be beneficial.

d. Pharmacotherapy to manage anxiety or depression, when present. Examples include beta blockers (e.g., 20 to 80 mg of propranolol [Inderal] three times daily), benzodiazepines (e.g., 0.5 mg of clonazepam twice daily), and SSRIs (e.g., 50 to 100 mg of sertraline at bedtime).

C. Dependent personality disorder

1. Definition. The patient is predominantly dependent and submissive.

2. Diagnosis, signs, and symptoms. See Table 19–10.

a. Patients subordinate needs and responsibilities to those of others and delegate decisions to others. They may tolerate abusive relationships.

b. They lack self-confidence and require advice and reassurance.

c. They are intolerant of being alone and tend to require excessive supervision at work.

d. They are passive, with difficulty expressing disagreement.

3. Epidemiology

a. The disorder is more prevalent in women than in men.

b. The disorder is common, possibly accounting for 2.5% of all personality disorders.

4. Etiology. Chronic physical illness, separation anxiety, or parental loss in childhood may predispose.

5. Psychodynamics

a. Unresolved separation issues are present.

b. The dependent stance is a defense against aggression.

TABLE 19–10
DSM-IV-TR DIAGNOSTIC CRITERIA FOR DEPENDENT PERSONALITY DISORDER

A pervasive and excessive need to be taken care of that leads to submissive and clinging behavior and fears of separation, beginning by early adulthood and present in a variety of contexts, as indicated by five (or more) of the following:
  (1) has difficulty making everyday decisions without an excessive amount of advice and reassuance from others
  (2) needs others to assume responsibility for most major areas of his or her life
  (3) has difficulty expressing disagreement with others because of fear of loss of support or approval
      Note: Do not include realistic fears of retribution
  (4) has difficulty initiating project or doing things on his or her own (because of a lack of self-confidence in judgment or abilities rather than a lack of motivation or energy)
  (5) goes to excessive lengths to obtain nurturance and support from others, to the point of volunteering to do things that are unpleasant
  (6) feels uncomfortable or helpless when alone because of exaggerated fears of being unable to care for himself or herself
  (7) urgently seeks another relationship as a source of care and support when a close relationship ends
  (8) is unrealistically preoccupied with fears of being left to take care of himself or herself

From American Psychiatric Association. *Diagnostic and Statistical Manual of Mental Disorders,* text revision, 4th ed. Washington, DC: American Psychiatric Association, 2000, with permission.

6. **Differential diagnosis**
    a. Agoraphobia—the patient is afraid of leaving or being away from home.
    b. Dependent features, short of dependent personality disorder, are common in other personality disorders.
7. **Course and prognosis**
    a. The course is variable.
    b. Depressive complications are possible if a relationship is lost. The prognosis can be favorable with treatment.
    c. The patient may not be able to tolerate the "healthy" step of leaving an abusive relationship.
8. **Treatment.** Patients have a tendency to regress, with fear of abandonment.
    a. Insight-oriented or supportive psychotherapy, depending on ego strength.
    b. Behavior therapy, assertiveness training, family therapy, and group therapy also are useful.
    c. Pharmacotherapy is useful for treating specific symptoms (e.g., 0.5 mg of clonazepam twice daily for anxiety and 50 to 100 mg of sertraline at bedtime for anxiety and depression).

V. **Other personality disorders**
  A. **Passive-aggressive personality disorder**
    1. **Definition.** The patient shows obstructionism, procrastination, stubbornness, and inefficiency.
    2. **Diagnosis, signs, and symptoms.** See Table 19–11.
        a. Resists demands for adequate performance.
        b. Finds excuses for delay and finds fault.
        c. Lacks assertiveness.
    3. **Epidemiology.** Unknown.

TABLE 19–11
DSM-IV-TR RESEARCH CRITERIA FOR PASSIVE-AGGRESSIVE PERSONALITY DISORDER

A. A pervasive pattern of negativistic attitudes and passive resistance to demands for adequate performance, beginning by early adulthood and present in a variety of contexts, as indicated by four (or
more) of the following:
  (1) passively resists fulfilling routine social and occupational tasks
  (2) complains of being misunderstood and unappreciated by others
  (3) is sullen and argumentative
  (4) unreasonably criticizes and scans authority
  (5) expresses envy and resentment toward those apparently more fortunate
  (6) voices exaggerated and persistent complaints of personal misfortune
  (7) alternates between hostile defiance and contrition
B. Does not occur exclusively during major depressive episodes and is not better accounted for by dysthymic disorder.

From American Psychiatric Association. *Diagnostic and Statistical Manual of Mental Disorders,* text revision, 4ᵗʰ ed. Washington, DC: American Psychiatric Association, Copyright 2000, with permission.

4. Etiology
  a. May involve learned behavior and parental modeling.
  b. Early difficulties with authority common.

5. Psychodynamics
  a. Conflicts regarding authority, autonomy, and dependence.
  b. Submission, defiance, and aggression.

6. Differential diagnosis
  a. **Histrionic and borderline personality disorders**—the patient's be-
    havior is more flamboyant, dramatic, and openly aggressive than in
    passive-aggressive personality disorder.
  b. **Antisocial personality disorder**—the patient's defiance is overt.
  c. **Obsessive-compulsive personality disorder**—the patient is overtly
    perfectionistic and submissive.

7. Course and prognosis. Possible complications are depressive disor-
ders and alcohol abuse. Prognosis is guarded.

8. Treatment
  a. The major difficulty lies in the patient's covert opposition to inter-
    ventions by a psychiatrist. The therapeutic goal is to make the patient
    conscious of oppositionalism.
  b. Supportive psychotherapy may be useful if the patient is willing and
    can comply.
  c. Assertiveness training may be helpful.

B. Depressive personality disorder
1. Definition. Patients are pessimistic, anhedonic, duty-bound, self-
doubting, and chronically unhappy.
2. Diagnosis, signs, and symptoms. See Table 19–12.
  a. The patient is often quiet, introverted, and passive.
  b. Pessimistic, critical of others, and often brooding.
3. Epidemiology
  a. The disorder is thought to be common, but no hard data are available.
  b. Probably occurs equally in men and women.
  c. Probably occurs in families with depression.
4. Etiology. The causes may involve early loss or poor parenting.

TABLE 19–12
DSM-IV-TR RESEARCH CRITERIA FOR DEPRESSIVE PERSONALITY DISORDER

A. A pervasive pattern of depressive cognitions and behaviors beginning by early adulthood and present in a variety of contexts, as indicated by five (or more) of the following:
  (1) usual mood is dominated by dejection, gloominess, cheerlessness, joylessness, unhappiness
  (2) self-concept centers around beliefs of inadequacy, worthlessness, and low self-esteem
  (3) is critical, blaming, and derogatory toward self
  (4) is brooding and given to worry
  (5) is negativistic, critical, and judgmental toward others
  (6) is pessimistic
  (7) is prone to feeling guilty or remorseful
B. Does not occur exclusively during major depressive episodes and is not better accounted for by dysthymic disorder.

From American Psychiatric Association. *Diagnostic and Statistical Manual of Mental Disorders,* text revision, 4th ed. Washington, DC: American Psychiatric Association, Copyright 2000, with permission.

5. Psychodynamics
  a. Low self-esteem. Guilt.
  b. Self-punishing.
  c. Early loss of love object.

6. Differential diagnosis
  a. Dysthymic disorder—fluctuations in mood are greater than in depressive personality disorder.
  b. Avoidant personality disorder—the patient tends to be more anxious than depressed.

7. Course and prognosis. A risk for dysthymic disorder and major depressive disorder is thought to be likely.

8. Treatment
  a. Insight-oriented or supportive psychotherapy, depending on ego strength.
  b. Cognitive therapy, group therapy, and interpersonal therapy may be useful.
  c. Pharmacotherapy—SSRIs (e.g., 100 mg of sertraline a day) or sympathomimetics (e.g., 5 to 15 mg of methylphenidate a day) may be helpful.

C. Sadistic personality disorder. Relationships among these patients are dominated by cruel or demeaning behavior. The disorder is clinically rare; it is perhaps more common in forensic settings. It is often related to parental abuse.

D. Self-defeating personality disorder. Patients direct their lives toward bad outcomes; they reject help or good outcomes and have a dysphoric response to good outcomes. The features occur frequently in other personality disorders, but the occurrence of this disorder by itself may be uncommon.

E. Personality disorder not otherwise specified. This diagnosis is made if the patient has a personality disorder with mixed features of other personality disorders.

For more detailed discussion of this topic, see Personality Disorders, Ch 24, p 1723, in CTP/VII.

20

Suicide, Violence, and Other Psychiatry Emergencies

I. Suicide

A. Definition

1. Intentional self-inflicted death (from the Latin words meaning *one's own* and *to kill*).
2. Identification of the potentially suicidal patient is among the most difficult tasks in psychiatry.
3. Patients who repeatedly attempt to harm themselves are said to show parasuicidal behavior.

B. Incidence and prevalence

1. About 35,000 persons commit suicide per year in the United States.
2. The rate is 12 persons per 100,000.
3. About 250,000 persons attempt suicide per year.
4. The United States is at the midpoint worldwide in numbers of suicides (e.g., 25 persons per 100,000 in Scandinavian countries). The rate is lowest in Spain and Italy.

C. Associated factors. Table 20–1 lists high- and low-risk factors in the evaluation of suicide risk.

1. **Sex.** Men commit suicide three times more often than women. Women attempt suicide four times more often than men.
2. **Method.** Men use more violent methods than women (e.g., guns vs. drugs).
3. **Age.** Rates increase with age.
   a. Among men, the suicide rate peaks after age 45; among women, it peaks after age 65.
   b. Older persons attempt suicide less often but are more successful.
   c. After age 75, the rate rises in both sexes.
   d. Currently, the most rapid rise is among male 15- to 24-year-olds.
4. **Race.** Two of every three suicides are committed by male white persons. The risk is lower in nonwhites. The risk is high in Native Americans and Inuits.
5. **Religion.** Rate highest in Protestants; lowest in Catholics, Jews, and Muslims.
6. **Marital status.** Rate higher in single persons than in married persons. High in divorced persons. Death of spouse increases risk.
7. **Physical health.** Medical or surgical illness is a high-risk factor, especially if associated with pain or chronic or terminal illness (Table 20–2).

8. Mental illness

a. Fifty percent of all persons who commit suicide are depressed. Fifteen percent of depressed patients kill themselves.

b. Ten percent of persons who commit suicide are schizophrenic with prominent delusions.

c. A substance use disorder increases risk, especially if the person is also depressed.

TABLE 20–1
EVALUATION OF SUICIDE RISK

Variable	High Risk	Low Risk
Demographic and social profile		
Age	Over 45 years	Below 45 years
Sex	Male	Female
Marital status	Divorced or widowed	Married
Employment	Unemployed	Employed
Interpersonal relationship	Conflictual	Stable
Family background	Chaotic or conflictual	Stable
Health		
Physical	Chronic illness	Good health
	Hypochondriac	Feels healthy
	Excessive substance intake	Low substance use
Mental	Severe depression	Mild depression
	Psychosis	Neurosis
	Severe personality disorder	Normal personality
	Substance abuse	Social drinker
	Hopelessness	Optimism
Suicidal activity		
Suicidal ideation	Frequent, intense, prolonged	Infrequent, low intensity, transient
Suicide attempt	Multiple attempts	First attempt
	Planned	Impulsive
	Rescue unlikely	Rescue inevitable
	Unambiguous wish to die	Primary wish for change
	Communication internalized (self-blame)	Communication externalized (anger)
	Method lethal and available	Method of low lethality or not readily available
Resources		
Personal	Poor achievement	Good achievement
	Poor insight	Insightful
	Affect unavailable or poorly controlled	Affect available and appropriately controlled
Social	Poor rapport	Good rapport
	Socially isolated	Socially integrated
	Unresponsive family	Concerned family

From Adam K. Attempted suicide. *Psychiatric Clin North Am* 1985;8:183, with permission.

TABLE 20–2
MEDICAL AND MENTAL DISORDERS ASSOCIATED WITH INCREASED SUICIDE RISK

- Acquired immune deficiency syndrome (AIDS)
- Amnesia
- Attention-deficit/hyperactivity disorder (ADHD)
- Bipolar disorder
- Borderline personality disorder
- Delirium
- Dementia
- Dysthymic disorder
- Eating disorders
- Impulse-control disorders
- Learning disability
- Major depression
- Panic disorder
- Posttraumatic stress disorder
- Schizoaffective disorder
- Schizophrenia
- Substance use disorders

   d. Borderline personality disorder is associated with a high rate of para-suicidal behavior.
   e. Dementia, delirium, panic states increase risk.

9. Other risk factors
   a. Unambiguous wish to die.
   b. Unemployment.
   c. Sense of hopelessness.
   d. Rescue unlikely.
   e. Hoarding pills.
   f. Possession of firearms.
   g. Family history of suicide.
   h. Fantasies of reunion with deceased loved ones.

D. Management of the suicidal patient. A general strategy for evaluating suicidal patients is presented in Table 20–3.

1. Do not leave a suicidal patient alone; remove any potentially dangerous objects from the room.

2. Assess whether the attempt was planned or impulsive. Determine the lethality of the method, the chances of discovery (whether the patient was alone or notified someone), and the reaction to being saved (whether the patient is disappointed or relieved). Also determine whether the factors that led to the attempt have changed.

3. Patients with severe depression may be treated on an outpatient basis if their families can supervise them closely and if treatment can be initiated rapidly. Otherwise, hospitalization is necessary.

4. The suicidal ideation of alcoholic patients generally remits with abstinence in a few days. If depression persists after the physiological signs of

---

TABLE 20–3
GENERAL STRATEGY IN EVALUATING PATIENTS

I. Protect yourself
   A. Know as much as possible about the patients before meeting them.
   B. Leave physical restraint procedures to those who are trained to handle them.
   C. Be alert to risks for impending violence.
   D. Attend to the safety of the physical surroundings (e.g., door access, room objects).
   E. Have others present during the assessment if needed.
   F. Have others in the vicinity.
   G. Attend to developing an alliance with the patient (e.g., do not confront or threaten patients with paranoid psychoses).

II. Prevent harm
   A. Prevent self-injury and suicide. Use whatever methods are necessary to prevent patients from hurting themselves during the evaluation.
   B. Prevent violence toward others. During the evaluation, briefly assess the patient for the risk of violence. If the risk is deemed significant, consider the following options:
      1. Inform the patient that violence is not acceptable.
      2. Approach the patient in a nonthreatening manner.
      3. Reassure and calm the patient or assist in reality testing.
      4. Offer medication.
      5. Inform the patient that restraint or seclusion will be used if necessary.
      6. Have teams ready to restrain the patient.
      7. When patients are restrained, always closely observe them, and frequently check their vital signs. Isolate restrained patients from agitating stimuli. Immediately plan a further approach—medication, reassurance, medical evaluation.

III. Rule out cognitive disorders
IV. Rule out impending psychosis.

alcohol withdrawal have resolved, a high suspicion of major depression is warranted. All suicidal patients who are intoxicated by alcohol or drugs must be reassessed when they are sober.

5. Suicidal ideas in schizophrenic patients must be taken seriously, as they tend to use violent, highly lethal, and sometimes bizarre methods.

6. Patients with personality disorders benefit mostly from empathic confrontation and assistance in solving the problem that precipitated the suicide attempt and to which they have usually contributed.

7. Long-term hospitalization is recommended for conditions that contribute to self-mutilation; brief hospitalization does not usually affect such habitual behavior. Parasuicidal patients may benefit from long-term rehabilitation, and brief hospitalization may be necessary from time to time, but short-term treatment cannot be expected to alter their course significantly.

E. Dos and don'ts in dealing with suicide

1. *Do* ask about suicidal ideas, especially plans to harm oneself. Asking about suicide does not plant the idea.

2. *Don't* hesitate to ask patients if they "want to die." A straightforward approach is the most effective.

3. *Do* conduct the interview in a safe place. Patients have been known to throw themselves out of a window.

4. *Don't* offer false reassurance (e.g., "Most people think about killing themselves at some time").

5. *Do* ask about past suicide attempts, which can be related to future attempts.

6. *Do* ask about access to firearms; access to weapons increases the risk in a suicidal patient.

7. *Don't* release patients from the emergency department if you are not certain that they will not harm themselves.

8. *Do* not assume that family or friends will be able to watch a patient 24 hours a day. If that is required, do admit the patient to the hospital.

II. Violence

A. Definition

1. Intentional act of doing bodily harm to another person.

2. Includes assault, rape, robbery, and homicide.

3. Physical and sexual abuse of adults, children, and the elderly are included in violent acts.

B. Incidence and prevalence

1. About 8 million violent acts are committed each year in the United States.

2. Lifetime risk of becoming a homicide victim is about 1 in 85 for men, 1 in 280 for women. Men are the victims of violence more often than women.

C. Disorders associated with violence. The psychiatric conditions most commonly associated with violence include such psychotic disorders as schizophrenia and mania (particularly if the patient is paranoid or is experiencing command hallucinations), intoxication with alcohol and drugs,

withdrawal from alcohol and sedative-hypnotics, catatonic excitement, agitated depression, personality disorders characterized by rage and poor impulse control (e.g., borderline and antisocial personality disorders), and cognitive disorders (especially those associated with frontal and temporal lobe involvement).

D. Predicting violent behavior.   See Table 20–4. Best predictors are past acts of violence. Look for the following:

1. Very recent acts of violence, also destruction of property.
2. Menacing verbal or physical threats.
3. Carrying weapons or other objects that might be used as weapons (e.g., forks, ashtrays).
4. Progressive psychomotor agitation.
5. Alcohol or drug intoxication.
6. Paranoid features in a psychotic patient.
7. Violent command auditory hallucinations.
8. Brain disease (e.g., tumors, dementia [global or with frontal lobe findings; violence less common with temporal lobe findings]).
9. Catatonic excitement.
10. Mania.
11. Agitated depression.
12. Patients with personality disorders who are prone to rage, violence, or impulsivity.
13. History of cruelty to animals.

E. Evaluation and management

1. Protect yourself. Assume that violence is always a possibility, and be on guard for a sudden violent act. Never interview an armed patient. The patient should always surrender the weapon to a security guard. Know as much as possible about the patient before the interview. Never interview a potentially violent patient alone or in an office with the door

TABLE 20–4
ASSESSING AND PREDICTING VIOLENT BEHAVIOR

Signs of impending violence:
Recent acts of violence, including property violence.
Verbal or physical threats (menacing).
Carrying weapons or other objects that may be used as weapons (e.g., forks, ashtrays).
Progressive psychomotor agitation.
Alcohol or other substance intoxication.
Paranoid features in a psychotic patient.
Command violent auditory hallucinations—some but not all patients are at high risk.
Brain diseases, global or with frontal lobe findings; less commonly with temporal lobe findings (controversial).
Catatonic excitement.
Certain manic episodes.
Certain agitated depressive episodes.
Personality disorders (rage, violence, or impulse dyscontrol).

Assess the risk for violence:
Consider violent ideation, wish, intention, plan, availability of means, implementation of plan, wish for help.
Consider demographics—sex (male), age (15 to 24), socioeconomic status (low), social supports (few).
Consider the patient's history: violence, nonviolent antisocial acts, impulse dyscontrol (e.g., gambling, substance abuse, suicide or self-injury, psychosis).
Consider overt stressors (e.g., marital conflict, real or symbolic loss).

closed. Consider removing neckties, necklaces, and other articles of clothing or jewelry you are wearing that the patient can grab or pull. Stay within sight of other staff members. Leave physical restraint to staff members who are trained in that. Do not give the patient access to areas where weapons may be available (e.g., a crash cart or a treatment room). Do not sit close to a paranoid patient, who may feel threatened. Keep yourself at least an arm's length away from any potentially violent patient. Do not challenge or confront a psychotic patient. Be alert to the signs of impending violence. Always leave yourself a route of rapid escape in case the patient attacks you. Never turn your back on the patient.

2. Signs of impending violence include recent violent acts against people or property, clenched teeth and fists, verbal threats (menacing), possession of weapons or objects potentially usable as weapons (e.g., fork, ice pick, ashtray), psychomotor agitation (considered to be an important indicator), alcohol or drug intoxication, paranoid delusions, and command hallucinations.

3. Be sure that enough staff members are on hand to restrain the patient safely. Call for staff assistance before the patient's agitation has escalated. Often, a show of force through the presence of several able-bodied staff members is sufficient to prevent a violent act.

4. Physical restraint should be applied only by persons with appropriate training. Patients with suspected phencyclidine intoxication should not be physically restrained (limb restraints especially should be avoided) because they may injure themselves. Usually, a benzodiazepine or an antipsychotic is given immediately after physical restraints have been applied to provide a chemical restraint, but the choice of drug depends on the diagnosis. Provide a nonstimulating environment.

5. Perform a definitive diagnostic evaluation. The patient's vital signs should be assessed, a physical examination performed, and a psychiatric history obtained. Evaluate the patient's risk for suicide and create a treatment plan that provides for the management of potential subsequent violence. Elevated vital signs may suggest withdrawal from alcohol or sedative-hypnotics.

6. Explore possible psychosocial interventions to reduce the risk for violence. If violence is related to a specific situations or person, try to separate the patient from that situation or person. Try family interventions and other modifications of the environment. Would the patient still be potentially violent while living with other relatives?

7. Hospitalization may be necessary to detain the patient and prevent violence. Constant observation may be necessary, even on a locked inpatient psychiatric ward.

8. If psychiatric treatment is not appropriate, you may involve the police and the legal system.

9. Intended victims must be warned of the continued possibility of danger (e.g., if the patient is not hospitalized).

F. Dos and don'ts in dealing with violent patients

1. If the patient is brought to the emergency department by police with restraining devices (e.g. handcuffs), *don't* immediately remove them.
2. *Do* conduct the interview in a safe environment with attendants on call should the patient become agitated.
3. *Don't* position yourself so that you can be blocked by the patient from exiting the examination room.
4. *Don't* interview a patient if sharp or potentially dangerous objects are in the interview room (e.g., a letter opener on a desk).
5. *Do* trust your feelings. If you feel apprehensive or fearful, terminate the interview.
6. *Do* ask about past attempts at violence (including cruelty to animals). They are predictors for future violent events.
7. *Don't* hesitate to admit a patient for observation if there is any question of his or her being a danger to others.

G. History and diagnosis.
Risk factors for violence include a statement of intent, formulation of a specific plan, available means, male sex, young age (15 to 24 years), low socioeconomic status, poor social support system, past history of violence, other antisocial acts, poor impulse control, history of suicide attempts, and recent stressors. A history of violence is the best predictor of violence. Additional important factors include a history of childhood victimization; a childhood history of the triad of bed-wetting, fire setting, and cruelty to animals; a criminal record; military or police service; reckless driving; and a family history of violence.

H. Drug treatment

1. Drug treatment depends on the specific diagnosis.
2. Benzodiazepines and antipsychotics are used most often to tranquilize a patient. Fluphenazine (Prolixin), thiothixene (Navane), trifluoperazine (Stelazine), or haloperidol (Haldol) all given at a dose of 5 mg by mouth or intramuscularly; 2 mg of risperidone (Risperdal) by mouth; or 2 mg of lorazepam (Ativan) by mouth or intramuscularly may be tried initially.
3. If the patient is already taking an antipsychotic, give more of the same drug. If the patient's agitation has not decreased in 20 to 30 minutes, repeat the dose.
4. Avoid antipsychotics in patients who are at risk for seizures.
5. Benzodiazepines may be ineffective in patients who are tolerant, and they may cause disinhibition, which can potentially exacerbate violence.
6. For patients with epilepsy, first try an anticonvulsant (e.g., carbamazepine [Tegretol] or gabapentin [Neurontin]) and then a benzodiazepine (e.g., clonazepam [Klonopin]). Chronically violent patients sometime respond to beta-blockers (e.g., propranolol [Inderal]).

III. Other psychiatric emergencies

A psychiatric emergency is a disturbance in thoughts, feelings, or actions that requires immediate treatment. It may be caused or accompanied by a medical or

TABLE 20–5
COMMON PSYCHIATRIC EMERGENCIES

Syndrome or Presenting Symptom	Emergency Problem	Emergency Treatment Issues
Abuse of child or adults	Is there another explanation? Protect from further injury.	Management of medical problems; psychiatric evaluation; notification of protective services.
AIDS	Unrealistic or obsessive concern about having contracted the illness; changes in behavior secondary to organic effects; symptoms of depression or anxiety in someone who has the illness; grief over the loss of a friend or lover from AIDS.	Explore the patient's primary concern; if there is a realistic possibility of the patient's having contracted the virus, arrange for counseling and HIV titer; rule out an organic component in the HIV-positive patient; facilitate grieving for the patient who has suffered a loss by identifying the depression and referring for brief psychotherapy treatment or AIDS-support group.
Adjustment disorder	Agitation, sleep disorder, or depression; substance abuse; anxiety.	Explore briefly the meaning of the loss that has precipitated the adjustment reaction; refer for brief focused therapy; do not prescribe medications for the symptoms of adjustment disorder in the emergency department, as many of the symptoms abate once the patient is aware of their origins and has a chance to deal with the associated feelings.
Adolescent crisis	Suicidal ideation or attempts, running-away behaviors, drug use, pregnancy, psychosis, assaultive behavior toward family members, eating disorders.	Family crisis intervention is ideal if that can be accomplished; for the adolescent who is completely estranged from the family, inquire about an interested adult relative or friend who can be involved; evaluate for sexual or other physical abuse; evaluate for suicidal ideation; refer to adolescent crisis services if those are available; consider hospitalization if necessary.
Agoraphobia	Determination of the reason for the patient's emergency department visit.	Agoraphobia is a long-standing problem; refer the patient for psychiatric treatment; do not prescribe medications in the emergency department unless there will be continuity of care in follow-up.
Akathisia	Is this a new onset? Is the patient on maintenance antipsychotics?	Determine the causative agent; diphenhydramine (Benadryl) orally or intravenously, or benztropine (Cogentin) orally or intramuscularly. Explain to patient and family the cause of the symptom.
Alcohol-related emergencies	Confusion; psychosis; assaultive behavior; suicidal ideation or behavior; hallucinations.	Determine blood alcohol concentration; concentrations above 300 mg/dL suggest fairly long-standing alcohol abuse; assess the need for emergency intervention; antipsychotic agents as needed for psychotic symptoms; confront the patient about the degree of alcohol abuse and hold in emergency department until level decreases sufficiently for an appropriate assessment of suicidality and judgment; refer to an alcohol treatment program.

TABLE 20-5—*continued*

Syndrome or Presenting Symptom	Emergency Problem	Emergency Treatment Issues
Alcohol idiosyncratic intoxication	Marked aggressive or assaultive behavior; "the patient just isn't himself (or herself)!"	Rule out organic cause; benzodiazepines as needed to calm the patient; decrease external stimulation and restrain the patient, if necessary; after a determination is made that the patient can be safely discharged, warn the patient about the likelihood that the idiosyncratic reaction will recur with further drinking.
Alcohol withdrawal	Irritability, shakiness; confusion and disorientation; abnormal vital signs, including tachycardia, hyperthermia, and hypertension.	Benzodiazepines as needed to reduce symptoms; observe patient closely and monitor vital signs over several hours to detect onset of delirium tremens; when the patient is ready for discharge, inform the patient firmly about the diagnosis of alcohol dependence and refer for treatment.
Korsakoff's syndrome, Wernicke's encephalopathy	Confusion, amnesia; multiple organic symptoms, including ataxia, confusion, and disturbances of eye muscles.	Determine onset if possible; institute treatment with thiamine; determine capacity for patient to care for self; hospitalize, if necessary; inform the patient firmly about the diagnosis of alcoholism.
Amnesia	Identification; differential diagnosis, particularly of an organic component.	Explore circumstances in which patient came to the emergency department; consider an amobarbital (Amytal) interview; evaluate patient to rule out organic cause.
Amphetamine, cocaine, or amphetamine-like intoxication	Psychosis; agitation or assaultive behavior; paranoia.	Decrease stimulation, consider restraints and antipsychotics to control behavior; consider hospitalization as amphetamine-induced psychotic disorder may persist for weeks to months; cocaine withdrawal may produce suicidal feelings.
Anxiety, acute	Differential diagnosis, particularly of medical or substance induced cause; management of the acute symptomatology.	Explore patient's capacity for insight regarding the precipitant; refer for outpatient psychiatric treatment; avoid prescribing medications from the emergency department because the principal agents that are effective are also commonly abused.
Borderline personality disorder	Determination of the immediate need for the emergency department visit; determination of the patient's agenda.	Evaluate for acute suicidal ideation; consider hospitalization if clinician is uncomfortable; state limits as clearly as able to enforce; state clear follow-up plan.
Catatonia	Differential diagnosis of an organic cause; management of the acute symptoms.	Rule out organic causes; consider rapid tranquilization if the emergency department has the capacity to monitor the patient over several hours.
Delirium, dementia	Fluctuating sensorium; determine acuity; differential diagnosis; need for physical restraint while the patient is evaluated.	Evaluate patient for organic cause; remember that prescribed medications are very common causes for acute cognitive disorders.

continued

TABLE 20-5—*continued*

Syndrome or Presenting Symptom	Emergency Problem	Emergency Treatment Issues
Delusions	Degree to which delusional beliefs interfere with the patient's ability to negotiate activities of daily living; degree to which the patient's response to these delusional beliefs is likely to cause problems for the patient.	Explore the time of onset, the pervasiveness of the delusions, and the degree to which the delusional beliefs interfere with the patient's daily functioning, particularly if there is anything to suggest that the patient might try to harm self or others because of these delusions; rule out organic causes; refer for ongoing treatment, or hospitalize if there is an immediate life threat or need for further organic evaluation.
Depression	Recognition of the diagnosis; onset; risk of suicide; assessment of the need to protect the patient.	Explore onset of symptoms; evaluate for suicidal ideation; evaluate non-psychiatric causes, drug-related depression; consider hospitalization if the patient does not respond to the interpersonal interaction of the emergency evaluation or seems hopeless or helpless even after the evaluation; tell the patient the presumptive diagnosis and refer for treatment; initiation of pharmacological treatment for depression should not take place from an emergency department unless there will be continuity of care for the patient in the same system.
Dystonia, acute	Patient's psychological and physical discomfort; identification of causative agent.	Determine the causative agent; treat with diphenhydramine or benzitropine and contact the agency or therapist that prescribed the medication for follow-up care; refer the patient back to treating agency after explaining the cause of the symptoms.
Family crises; marital cases	Determination of danger to members of the family; resolution of the crisis sufficiently to get the couple or family out of the emergency department.	Offer an opportunity for the family unit to meet briefly to explore the issue that brought them to the emergency department; do not make any recommendations that seem self-evident because there is always more than meets the eye when a crisis propels a family to use an emergency department as an intervention; rule out issues of domestic violence, child abuse, or substance abuse; refer as appropriate.
Geriatric crises	Identification of contributory medical or pharmacological problems; identification of family agenda.	Determine acuity; try to uncover the family agenda; rule out organicity, especially as it relates to the reason for the emergency department visit now; rule out elder abuse; refer as appropriate.

TABLE 20–5—*continued*

Syndrome or Presenting Symptom	Emergency Problem	Emergency Treatment Issues
Grief and bereavement	Identification of an excessive or pathological reaction; determination of the need for professional referral; facilitation of the grieving process in the emergency department.	Explore any extreme or pathological reactions to the loss, especially undue use of medications, drugs, or alcohol; rule out major depressive disorder; acknowledge the validity of the feelings, and refer for appropriate treatment or to support groups as necessary; avoid prescribing any medications from the emergency department unless there is the capacity for continuity of care and follow-up.
Hallucinations	Onset; differential diagnosis, particularly for a medical or substance-related cause.	Evaluate for possible organic cause, especially for visual, tactile, or olfactory hallucinations; assess for suicidal or homicidal content and consider hospitalization or referral for immediate care, if indicated.
High fever	Potential life threat; determine cause; potential offenders include lithium, anticholinergics, agranulocytosis induced by clozapine (Clozaril) or phenothiazines: neuroleptic malignant syndrome.	Emergency treatment for high fever; stop offending medication and treat underlying cause.
Homicidal and assaultive behavior	Danger to staff and other patients; determination of risk for suicide; cause of the behavior.	Determine whether there is an acute psychiatric condition determining the homicidal or assaultive behavior; use sufficient personnel and restraints to ensure the safety of staff and other patients; rule out medical or substance-related components.
Homosexual panic	Circumstances precipitating the behavior; emergency department capacity to accommodate patient's immediate need.	Allow the patient room and an opportunity to talk; medication, including benzodiazepines or antipsychotics, may be needed to calm the patient; be particularly cautious about any physical assessment of the patient.
Hyperventilation	Physical symptoms; patient's anxiety with respect to the symptoms.	Explain briefly to the patient how the symptoms are caused by hyper-ventilation; instruct the patient to breathe into a paper bag for several minutes; it may be useful to encourage the patient to hyperventilate again in the clinician's presence to confirm the cause of the symptoms.
Insomnia	Determination of an acute precipitant; identification of the patient's primary concern.	Determine the cause of the symptoms; rule out depression or incipient psychosis; refer as appropriate; do not prescribe medications from the emergency department for the condition.
Lithium (Eskalith) toxicity	Medical instability; contributing medical conditions.	Monitor for significant medical instability and consider hospitalization; stop lithium immediately; institute supportive measures as indicated.

continued

TABLE 20-5—*continued*

Syndrome or Presenting Symptom	Emergency Problem	Emergency Treatment Issues
Mania	Danger to self or others; need for restraints before behavior escalates out of control in the emergency department.	Reduce stimulation and consider the use of restraints; rule out organic cause if there is no history of a bipolar disorder or if the symptoms are significantly worse; consider hospitalization, especially if patient is unable to appreciate need for treatment.
Neuroleptic malignant syndrome	Medical instability; correct identification of the problem; need for rapid response.	Institute life support measures as indicated; the illness can progress rapidly; hospitalize; make clear to the receiving physicians the presumptive diagnosis.
Opioid intoxication or withdrawal	Correct identification of the problem.	Administer naloxone (Narcan) for overdose; opiate withdrawal is not life-threatening, and patient may be treated symptomatically for relief of discomfort; refer to proper treatment program.
Panic reactions	Identification of an acute precipitant; response to the patient's need for immediate relief.	Talk the patient down; look for an organic cause, especially for a first episode; attempt to identify the acute precipitant, but it is a chronic problem that must be referred for adequate management; there is some evidence that encouraging the patient to face the precipitating stimulus again as soon as possible minimizes the long-term disability associated with panic reactions.
Paranoia	Underlying psychosis; possible organic cause.	Consider an underlying psychosis; stimulant abuse is the most common organic cause for paranoid symptoms; refer the patient as appropriate, or consider hospitalization if the paranoia poses a threat to the patient's life or to other's; suicidal behavior is not uncommon in acute paranoia.
Parkinsonism	Identification of the cause (i.e., idiopathic vs. side effects of medication).	Prescribe an antiparkinsonian agent and refer the patient to the original prescribing physician or to a neurologist or psychiatrist as indicated.
Phencyclidine intoxication	Identification of causative agent; danger to self or others.	Reduce stimulation, observe for significant physiological disturbances, such as temperature elevation; avoid antipsychotics; hospitalize, if necessary, to protect the patient during intoxication, which may last for several days.
Phobias	Reason for current emergency department visit.	Assess onset of symptoms and the degree to which they are interfering with the patient immediately; refer for long-term management, probably to a behavioral treatment program.
Photosensitivity or rash	Confirm cause (phenothiazines).	Advise patient of necessary precautions (sunscreen, hat, avoidance of strong sunlight).
Posttraumatic stress disorder	Identification of the precipitant; identification of symptoms that are particularly disruptive to normal functioning, such as substance abuse, sleep disturbances, isolation.	Assess onset of symptoms; try to identify the precipitant for the current visit; refer to a brief treatment program if a specific precipitant can be identified.

TABLE 20–5—*continued*

Syndrome or Presenting Symptom	Emergency Problem	Emergency Treatment Issues
Priapism	Discomfort, anxiety; determine whether patient is on trazodone (Desyrel).	Discontinue trazodone; consult urologist if symptom persists.
Psychosis	Acuity; differential diagnosis; danger to self or others from suicidal ideation or psychotic ideation.	Evaluate for, organic cause; explore possible precipitants; take whatever measure are indicated to protect the patient and others, consider rapid neuroleptization if medical or substance-related cause can be clearly ruled out.
Rape	Identification of any extreme features of the assault; need for support; medical components.	Be sure that all medical and forensic issues have been addressed, such as chain of evidence, prevention of pregnancy, and sexually transmitted disease; facilitate the patient's exploration of feelings about the assault; facilitate access to rape crisis counseling.
Repeaters	Reason for the return visit; emergency issues; danger to self or others; reason for failure of prior management or referral.	Once genuine reasons for a return visit have been ruled out, review how the emergency department may be encouraging the patient to use such a method of receiving care and attention rather than more traditional channels; consider substance abuse or medical condition as possible overlooked conditions.
Schizophrenia	Onset; reason for current emergency department visit; question whether there is a breakdown of long-term case management.	Determine reason for use of the emergency department rather than the patient's identified treatment program; contact program before making any decisions about treatment or hospitalization; consider suicide potential.
Sedative intoxication	Medical management; exploration of motivation (was it a suicidal act?) for intoxication.	Initiate treatment as indicated; consider suicidal intent even if patient denies it.
Seizures	Patient safety; determination of cause.	Observe for postictal confusion; discontinue or lower seizure-inducing medication; refer or hospitalize for comprehensive evaluation.
Substance abuse	Onset; reason for use of the emergency department; identification of agent; level of need for treatment (intoxication, withdrawal, or desire for abstinence).	Institute treatment as indicated for medically unstable patients; refer all others to formal treatment programs and do not institute treatment in the emergency department.
Suicidal behavior	Seriousness of intent; seriousness of attempt; need for medical intervention; need for hospitalization.	Consider hospitalization, particularly if patient has made prior attempts; has a family history of suicide; has had a significant recent loss, particularly by suicide; and does not seem to respond to the interpersonal interaction with the physician; hospitalize if uneasy.
Suicide thoughts or threats	Seriousness of intent; ability of patient to control thoughts; determination of usefulness of prior or current psychiatric treatment.	As above.

continued

TABLE 20-5—*continued*

Syndrome or Presenting Symptom	Emergency Problem	Emergency Treatment Issues
Tardive dyskinesia	Patient's discomfort; reason for emergency department visit; question whether there has been a breakdown of outpatient management.	This is a long-term problem, not an acute one; reduction of antipsychotic often increases the symptoms of tardive dyskinesia; refer the patient for appropriate psychiatric treatment.
Tremor	New onset? Determine cause, such as lithium toxicity, tardive dyskinesia, substance withdrawal, anxiety.	Treat according to cause.
Violence	Danger to others; determination of underlying psychiatric basis for behavior.	Use sufficient strength, in terms of numbers and competence of staff, and restraints to control the behavior quickly; delay or hesitation may escalate the violence; assess, and treat the patient as indicated according to the underlying cause; file charges if there has been any damage or injury because of the patient's behavior.

Table by Beverly J. Fauman, M.D.

surgical condition that requires timely evaluation and treatment. Emergencies can occur in any location—home, office, street, and medical, surgical, and psychiatric units. Under ideal conditions, the patient will be brought to the psychiatric emergency unit, where physicians and psychiatrists who specialize in emergency medicine can evaluate the situation and institute treatment. Table 20-5 lists a broad range of conditions that fall into the category of psychiatric emergencies.

For more detailed discussion of this topic, see Psychiatric Emergencies, Ch 29, p 2031, in CTP/VII.

21

Infant, Child, and Adolescent Disorders

I. Principles of child and adolescent diagnostic assessment

A comprehensive evaluation of a child or adolescent is intended to develop a formulation of the child's overall functioning based on genetic contributions, maturational patterns, environmental factors, and adaptation to the environment. As developmental level and age increase, the evaluation focuses on the psychiatrist's direct interaction with the child. Thus, with adolescents, it is appropriate to include the adolescent in the initial interview, either alone or with parents or caregivers. Psychiatrists do not usually see young children alone in the first contact; it is difficult for a young child to synthesize his or her history.

A comprehensive evaluation of a child includes the following: (1) clinical interviews with the parents, child, and family; (2) obtaining information regarding the child's current school functioning; and (3) a standardized assessment of the child's intellectual functioning and academic achievement. The examiner should also make sure that the following areas are covered:

A. Supplement data from patient interviews with information from family members, guardians, teachers, and outside agencies.

B. Understand normal development so as to understand fully what constitutes abnormality at a given age. Table 21–1 presents developmental milestones.

C. Be familiar with the current diagnostic criteria of disorders so as to guide anamnesis on the mental status examination.

D. Understand the family psychiatric history, which is necessary given the genetic predispositions and environmental influences associated with many disorders.

II. Child development

Development results from the interplay of maturation of the CNS, neuromuscular apparatus, and endocrine system and various environmental influences (e.g., parents and teachers, who can either facilitate or thwart a child's attainment of his or her developmental potential). This potential is specific to each person's given genetic predisposition to (1) intellectual level and (2) mental disorders, temperament, and probably certain personality traits.

Development is continuous and lifelong but is most rapid in early life. The neonatal brain weighs 350 g, almost triples in weight by 18 months, and at 7 years is very close to the adult weight of 1,350 g. Whereas neurogenesis is virtually complete at birth, the arborization of axons and dendrites continues for many years. This and synaptogenesis appear to be influenced by the environ-

TABLE 21-1
LANDMARKS OF NORMAL BEHAVIORAL DEVELOPMENT

Age	Motor and Sensory Behavior	Adaptive Behavior	Personal and Social Behavior
Birth to 4 weeks	Hand to mouth reflex, grasping reflex Rooting reflex (puckering lips in response to perioral stimulation); Moro reflex (digital extension when startled); sucking reflex; Babinski reflex (toes spread when sole of foot touched) Differentiates sounds (orients to human voice) and sweet and sour tastes Visual tracking Fixed focal distance of 8 inches Makes alternating crawling movements Moves head laterally when placed in prone position	Anticipatory feeding-approach behavior of 4 days Responds to sound of rattle and bell Regards moving objects momentarily	Responsiveness to mother's face, eyes, and voice within first few hours of life Endogenous smile Independent play (until 2 years) Quiets when picked up Impassive face
4 weeks	Tonic neck reflex positions predominate Hands fisted Head sags but can hold head erect for a few seconds Visual fixation, stereoscopic vision (12 weeks)	Follows moving objects to the midline Shows no interest and drops objects immediately	Regards face and diminishes activity Responds to speech Smiles preferentially to mother
16 weeks	Symmetrical postures predominate Holds head balanced Head lifted 90 degrees when prone on forearm Visual accommodation	Follows a slowly moving object well Arms activate on sight of dangling object	Spontaneous social smile (exogenous) Aware of strange situations
28 weeks	Sits steadily, leaning forward on hands Bounces actively when placed in standing position	One-hand approach and grasp of toy Bangs and shakes rattle Transfers toys	Takes feet to mouth Pats mirror image Starts to imitate mother's sounds and actions
40 weeks	Sits alone with good coordination Creeps Pulls self to standing position Points with index finger	Matches two objects at midline Attempt to imitate scribble	Separation anxiety manifest when taken away from mother Responds to social play, such as pat-a-cake and peekaboo Feeds self cracker and holds own bottle
52 weeks	Walks with one hand held Stands alone briefly	Seeks novelty	Cooperates in dressing
15 months	Toddles Creeps up stairs		Points or vocalizes wants Throws objects in play or refusal

Age	Gross motor	Fine motor/adaptive	Personal/social
18 months	Coordinated walking, seldom falls Hurls ball Walks up stairs with one hand held	Builds a tower of three or four cubes Scribbles spontaneously and imitates a writing stroke	Feeds self in part, spills Pulls toy on string Carries or hugs a special toy, such as a doll Imitates some behavioral patterns with slight delay
2 years	Runs well, no falling Kicks large ball Goes up and down stairs alone Fine motor skills increase	Builds a tower of six or seven cubes Aligns cubes, imitating train Imitates vertical and circular strokes Develops original behaviors	Pulls on simple garment Domestic mimicry Refers to self by name Says "no" to mother Separation anxiety begins to diminish Organized demonstrations of love and protest Parallel play (plays side by side but does not interact with other children)
3 years	Rides tricycle Jumps from bottom steps Alternates feet going up stairs	Builds tower of nine or 10 cubes Imitates a three-cube bridge Copies a circle and a cross	Puts on shoes Unbuttons buttons Feeds self well
4 years	Walks down stairs one step to a tread Stands on one foot for five to eight seconds	Copies a cross Repeats four digits Counts three objects with correct pointing	Understands taking turns Washes and dries own face Brushes teeth Associative or joint play (plays cooperatively with other children)
5 years	Skips, using feet alternately Usually has complete sphincter control Fine coordination improves	Copies a square Draws a recognizable human with a head, a body, limbs Counts 10 objects accurately Prints name	Dresses and undresses self Prints a few letters Plays competitive exercise games
6 years	Rides two-wheel bicycle	Copies triangle	Ties shoelaces

Adapted from Arnold Gessell M.D., and Stella Chess M.D.

TABLE 21–2
A SYNTHESIS OF DEVELOPMENTAL THEORISTS

Age (years)	Margaret Mahler	Sigmund Freud	Erik Erikson	Jean Piaget	Comments
0–1	Normal autistic phase (birth to 4 weeks) • State of half-sleep, half-wake • Major task of phase is to achieve homeostatic equilibrium with the environment Normal symbiotic phase (3–4 weeks to 4–5 months) • Dim awareness of caretaker, but infant still functions as if he or she and caretaker are in state of undifferentiation or fusion • Social smile characteristic (2–4 months) The subphases of separation–individuation proper First subphase: differentiation (5–10 months) • Process of hatching from autistic shell (i.e., developing more alert sensorium that reflects cognitive and neurological maturation) • Beginning of comparative scanning, (i.e., comparing what is and what is not mother)	Oral phase (birth to 1 year) • Major site of tension and gratification is the mouth, lips, tongue—includes biting and sucking activities	Basic trust vs. basic mistrust (oral sensory) (birth to 1 year) • Social mistrust demonstrated via ease of feeding, depth of sleep, bowel relaxation • Depends on consistency and sameness of experience provided by caretaker • Second 6 months teething and biting move infant "from getting to taking" • Weaning leads to "nostalgia for lost paradise" • If basic trust is strong, child maintains hopeful attitude	Sensorimotor phase (birth to 2 years) • Intelligence rests mainly on actions and movements coordinated under schemata (Schemata is a pattern of behavior in response to a particular environmental stimulus.) • Environment is mastered through assimilation and accommodation (Assimilation is the incorporation of new environmental stimuli; accommodation is the modification of behavior to adapt to new stimuli.) • Object permanence is achieved by age 2 years. Object still exists in mind if disappears from view: search for hidden object • Reversibility in action begins.	In contrast to Mahler, other observers of mother–infant pairs are impressed with a mutuality and complementarity (not autism or fusion), which provides a groundwork for relatedness and language development, as if there were a prewiring for these abilities. Piaget and others emphasize the infant's active striving to manipulate the inanimate environment. This supplements Freud's work because the infant and young child's motivation for behavior is not simply to relieve drive tension and attain oral, anal, and phallic gratification.

1-2	• Characteristic anxiety: stronger anxiety, which involves curiosity and fear (most prevalent around 8 months) Second subphase: practicing (10–16 months) • Beginning of this phase marked by upright locomotion—child has new perspective and also mood of elation • Mother used as home base • Characteristic anxiety: separation anxiety Third subphase: rapprochement (16–24 months) • Infant now a toddler—more aware of physical separateness, which dampens mood of elation • Child tries to bridge gap between self and mother—concretely seen as bringing objects to mother • Mother's efforts to help toddler often not perceived as helpful, temper tantrums typical • Characteristic event: rapprochement crisis, wanting to be soothed by mother and yet not able to accept her help	Anal phase (1–3 years) • Anus and surrounding area major source of interest • Acquisition of voluntary sphincter control (toilet training)	Autonomy vs. shame and doubt (muscular-anal) (1–3 years) • Biologically includes learning to walk, feed self, talk • Muscular maturation sets stage for "holding on and letting go" • Need for outer control, firmness of caretaker before development of autonomy • *Shame* occurs when child is overtly self-conscious via negative exposure • *Self-doubt* can evolve if parents overtly shame child (e.g., about elimination)	Preoperational phase (2–7 years) • Appearance of *symbolic* functions, associated with language acquisition • *Egocentrism*: child understands everything exclusively from own perspective • Thinking is illogical and magical • Nonreversible thinking with absence of conversation — *Animism*: belief that inanimate objects are alive (i.e., have feelings and intentions) —"*Imminent justice*" belief that punishment for bad deeds is inevitable	Supplementing the work of Freud and Mahler, theorists have postulated that severe problems in mother–infant/toddler interactions contribute to the formation of pathological character traits, gender identity disorder, or personality disorders. Angry, frustrating, narcissistic caretakers often produce angry, needy children and adults who cannot tolerate the normal frustrations and disappointments in relationships and whose character formation is grossly distorted.

continued

TABLE 21-2—*continued*

Age (years)	Margaret Mahler	Sigmund Freud	Erik Erikson	Jean Piaget	Comments
	• Symbol of rapprochement: child standing on threshold of door not knowing which way to turn, helpless frustration • Resolution of crisis occurs as child's skills improve and child able to get gratification from doing things on own				
2–3	Fourth subphase: consolidation and object constancy (24–36 months) • Child better able to cope with mother's absence and engage substitutes • Child can begin to feel comfortable with mother's absences by knowing she will return • Gradual internalization of image of mother as reliable and stable • Through increasing verbal skills and better sense of time, child can tolerate delay and endure separations				

3–4	Phallic-oedipal phase (3–5 years) • Genital focus of interest, stimulation, and excitement • Penis is organ of interest for both sexes • Genital masturbation common	Initiative vs. guilt (locomotor genital) (3–5 years) • *Initiative* arises in relation to tasks for the sake of activity, both motor and intellectual • *Guilt* may arise over goals contemplated (especially aggressive) • Desire to mimic adult world; involvement in oedipal struggle leads to resolution via social role identification • Sibling rivalry frequent	Researchers have amended Freud's work. Children of both sexes explore and are aware of their own genitals during the second year of life and, with proper parental reinforcement, begin to correctly identify themselves as girls or boys. Penis envy is neither universal nor normative. Freud emphasized problems with oedipal resolution in psychopathogenesis. His theory accounts for only a part of psychopathology.
4–5	• Intense preoccupation with *castration anxiety* (fear of genital loss or injury) • *Penis envy* (discontent with one's own genitals and wish to possess genitals of male) seen in girls in this phase • *Oedipus complex* universal: child wishes to have sex with and marry parent of opposite sex and simultaneously be rid of parent of same sex		
5–6	Latency phase (from 5–6 years to 11–12 years) • State of relative quiescence of sexual drive with resolution of oedipal complex • Sexual drives channeled into more socially appropriate aims (i.e., schoolwork and sports)		Contrary to Freud, the onset of latency (school age or middle childhood) is now considered primarily a consequence of changes in the CNS and less dependent on the nondemonstrable quiescence and sublimation of sexual drive. During the years 6–8 changes in the CNS are reflected in developmental progress, of continued

TABLE 21–2—continued

Age (years)	Margaret Mahler	Sigmund Freud	Erik Erikson	Jean Piaget	Comments
6–11		• Formation of *superego*, one of three psychic structures in mind responsible for moral and ethical development, including conscience • Other two psychic structures are *ego*, a group of functions mediating between drives and the external environment, and *id*, repository of sexual and aggressive drives • The id is present at birth, and the ego develops gradually from rudimentary structure present at birth	Industry vs. inferiority (latency) (6–11 years) • Child is busy building, creating, accomplishing • Receives systematic instruction as well as fundamentals of technology • Danger of sense of inadequacy and inferiority if child despairs of his or her tools/skills and status among peers • Socially decisive age	Concrete (operational) phase (7–11 years) • Emergence of logical (cause–effect) thinking, including reversibility and ability to sequence and serialize • Understanding of part–whole relationships and classifications • Child able to take other's point of view • Conservation of number, length, weight, and volume	perceptual-sensory-motor functioning and thought processes. In Piaget's framework, it is the transition from the preoperational to the concrete (operational) phase. Compared with preschoolers, latency children are capable of greater learning, independent functioning, and socialization. Friendships develop with less dependence on parents (and less preoccupation with intrafamilial oedipal rivalries). Superego development is today considered more prolonged gradual and less related to oedipal resolution.
11+		Genital phase (from 11–12 years and beyond) • Final stage of psychosexual development—begins with puberty and the biological capacity for orgasm but also involves the capacity for true intimacy	Identity vs. role diffusion (11 years through end of adolescence) • Struggle to develop ego *identity* (sense of inner sameness and continuity) • Preoccupation with appearance, hero worship, ideology • *Group identity* (peers) develops	Formal (abstract) phase (11 years through end of adolescence) • Hypothetical-deductive reasoning, not only on basis of objects but also on basis of hypotheses or propositions • Capable of thinking about one's thoughts	The interplay of child and caretaker is emphasized in the attachment theory of John Bowlby. Mary Ainsworth developed the "strange situation" protocol for examining infant-caretaker separations. "Goodness of fit" between child and caretaker is also stressed in the work on

- Danger of *role confusion*, doubts about sexual and vocational identity
- *Psychosocial moratorium,* stage between morality learned by the child and the ethics to be developed by the adult

- Combinative structures emerge, permitting flexible grouping of elements in a system
- Ability to use two systems of reference simultaneously
- Ability to grasp concept of probabilities

temperament by Chess and Thomas. Infants have inborn differences in certain, behavioral dimensions, such as activity level, approach or withdrawal, intensity of reaction. How parents respond to these behaviors influence development. Lawrence Kohlberg, who was influenced by Piaget, described three levels of moral development: preconventional, in which moral decisions are made to avoid punishment; conventional role conformity, with decisions made to maintain friendships; and in adolescence self-accepted moral principles, (i.e., voluntary compliance with ethical principles).

Adapted from Sylvia Karasu, M.D., and Richard Oberfield, M.D.

ment. Because of brain plasticity, some connections are strengthened and others are developed in response to environmental input. Myelinization continues for decades.

The most cited theorists in child development have been Sigmund Freud, Margaret Mahler, Erik Erikson, and Jean Piaget; their work is outlined in Table 21–2.

III. Mental retardation (MR)

A. Diagnosis. (Code on Axis II.) See Table 21–3. In about 85% of persons with MR, the condition is mild, and they are considered educable, being able to attain about a grade 6 education. About 10% have a moderate type and are considered trainable, being able to attain about a grade 2 education; about 3–4% have a severe type; and about 1–2% have a profound type.

B. Epidemiology and etiology. MR occurs in 1% of the population. The male-to-female ratio is 1.5:1. The cause is organic or psychosocial and is known in 50–70% of cases.

1. Genetic

a. Inborn errors of metabolism (e.g., phenylketonuria, Tay-Sachs disease).

b. Chromosomal abnormalities. Down syndrome (trisomy 21), 1 in 700 live births. Typical facies, hypotonia, hyperreflexia, cardiac malformations, gastrointestinal anomalies. Mostly moderate to severe retardation. Fragile X syndrome, 1 in 1,000 male births. Postpubertal macroorchidism; large head and ears; long, narrow face. (Facial features and cognitive dysfunction are seen in some female carriers.) Retardation ranges from mild to severe. High rates of attention-deficit/hyperactivity disorder (ADHD), learning disorders, and pervasive developmental disorder.

2. Psychosocial. Mild MR may be caused by chronic lack of intellectual stimulation.

TABLE 21–3
DSM-IV-TR DIAGNOSTIC CRITERIA FOR MENTAL RETARDATION

A. Significantly subaverage intellectual functioning: on I.Q. of approximately 70 or below on an individually administered I.Q. test (for infants, a clinical judgment of significantly subaverage intellectual functioning).

B. Concurrent deficits or impairments in present adaptive functioning (i.e., the person's effectiveness in meeting the standards expected for his or her age by his or her cultural group) in at least two of the following areas: communication, self-care, home living, social/interpersonal skills, use of community resources, self-direction, functional academic skills, work, leisure, health, and safety.

C. The onset is before age 18 years.

Code based on degree of severity reflecting level of intellectual impairment:

Mild mental retardation:	I.Q. level 50–55 to approximately 70
Moderate mental retardation:	I.Q. level 35–40 to 50–55
Severe mental retardation:	I.Q. level 20–25 to 35–40
Profound mental retardation:	I.Q. level below 20 or 25

Mental retardation, severity unspecified: when there is strong presumption of mental retardation but the person's intelligence is untestable by standard tests.

From American Psychiatric Association. *Diagnostic and Statistical Manual of Mental Disorders*, text revision, 4th ed. Washington, DC: American Psychiatric Association, Copyright 2000, with permission.

3. **Other.** Sequelae of infection, toxin, or brain trauma sustained prenatally, perinatally, or later (e.g., congenital rubella or fetal alcohol syndrome [microcephaly, midfacial hypoplasia, short palpebral fissure, pectus excavatum, possible cardiac defects, short stature]).

C. **General considerations.** No behavior or personality is typical. Poor self-esteem is common. Thinking tends to be concrete and egocentric. One third to two thirds of MR patients have concomitant mental disorders that run the gamut of DSM-IV-TR disorders.

D. **Treatment**
   1. **Educational.** Special schools or classes providing (as needed) remediation, tutoring, vocational training, social skills training.
   2. **Pharmacological.** See Table 21–4.
      a. A concomitant mental disorder, such as ADHD or depression, may require treatment with stimulants or antidepressants, respectively.
      b. Agitation, aggression, and tantrums often respond to antipsychotics. Atypical antipsychotics (e.g., risperidone [Risperdal], olanzapine [Zyprexa]) are preferred because they are less likely to cause extrapyramidal symptoms and dyskinesia. Low-dosage, high-potency drugs (e.g., haloperidol [Haldol]) are preferred to high-dosage, low-potency drugs (e.g., chlorpromazine [Thorazine]) which are more cognitively dulling. Many institutionalized MR patients are poorly monitored on medication.
      c. Lithium (Eskalith) is useful for aggressive or self-abusive behaviors.
      d. Carbamazepine (Tegretol), valproate (Depakene), and propranolol (Inderal) can be tried for aggressive behavior or tantrums. Their efficacy is less proven than that of antipsychotics and lithium.
   3. **Psychological**
      a. Behavior therapy.
      b. Parental and family counseling.
      c. Individual supportive psychotherapy. Awareness of inadequacies can breed low self-esteem.
      d. Mildly impaired persons with good verbal skills may profit from other psychotherapies for concomitant disorders.
      e. Activity groups improve socialization.

IV. **Pervasive developmental disorders**

A. **Diagnosis, signs, and symptoms.** (Code on Axis I.) See Tables 21–5 through 21–8.

B. **General considerations**
   1. **Autistic disorder.** Autistic disorder affects 4 in 10,000 persons. The male-to-female ratio is 3:1. Children with autistic disorder can function well or poorly, depending on I.Q., amount and communicativeness of language, and severity of other symptoms. Of these children, 70% have I.Q.s below 70 and 50% have I.Q.s below 50 to 55. Concordance is higher in monozygotic than in dizygotic twins; at least 2–4% of siblings are afflicted, and language and learning problems are increased in

TABLE 21-4
COMMON PYSCHOACTIVE DRUGS IN CHILDHOOD AND ADOLESCENCE

Drug	Indications	Dosage	Adverse Reactions and Monitoring
Antipsychotics—also known as *major tranquilizers, neuroleptics* Divided into (1) high-potency, low-dosage (e.g. haloperidol (Haldol), pimozide (Orap), trifluoperazine (Stelazine), thiothixene (Navane); (2) low-potency high-dosage (more sedating) (e.g., chlorpromazine (Thorazine); and (3) atypicals (e.g., risperidone (Risperdal), olanzapine (Zyprexa), quetiapine (Seroquel), and clozapine (Clozaril)).	Psychoses; agitated self-injurious behaviors in MR, PDDs, CD, and Tourette's disorder— haloperidol and pimozide. Clozapine—refractory schizophrenia in adolescence.	All can be given in two to four divided doses or combined into one dose after gradual buildup. Haloperidol—child 0.5-6 mg/d, adolescent 0.5-16 mg/d. Clozapine—dosage not determined in children; < 600 mg/d in adolescents. Risperidone—1-3 mg/d. Olanzapine— 2.5-10 mg/d. Quetiapine— 25-500 mg/d.	Sedation, weight gain, hypotension, lowered seizure threshold, constipation, extrapyramidal symptoms, jaundice, agranulocytosis, dystonic reaction, tardive dyskinesia. Hyperprolactenemia with atypicals except quetiapine. Monitor blood pressure, CBC count, LFTs and prolactia if indicated. With thioridazine, pigmentary retinopathy is rare but dictates ceiling of 800 mg in adults and proportionally lower in children; with clozapine, weekly WBC counts for development of agranulocytosis and EEG monitoring because of lowering of seizure threshold.
Stimulants Dextroamphetamine (Dexedrine) and amphetamine- dextroamphetamine (Adderall) FDA-approved for children 3 years and older Methylphenidate (Ritalin, Concerta) and pemoline (Cylert)— FDA-approved for children 6 years and older	In ADHD for hyperactivity, impulsivity, and inattentiveness. Narcolepsy.	Dextroamphetamine and methylphenidate are generally given at 8 AM and noon. Dextroamphetamine— about half the dosage of methylphenidate. Methylphenidate— 10-60 mg/d or up to about 0.5 mg/kg per dose. Adderall—about half the dosage of methylphenidate.	Insomnia, anorexia, weight loss (possibly growth delay), rebound hyperactivity, headache, tachycardia, precipitation or exacerbation of tic disorders. With pemoline, monitor LFTs, as hepatoxicity and liver failure are possible.
Mood stabilizers Lithium—considered an antimanic drug; also has antiaggresis on properties	Studies support use in MR and CD for aggressive and self-injurious behaviors; can be used for same in PDD; also indicated for early-onset bipolar disorder.	600-2,100 mg in two or three divided doses; keep blood levels to 0.4-1.2 mEq/L.	Nausea, vomiting, polyuria, headache, tremor, weight gain, hypothyroidism. Experience with adults suggests renal function monitoring.
Divalproex (Depakote)	Bipolar disorder, aggression.	Up to about 20 mg/kg per day; therapeutic blood level range appears to be 50-100 µg/mL.	Monitor CBC count and LFTs for possible blood dycrasias and hepatotoxicity.

TABLE 21-4—continued

Drug	Indications	Dosage	Adverse Reactions and Monitoring
Carbamazepine (Tegretol)—an anticonvulsant	Aggression or dyscontrol in MR or CD. Bipolar disorder.	Start with 10 mg/kg per day, can build to 20–30 mg/kg per day; therapeutic blood level range appears to be 4–12 mg per day.	Nausea, vomiting, sedation, hair loss, weight gain, possibly polycystic ovaries. Drowsiness, nausea, rash, vertigo, irritability. Monitor CBC count and LFTs for possible blood dyscrasias and hepatotoxicity; must obtain blood concentrations.
Antidepressants			
Tricyclic antidepressants— imipramine (Tofranil), nortriptyline (Pamelor), clomipramine (Anafranil)	Major depressive disorder, separation anxiety disorder, bulimia nervosa, enuresis; sometimes used in ADHD, sleepwalking disorder, and sleep terror disorder. Clomipramine is effective in childhood OCD and sometimes in PDD.	Impramine—start with divided doses totaling about 1.5 mg/kg per day; can build up to not more than 5 mg/kg per day and eventually combine in one dose, which is usually 50–100 mg before sleep. Clomipramine—start at 50 mg/d; can raise to not more than 3 mg/kg per day or 200 mg/d.	Dry mouth, constipation, tachycardia, arrythmia.
Selective serotonin reuptake inhibitors— fluoxetine (Prozac), sertraline (Zoloft), fluvoxamine (Luvox), paroxetine (Paxil), citalopram (Celexa)	OCD; may be useful in major depressive disorder, anorexia nervosa, bulimia nervosa, repetitive behaviors in MR or PDD.	Less than adult dosages.	Nausea, headache, nervousness, insomnia, dry mouth, diarrhea, drowsiness, disinhibition.
Bupropion (Wellbutrin)	ADHD.	Start low and titrate up to between 100 and 250 mg/d.	Disinhibition, insomnia, dry mouth, gastrointestinal problems, tremor, seizures.
Anxiolytics			
Benzodiazepines			
Clonazepam (Klonopin)	Panic disorder, generalized anxiety disorder.	0.5 mg–2.0 mg/d.	Drowsiness, disinhibition.
Alprazolam (Xanax)	Separation anxiety disorder.	Up to 1.5 mg/d.	Drowsiness, disinhibition.
Buspirone (BuSpar)	Various anxiety disorders.	15–90 mg/d.	Dizziness, upset stomach.
α_2-Adrenergic receptor agonists			
Clonidine (Catapres)	ADHD, Tourette's disorder, aggression.	Up to 0.4 mg/d.	Bradycardia, arrhythmia, hypertension, withdrawal hypotension.

continued

TABLE 21–4—continued

Drug	Indications	Dosage	Adverse Reactions and Monitoring
Guanfacine (Tenex)	ADHD.	0.5–3.0 mg/d.	Same as with clonidine plus headache, stomachache.
β-Adrenergic receptor antagonist (beta blocker)			
Propranolol (Inderal)	Explosive aggression.	Start at 20–30 mg/d and titrate.	Monitor for bradycardia, hypotension, bronchoconstriction. Contraindicated in asthma and diabetes.
Other agents			
Naltrexone (ReVia)	Hyperactivity or self-injurious behavior in autism or MR.	0.5–1.0 mg/kg per day.	Drowsiness, vomiting, anorexia, headache, nasal congestion, hyponatremic seizures.
Desmopressin (DDAVP)	Nocturnal enuresis.	20–40 μg intranasally.	Headache, nasal congestion, hyponatremic seizures (rare).

MR, mental retardation; PDD, pervasive development disorder; CD, conduct disorder; CBC, complete blood cell; LFT, liver function test; WBC, white blood cell; ADHD, attention-deficit/hyperactivity disorder; OCD, obsessive-compulsive disorder.

TABLE 21–5
DSM-IV-TR DIAGNOSTIC CRITERIA FOR AUTISTIC DISORDER

A. A total of six (or more) items from (1), (2), and (3), with at least two from (1), and one each from (2) and (3).
  (1) qualitative impairment in social interaction, as manifested by at least two of the following:
    (a) marked impairment in the use of multiple nonverbal behaviors such as eye-to-eye gaze, facial expression, body postures, and gestures to regulate social interaction
    (b) failure to develop peer relationships appropriate to developmental level
    (c) a lack of spontaneous seeking to share enjoyment, interests, or achievements with other people (e.g., by showing, bringing, or pointing out objects of interest)
    (d) lack of social or emotional reciprocity
  (2) qualitative impairments in communication as manifested by at least one of the following:
    (a) delay in, or total lack of, the development of spoken language (not accompanied by an attempt to compensate through alternative modes or communication such as gesture or mime)
    (b) in individuals with adequate speech, marked impairment in the ability to initiate or sustain a conversation with others
    (c) stereotyped and repetitive use of language or idiosyncratic language
    (d) lack of varied, spontaneous make-believe play or social imitative play appropriate to developmental level
  (3) restricted repetitive and stereotyped patterns of behavior, interests, and activities, as manifested by at least one of the following:
    (a) encompassing preoccupation with one or more stereotyped and restricted patterns of interest that is abnormal either in intensity or focus
    (b) apparently inflexible adherence to specific, nonfunctional routines or rituals
    (c) stereotyped and repetitive motor mannerisms (e.g., hand or finger flapping or twisting, or complex whole-body movements)
    (d) persistent preoccupation with parts of objects
B. Delays or abnormal functioning in at least one of the following areas, with onset prior to age 3 years: (1) social interaction, (2) language as used in social communication, or (3) symbolic at imaginative play.
C. The disturbance is not better accounted for by Rett's disorder or childhood disintegrative disorder.

From American Psychiatric Association. Diagnostic and Statistical Manual of Mental Disorders, text revision, 4th ed. Washington, DC: American Psychiatric Association, Copyright 2000, with permission.

the families of autistic children. Associated genetic disorders include tuberous sclerosis and fragile X syndrome. Prenatal and perinatal insults are increased, but these may be insufficient to cause the disorder without a genetic predisposition. No site of organic damage is specific to autistic disorder. Cortical, cerebellar, brainstem, and immunologic abnormalities have been implicated in subgroups based on findings from electroencephalogram (EEG), computed tomography (CT), magnetic resonance imaging (MRI), autopsy, and positron emission tomography (PET) studies. Subgroups have abnormal levels of neurotransmitters or their metabolites in blood or CSF.

TABLE 21–6
DIAGNOSTIC CRITERIA FOR RETT'S DISORDER

A. All of the following:
  (1) apparently normal prenatal and perinatal development
  (2) apparently normal psychomotor development through the first 5 months after birth
  (3) normal head circumference at birth
B. Onset of all of the following after the period of normal development:
  (1) deceleration of head growth between ages 5 and 48 months
  (2) loss of previously acquired purposeful hand skills between ages 5 and 30 months with the subsequent development of stereotyped hand movements (e.g., hand-wringing or hand washing)
  (3) loss of social engagement early in the course (although often social interaction develops later)
  (4) appearance of poorly coordinated gait or trunk movements
  (5) severely impaired expressive and receptive language development with severe psychomotor retardation

From American Psychiatric Association. *Diagnostic and Statistical Manual of Mental Disorders.* Text revision, 4th ed. Washington, DC: American Psychiatric Association: Copyright 2000, with permission.

TABLE 21–7
DSM-IV-TR DIAGNOSTIC CRITERIA FOR ASPERGER'S DISORDER

A. Quantitative impairment in social interaction, as manifested by at least two of the following:
  (1) marked impairment in the use of multiple nonverbal behaviors such as eye-to-eye gaze, facial expression, body postures, and gestures to require social interaction
  (2) failure to develop peer relationship appropriate to developmental level
  (3) a lack of spontaneous seeking to share enjoyment, interests, or achievements with other people (e.g., by a lack of showing, bringing, or pointing out objects of interest to other people)
  (4) lack of social or emotional reciprocity
B. Restricted repetitive and stereotyped patterns of behavior, interests, and activities, as manifested by at least one of the following:
  (1) encompassing preoccupation with one or more stereotyped and restricted patterns of interest that is abnormal either in intensity or in focus
  (2) apparently inflexible adherence to specific, nonfunctional routines or rituals
  (3) stereotyped and repetitive motor mannerisms (e.g., hand or finger flapping or twisting, or complex whole-body movements)
  (4) persistent preoccupation with parts of objects
C. The disturbance causes clinically significant impairment in social, occupational, or other important areas in functioning.
D. There is no clinically significant general delay in language (e.g., single words used by age 2 years, communicative phrases used by age 3 years).
E. There is no clinically significant delay in cognitive development or in the development of age-appropriate self-help skills, adaptive behavior (other than in social interaction), and curiosity about the environment in childhood.
F. Criteria are not met for another specific pervasive developmental disorder or schizophrenia.

From American Psychiatric Association. *Diagnostic and Statistical Manual of Mental Disorders,* text revision, 4th ed. Washington, DC: American Psychiatric Association, Copyright 2000, with permission.

TABLE 21–8
DSM-IV-TR DIAGNOSTIC CRITERIA FOR CHILDHOOD DISINTEGRATIVE DISORDER

A. Apparently normal development for at least the first 2 years after birth or manifested by the presence of age-appropriate verbal and nonverbal communication, social relationships, play, and adaptive behavior.
B. Clinically significant loss of previously acquired skills (before age 10 years) in at least two of the following areas:
   (1) expressive or receptive language
   (2) social skills or adaptive behavior
   (3) bowel or bladder control
   (4) play
   (5) motor skills
C. Abnormalities of functioning in at least two of the following areas:
   (1) qualitative impairment in social interaction (e.g., impairment in nonverbal behaviors, failure to develop peer relationships, lack of social or emotional reciprocity)
   (2) qualitative impairments in communication (e.g., delay or lack of spoken language, inability to initiate or sustain a conversation, stereotyped and repetitive use of language, lack of varied make-believe play)
   (3) restrictive, repetitive, and stereotyped patterns of behavior, interests, and activities, including motor stereotypes and mannerisms
D. The disturbance is not better accounted for by another specific pervasive developmental disorder or by schizophrenia.

From American Psychiatric Association. *Diagnostic and Statistical Manual of Mental Disorders*, text revision, 4th ed. Washington, DC: American Psychiatric Association, Copyright 2000, with permission.

   2. Asperger's disorder. Asperger's disorder is characterized by autistic-like behavior without significant delays in language or cognitive development. There are circumscribed interests. The cause is unknown, but family studies suggest a relation to autistic disorder. Prevalence is greater than that of autistic disorder.
   3. Rett's disorder. Rett's disorder is neurodegenerative. It probably has genetic basis, as it is seen only in girls; case reports indicate complete concordance in monozygotic twins.
   4. Childhood disintegrative disorder (also called *Heller's syndrome*). Distinguished by at least 2 years of normal development before deterioration to the clinical picture of autistic disorder. The cause is unknown, but this disorder is associated with other neurological conditions (e.g., seizure disorders, tuberous sclerosis, metabolic disorders).
C. Treatment
   1. Special education. Paramount. Much evidence suggests that early, intensive, special educational intervention is most beneficial. Thus, early diagnosis is important.
   2. Pharmacological. See Table 21–4.
      a. In nonsedating dosages for agitation, tantrums, aggression, and extreme hyperactivity, haloperidol has been effective in controlled studies. In a long-term study, dyskinesia occurred in 33% of children but resolved after cessation of the drug. Risperidone (Risperdal) and olanzepine (Zyprexa) have been beneficial in anecdotal reports.
      b. Selective serotonin reuptake inhibitors (SSRIs) (e.g., fluoxetine [Prozac] and fluvoxamine [Luvox]) are sometimes beneficial in reducing perseveration.
      c. Stimulants such as methylphenidate (Ritalin) can be tried to target inattentiveness or hyperactivity. However, they can increase agitation and stereotypies.

    d. Opioid antagonists (e.g., naltrexone [ReVia]) are being studied. The major rationale is to reduce interpersonal withdrawal by blocking endogenous opioids, as one does in addicts by blocking exogenous opioids. Self-injurious behaviors may also be targeted.

    e. Lithium, β-adrenergic receptor antagonists (beta blockers), and antiepileptic drugs may be useful.

    f. Anticonvulsants are used in Rett's disorder to control seizures.

  3. Psychological. Individual psychotherapy is generally useless, given the language and other cognitive impairments of these patients. Family support and counseling are crucial; parents should be told that autistic disorder does not result from a faulty upbringing. Parents often require strategies for dealing with the child and siblings. Associations and self-help groups exist for parents of children with autistic disorder.

V. Learning disorders, motor skills disorder, and communication disorders

    Learning disorders (**reading disorder, mathematics disorder, disorder of written expression**, and **learning disorder not otherwise specified**), motor skills disorder (**developmental coordination disorder**), and communication disorders (**expressive language disorder, mixed receptive-expressive language disorder, phonologic disorder, stuttering**) share many characteristics and comorbidities. The prevalence of learning and motor skills disorders in general is about 5%; estimates are 1% for stuttering and 1% for the other communication disorders. The male-to-female ratio is 2:1 to 4:1 in all the disorders, with the exceptions of written expression (unknown) and mathematics (prevalence possibly higher in girls than in boys).

  A. Diagnosis, signs, and symptoms. The criteria for the disorders are similar.

    1. Learning disorders. See Table 21–9.

    2. Motor skills disorder. See Table 21–10.

    3. Communication disorders. See Tables 21–11 through 21–14.

  B. General considerations. Learning, developmental coordination, and communication disorders often coexist with one another and with attention-deficit and disruptive behavior disorders. The family incidence is increased.

TABLE 21–9
DSM-IV-TR DIAGNOSTIC CRITERIA FOR READING DISORDER, MATHEMATICS DISORDER, OR DISORDER OF WRITTEN EXPRESSION

A. Reading achievement, mathematical ability, or writing skills, as measured by individually administered standardized tests (or functional assessments of writing skills), are substantially below those expected given the person's chronological age, measured intelligence, and age-appropriate education.

B. The disturbance in Criterion A significantly interferes with academic achievement or activities of daily living that require reading skills, mathematical ability, or the composition of written texts (e.g., writing grammatically contact sentences and organized paragraph).

C. If a sensory deficit is present, the difficulties are in excess of those usually associated with it.

From American Psychiatric Association. *Diagnostic and Statistical Manual of Mental Disorders*, text revision, 4th ed. Washington, DC: American Psychiatric Association, Copyright 2000, with permission.

TABLE 21–10
DSM-IV-TR DIAGNOSTIC CRITERIA FOR DEVELOPMENTAL COORDINATION DISORDER

A. Performance in daily activities that require motor coordination is substantially below that expected given the person's chronological age and measured intelligence. This may be manifested by marked delays in achieving motor milestones (e.g., walking, crawling, sitting), dropping things, "clumsiness," poor performance in sports, or poor handwriting.
B. The disturbance in Criterion A significantly interferes with academic achievement or activities of daily living.
C. The disturbance is not due to a general medical condition (e.g., cerebral palsy, hemiplegia, or muscular dystrophy) and does not meet criteria for a pervasive developmental disorder.
D. If mental retardation is present, the motor difficulties are in excess of those usually associated with it.

From American Psychiatric Association. *Diagnostic and Statistical Manual of Mental Disorders*, text revision, 4th ed. Washington, DC: American Psychiatric Association, Copyright 2000, with permission.

TABLE 21–11
DSM-IV-TR DIAGNOSTIC CRITERIA FOR EXPRESSIVE LANGUAGE DISORDER

A. The scores obtained from standardized individually administered measures of expressive language development are substantially below those obtained from standardized measures of both nonverbal intellectual capacity and receptive language development. The disturbance may be manifest clinically by symptoms that include having a markedly limited vocabulary, making errors in tense, or having difficulty recalling words or producing sentences with developmentally appropriate length or complexity.
B. The difficulties with expressive language interfere with academic or occupational achievement or with social communication.
C. Criteria are not met for mixed receptive-expressive language disorder or a pervasive developmental disorder.
D. If mental retardation, a speech-motor or sensory deficit, or environmental deprivation is present. The language difficulties are in excess of those usually associated with these problems.

From American Psychiatric Association. *Diagnostic and Statistical Manual of Mental Disorders*, text revision, 4th ed. Washington, DC: American Psychiatric Association, Copyright 2000, with permission.

TABLE 21–12
DSM-IV-TR DIAGNOSTIC CRITERIA FOR MIXED RECEPTIVE-EXPRESSIVE LANGUAGE DISORDER

A. The scores obtained from a battery of standardized individually administered measures of both receptive and expressive language development are substantially below those obtained from standardized measures of nonverbal intellectual capacity. Symptoms include those for expressive language disorder as well as difficulty understanding words, sentences, or specific types of words, such as spatial terms.
B. The difficulties with receptive and expressive language significantly interfere with academic or occupational achievement or with social communication.
C. Criteria are not met for a pervasive developmental disorder.
D. If mental retardation, a speech motor or sensory deficit, or environmental deprivation is present, the language difficulties are in excess of those usually associated with these problems.

From American Psychiatric Association. *Diagnostic and Statistical Manual of Mental Disorders*, text revision, 4th ed. Washington, DC: American Psychiatric Association, Copyright 2000, with permission.

TABLE 21–13
DSM-IV-TR DIAGNOSTIC CRITERIA FOR PHONOLOGICAL DISORDER

A. Failure to use developmentally expected speech sounds that are appropriate for age and dialect (e.g., errors in sound production, use, representation, or organization such as, but not limited to substitutions of one sound for another (use of /t/ for target /k/ sound) or omissions of sounds such as final consonants).
B. The difficulties in speech sound production interfere with academic or occupational achievement or with social communication.
C. If mental retardation, a speech-motor or sensory deficit, or environmental deprivation is present, the speech difficulties are in excess of those usually associated with these problems.

From American Psychiatric Association. *Diagnostic and Statistical Manual of Mental Disorders*, text revision, 4th ed. Washington, DC: American Psychiatric Association, Copyright 2000, with permission.

TABLE 21-14
DSM-IV-TR DIAGNOSTIC CRITERIA FOR STUTTERING

A. Disturbance in the normal fluency and time patterning of speech (inappropriate for the individual's age), characterized by frequent occurrences of one or more of the following:
   (1) sound and syllable repetitions
   (2) sound prolongations
   (3) interjections
   (4) broken words (e.g., pauses within a word)
   (5) available or silent blocking (filled or unfilled pauses in speech)
   (6) circumlocutions (word substitutions to avoid problematic words)
   (7) words produced with an excess of physical tension
   (8) monosyllabic whole-word repetitions (e.g., "I-I-I see him")
B. The disturbance in fluency interferes with academic or occupational achievement or with social communication.
C. If a speech-motor or sensory deficit is present, the speech difficulties are in excess of those usually associated with these problems.

From American Psychiatric Association. *Diagnostic and Statistical Manual of Mental Disorders*, text revision, 4th ed. Washington, DC: American Psychiatric Association, Copyright 2000, with permission.

Little is known about the neurobiology of these disorders. In reading disorder, a few studies (CT, MRI, and autopsy) have demonstrated a lack of normal hemispheric asymmetries in parietal or temporal lobes. Left-handedness and ambilaterality are increased in communication disorders (with the possible exception of phonologic disorder). Hearing impairment must be ruled out in communication disorders.

C. Treatment

1. **Remediation.** Remediation for learning disabilities is usually provided in school and depends on the severity of the condition. Most cases require no intervention or tutoring. Resource rooms or special class placement may be necessary. Speech therapy is often required for patients with communication disorders. No intervention or tutoring is required in milder cases.

2. **Psychological.** Lowered self-esteem, school failure, and dropping out are common in patients with these disorders. Therefore, psychoeducation is crucial, and school counseling or individual, group, or family therapy may be indicated.

3. **Pharmacological.** Only for an associated psychiatric disorder, such as ADHD. No evidence that medication directly benefits children with learning, motor skills, or communications disorders.

VI. Attention-deficit and disruptive behavior disorders

A. ADHD. Prevalence is probably 3–5%. The male-to-female ratio is 3:1 to 5:1.

1. **Diagnosis, signs, and symptoms.** See Table 21–15.

2. **General considerations.** ADHD, particularly the predominantly hyperactive-impulsive type, often coexists with conduct disorders or oppositional defiant disorder. ADHD also coexists with learning and communication disorders.

It is thought that ADHD reflects subtle but unclear neurological impairments. ADHD is associated with perinatal trauma and early malnutrition. The incidence is increased in parents and siblings, and concor-

TABLE 21-15
DSM-IV-TR DIAGNOSTIC CRITERIA FOR ATTENTION-DEFICIT/HYPERACTIVITY DISORDER

A. Either (1) or (2):
   (1) six (or more) of the following symptoms of inattention have persisted for at least 6 months to a degree that is maladaptive and inconsistent with developmental level:
   Inattention
      (a) often fails to give close attention to details or makes careless mistakes in schoolwork, work, or other activities
      (b) often has difficulty sustaining attention in tasks or play activities
      (c) often does not seem to listen when spoken to directly
      (d) often does not follow through on instructions and fails to finish schoolwork, chores, or duties in the workplace (not oppositional behavior or failure to understand instructions)
      (e) often has difficulty organizing tasks and activities
      (f) often avoids, dislikes, or is reluctant to engage in tasks that require sustained mental effort (such as schoolwork or homework)
      (g) often loses things necessary for tasks of activities (e.g., toys, school assignments, nails, books, or tools)
      (h) is often easily distracted by extraneous stimuli
      (i) is often forgetful in daily activities
   (2) six (or more) of the following symptoms of **hyperactivity-impulsivity** have persisted for at least 6 months to a degree that is maladaptive and inconsistent with developmental level:
   Hyperactivity
      (a) often fidgets with hands or feel or squirms in seat
      (b) often leaves seat in classroom or in other situations in which remaining seated is expected
      (c) often runs about or climbs excessively in situations in which it is inappropriate (in adolescents or adults, may be limited to subjective feelings of restlessness)
      (d) often has difficulty playing or engaging in leisure activities quietly
      (e) is often "on the go" or often acts as if "driven by a motor"
      (f) often talks excessively
   Impulsivity
      (g) often blunts out answers before questions have been completed
      (h) often has difficulty awaiting turn
      (i) often interrupts or intrudes on others (e.g., butts into conversations or games)
B. Some hyperactive-impulsive or inattentive symptoms that caused impairment was present before age 7 years.
C. Some impairment from the symptoms is present in two or more settings (e.g., of school (or work) and at home).
D. There must be clear evidence of clinically significant impairment in social academic, or occupational functioning.
E. The symptoms do not occur exclusively during the course of a pervasive developmental disorder, schizophrenia, or other psychotic disorder and are not better accounted for by another mental disorder (e.g., mood disorder, anxiety disorder, dissociative disorder, or a personality disorder).

Code based on type:
   Attention-deficit/hyperactivity disorder, combined type: if both Criteria A1 and A2 are met for the past 6 months.
   Attention-deficit/hyperactivity disorder, predominantly inattentive type: If Criterion A1 is met but Criterion A2 is not met for the past 6 months
   Attention-deficit/hyperactivity disorder, predominantly hyperactive-impulsive type: If Criterion A2 is met but Criterion A1 is not met for the past 6 months

Coding note: For individuals (especially adolescents and adults) who currently have symptoms that no longer meet full criteria, "in partial permission" should be specified.

From American Psychiatric Association. *Diagnostic and Statistical Manual of Mental Disorders,* text revision, 4th ed. Washington, DC: American Psychiatric Association, Copyright 2000, with permission.

dance is greater in monozygotic than in dizygotic twins. Children with ADHD are often temperamentally difficult. In neurotransmitter systems, the clearest evidence is of noradrenergic and dopaminergic dysfunction. Nonfocal (soft) neurological signs are common. Reduced frontal lobe disinhibition is supported by imaging studies; frontal lobe hypoperfusion and lower frontal lobe metabolic rates have been noted.

ADHD is probably not related to sugar intake; few patients (perhaps 5%) are affected by food additives. Of persons with ADHD, 20–25% continue to show symptoms into adolescence, and some into adulthood. Some, especially those with concomitant conduct disorder, become delinquent or later develop antisocial personality disorder.

3. Treatment.

    a. Pharmacological—see Table 21–4.

        (1) Stimulants reduce symptoms in about 75%; they improve self-esteem by improving the patient's rapport with parents and teachers. Stimulants decrease hyperactivity. Plasma levels are not useful.

            (a) Dextroamphetamine (Dexedrine) is approved by the FDA for children ages 3 years and older.

            (b) Methylphenidate (Ritalin) is FDA-approved for children ages 6 years and older. The 8 hour sustained-release preparations do not have any proven increased usefulness. Concerta, promoted as having a duration of 12 hours, is a new preparation. Early reports of a good side effect profile await replication.

            (c) The duration of action of amphetamine-dextroamphetamine (Adderall) appears to be longer than that of methylphenidate.

            (d) Modafinil (Provigil), used on narcolepsy, is being tried. It is long acting and appears to have a small abuse potential.

            (e) Pemoline (Cylert) is given in dosages of 18.75 to 37.5 mg/day. Its onset and duration of action are delayed, but the drug is of very limited use because of associated liver toxicity.

        (2) Clonidine (Catapres) and guanfacine (Tenex) are reported to reduce arousal in children with the disorder.

        (3) Antidepressants if stimulants fail; may be best in ADHD with comorbid depression or anxiety. Efficacy has been reported for imipramine (Tofranil) and desipramine (Norpramin), but four children died suddenly while taking desipramine. Bupropion (Wellbutrin) and venlafaxine (Effexor) are also reported to be useful for ADHD and appear to be safe.

        (4) Antipsychotics, lithium, or divalproex (Depakote) if other medications fail, but only for patients with severe symptoms and aggression (concomitant disruptive behavior disorder).

    b. Psychological—multimodality treatment is often necessary for child and family. May include medication, behavioral technique, individual psychotherapy, family therapy, and special education (especially with coexisting specific developmental disorder). These interventions are crucial in moderate or severe cases, given the risk for delinquency.

B. Conduct disorder. Prevalence ranges from 5–15% in studies. Accounts for many inpatient admissions in urban areas. The male-to-female ratio is 4:1 to 12:1.

    1. Diagnosis, signs, and symptoms. See Table 21–16.

TABLE 21–16
DSM-IV-TR DIAGNOSTIC CRITERIA FOR CONDUCT DISORDER

A. A repetitive and persistent pattern of behavior in which the basic rights of others or major age-appropriate societal norms or rules are violated, as manifested by the presence of three (or more) of the following criteria in the past 12 months, with at least one criterion present in the past 6 months:

Aggression to people and animals
  (1) often bullies, threatens, or intimidates others
  (2) often initiates physical fights
  (3) has used a weapon that can cause serious physical harm to others (e.g., a bat, brick, broken bottle, knife, gun)
  (4) has been physically cruel to people
  (5) has been physically cruel to animals
  (6) has stolen while confronting a victim (e.g., mugging, purse snatching, extortion, armed robbery)
  (7) has forced someone into sexual activity

Destruction of property
  (8) has deliberately engaged in fire setting with the intention of causing serious damage
  (9) has deliberately destroyed others property (other than by fire setting)

Deceitfulness or theft
  (10) has broken into someone else's house, building, or car
  (11) often lies to obtain goods or favors or to avoid obligations (i.e., "cons" others)
  (12) has stolen items of nontrivial value without confronting a victim (e.g., shoplifting, but without breaking and entering; forgery)

Serious violations of rules
  (13) often stays out at night despite parental prohibitions, beginning before age 13 years
  (14) has run away from home overnight at least twice while living in parental or parental surrogate home (or once without returning for a lengthy period)
  (15) is often truant from school, beginning before age 13 years

B. The disturbance in behavior causes clinically significant impairment in social, academic, or occupational functioning.

C. If the individual is age 18 years or older, criteria are not met for antisocial personality disorder.

Specify type based on age at onset:
  Childhood-onset type: onset of at least one criterion characteristic of conduct disorder prior to age 10 years
  Adolescent-onset type: absence of any criteria characteristic of conduct disorder prior to age 10 years
  Unspecified type: age of onset is not known

Specify severity:
  Mild: few if any conduct problems in excess of those required to make the diagnosis **and** conduct problems cause only minor harm to others
  Moderate: number of conduct problems and effect on others are intermediate between "mild" and "severe"
  Severe: many conduct problems in excess of those required to make the diagnosis or conduct problems cause considerable harm to others

From American Psychiatric Association. *Diagnostic and Statistical Manual of Mental Disorders,* text revision, 4th ed. Washington, DC: American Psychiatric Association, Copyright 2000, with permission.

2. **General considerations.** Conduct disorder is associated with family instability, including victimization by physical or sexual abuse. Propensity for violence correlates with child abuse, family violence, alcoholism, and signs of severe psychopathology (e.g., paranoia and cognitive or subtle neurological deficits). It is crucial to explore for these signs; findings can guide treatment.

Conduct disorder often coexists with ADHD and learning or communication disorders. Suicidal thoughts and acts and alcohol and drug abuse correlate with conduct disorder.

Some children with conduct disorder have low plasma levels of dopamine and β-hydroxylase. Abnormal serotonin levels have been implicated.

3. **Treatment**
   a. **Pharmacological**—see Table 21–4. Stimulants may reduce mild aggression in conduct disorder comorbid with ADHD. Lithium or haloperidol is of proven efficacy in targeting explosive, aggressive behavior in children with conduct disorder. However, the atypical antipsychotics also diminish aggression and have a better side effect profile than haloperidol. α-adrenergic agonists may help; β-adrenergic receptor antagonists deserve study.
   b. **Psychological**—multimodality, as in ADHD. May include medication, individual or family therapy, parenting classes, tutoring, or special class placement (for cognitive or conduct problems). It is crucial to discover and fortify any interests or talents to build resistance to the lure of crime. If the environment is noxious or if conduct disorder is severe, placement away from home may be indicated.

C. **Oppositional defiant disorder**
   1. **Diagnosis, signs, and symptoms.** See Table 21–17.
   2. **General considerations.** Oppositional defiant disorder can coexist with many disorders, including ADHD and anxiety disorders. It can result from parent–child struggles over autonomy; therefore, the occurrence increases in families with overly rigid parents and temperamentally active, moody, and intense children.
   3. **Treatment.**
      a. **Pharmacological**—drugs used for any comorbid disorder may be necessary, but only after careful consideration of benefits and risks and failure of other interventions.
      b. **Psychological**—behavioral interventions and family therapy are the interventions of choice. Behavior modification can be helpful.

VII. **Feeding and eating disorders of infancy or early childhood**
   A. **Pica.** Repeated ingestion of a nonnutritive substance that is inappropriate to the developmental level, for at least 1 month, by infants who do not meet the criteria for autistic disorder, schizophrenia, or Kleine-Levin syn-

TABLE 21–17
DSM-IV-TR DIAGNOSTIC CRITERIA FOR OPPOSITIONAL DEFIANT DISORDER

A. A pattern of negativistic, hostile, and defiant behavior lasting at least 6 months, during which four (or more) of the following are present:
   (1) often loses temper
   (2) often argues with adults
   (3) often actively defies or refuses to comply with adults' requests or rules
   (4) often deliberately annoys people
   (5) often blames others for his or her mistakes or misbehavior
   (6) is often touchy or easily annoyed by others
   (7) is often angry and resentful
   (8) is often spiteful or vindictive
   Note: Consider a criterion met only if the behavior occurs more frequently than is typically observed in individuals of comparable age and developmental level.
B. The disturbance in behavior causes clinically significant impairment in social, academic, or occupational functioning.
C. The behaviors do not occur exclusively during the course of a psychotic or mood disorder.
D. Criteria are not met for conduct disorder, and, if the individual is age 18 years or older, criteria are not met for antisocial personality disorder.

From American Psychiatric Association. *Diagnostic and Statistical Manual of Mental Disorders*, text revision, 4th ed. Washington, DC: American Psychiatric Association, Copyright 2000, with permission.

drome. The prevalence is unclear; studies report 10–32% in preschool children. It is associated with MR, neglect, and nutritional deficiency (e.g., iron or zinc). Lead or other poisonings can result. It usually stops in early childhood. Treatment involves testing for lead intoxication and treating if necessary. Because cravings for dirt and ice may relate to iron and zinc deficiencies, such deficiencies should be ruled out. Parent guidance may be necessary. Infrequently, aversive conditioning is necessary.

B. **Rumination disorder.** Repeated regurgitation, for at least 1 month, that follows a period of normal eating (in the absence of gastrointestinal illness) and is not secondary to anorexia nervosa or bulimia nervosa. Swallowed food is brought back into the mouth, ejected or rechewed, and swallowed. The child is in no distress. The condition is rare, with onset between 3 and 12 months of age. Immature, ungiving mothers who further reject because of the disorder may be associated with rumination. Little is known of the outcome, but it ranges from spontaneous remission, to malnutrition, to failure to thrive, to death. Gastrointestinal problems (e.g., pyloric stenosis, gastroesophageal reflux, hiatal hernia) must be ruled out. Treatment involves parental guidance and behavioral techniques.

C. **Feeding and eating disorder of infancy or early childhood.** Category for children who persistently eat inadequately for at least 1 month in the absence of a general medical condition or other causal mental condition, with resultant failure to gain weight and loss of significant weight. The onset is before 6 years of age. Because many children with the disorder are temperamentally difficult or developmentally delayed and their caregivers may lack patience or be neglectful, counseling of the caregivers is often crucial. Cognitive behavior interventions can be useful.

VIII. Tic disorders

A. **Tourette's disorder.** (Also known as *Gilles de la Tourette's syndrome.*) The prevalence is about 4 in 10,000 to 5 in 10,000; the mean age of onset is 7 years. The male-to-female ratio is 3:1.

1. **Diagnosis, signs, and symptoms.** See Table 21–18. Motor and vocal tics can be simple or complex. Simple tics generally are the first to appear. Examples:

   Simple motor tics—eye blinking, head jerking, facial grimacing.
   Simple vocal tics—coughing, grunting, sniffing.
   Complex motor tics—hitting self, jumping.

TABLE 21–18
DSM-IV-TR DIAGNOSTIC CRITERIA FOR TOURETTE'S DISORDER

A. Both multiple motor and one or more vocal tics have been present at some time during the illness, although not necessarily concurrently. (A tic is a sudden, rapid, recurrent, nonrhythmic, stereotyped motor movement or vocalization.)

B. The tics occur many times a day (usually in bouts) nearly every day or intermittently throughout a period of more than 1 year, and during this period there was never a tic-free period of more than 3 consecutive months.

C. The onset is before age 18 years.

D. The disturbance is not due to the direct physiological effects of a substance (e.g., stimulants) or a general medical condition (e.g., Huntington's disease or postviral encephalitis).

Complex vocal tics—coprolalia (use of vulgar words), palilalia (repeating own words), echolalia (repeating another's words).

2. **General considerations.** Evidence suggests a genetic transmission—familial increases in tic disorders, significantly greater concordance in monozygotic twins than in dizygotic twins. Evidence of neurobiological substrate-nonspecific EEG abnormalities and abnormal CT findings in many patients. Implications of dopamine abnormality: abnormal levels of homovanillic acid (dopamine metabolite) in CSF; stimulants, which are dopamine agonists, can worsen tics or precipitate their occurrence; dopamine antagonists generally cause tics to diminish. Tourette's disorder and other tic disorders must be differentiated from a multitude of other disorders and diseases (e.g., dyskinesias, Sydenham's chorea, Huntington's disease). Associated with Tourette's disorder: ADHD, learning problems, and obsessive-compulsive symptoms, of which the prevalence is increased in first-degree relatives. Social ostracism is frequent. If the condition is untreated, the course is usually chronic, with periods in which tics wax and wane.

3. **Treatment**
   a. **Pharmacological**—see Table 21–4.
      (1) Haloperidol—leads to improvement, often marked, in about 85% of patients; sometimes sedating dosages are required.
      (2) Pimozide (Orap)—is strongly antidopaminergic, like haloperidol; a small potential exists for slowing cardiac conduction.
      (3) Clonidine—α_2-adrenergic agonist; not as effective as haloperidol or pimozide but not associated with risk for tardive dyskinesia. Little evidence is available to implicate a noradrenergic mechanism in Tourette's disorder. The less sedating guanfacine can be tried.
   b. **Psychological**—counseling or therapy is often necessary for child, family, or both. The nature of Tourette's disorder, coping with it, and ostracism must be addressed. Group therapy may reduce social isolation.

B. **Chronic motor or vocal tic disorder.** Similar to Tourette's disorder; diagnostic criteria are the same, except that the patient has either single or multiple motor tics or vocal tics, not both. The condition is much more prevalent than Tourette's disorder, but it is less severe and generally causes less social impairment than Tourette's disorder. Genetically, chronic motor or vocal tic disorder and Tourette's disorder frequently occur in the same families. The neurobiology appears to be the same, and the treatment is identical to that for Tourette's disorder.

C. **Transient tic disorder.** The prevalence is unclear; nonrigorous surveys report that 5–24% of school children have some sort of tic. The male-to-female ratio is 3:1.

1. **Diagnosis, signs, and symptoms.** See Table 21–19.
2. **General considerations.** In most cases, the tics are psychogenic, increasing during stress and tending to remit spontaneously. In a few cases, chronic motor or vocal tic disorder or Tourette's disorder eventually develops.

3. **Treatment.** In mild cases, treatment may not be needed. In severe cases, behavioral techniques or psychotherapy is indicated. Medication used for other tic disorders is tried only in severe cases.

IX. Elimination disorders

A. **Encopresis.** The prevalence is about 1% of 5-year-old children; encopresis is more common in boys than in girls.

1. **Diagnosis, signs, and symptoms.** See Table 21–20.

2. **General considerations.** Rule out a physical disorder, such as aganglionic megacolon (Hirschsprung's disease). Inadequate toilet training can result in child–parent power struggles and functional encopresis. Some children appear to have abnormal anal sphincter contractions, which contribute to the condition. Some fear using the toilet. Impaction can develop in children with constipation and overflow incontinence, causing pain on defecation and anal fissures. Leakage is persistent. Those without constipation and overflow often have oppositional defiant or conduct disorders. Encopresis may be precipitated by the birth of a sibling or parental separation. Encopresis usually brings embarrassment and social ostracism. When encopresis is deliberate, the associated psychopathology is usually severe. About 25% of patients also have enuresis. Encopresis can last for years but usually resolves.

3. **Treatment.** The child may require individual psychotherapy to address the meaning of the encopresis and any embarrassment or os-

TABLE 21–19
DSM-IV-TR DIAGNOSTIC CRITERIA FOR TRANSIENT TIC DISORDER

A. Single or multiple motor and/or vocal tics (i.e., sudden, rapid, recurrent, nonrhythmic, stereotyped motor movements or vocalizations).
B. The tics occur many times a day, nearly every day for at least 4 weeks, but for no longer than 12 consecutive months.
C. The onset is before age 18 years.
D. The disturbance is not due to the direct physiological effects of a substance (e.g., stimulants) or a general medical condition (e.g., Huntington's disease or postviral encephalitis).
E. Criteria have never been met for Tourette's disorder or chronic motor or vocal tic disorder.

Specify if:
Single episode or **recurrent**

From American Psychiatric Association. *Diagnostic and Statistical Manual of Mental Disorders,* text revision, 4th ed. Washington, DC: American Psychiatric Association, Copyright 2000, with permission.

TABLE 21–20
DSM-IV-TR DIAGNOSTIC CRITERIA FOR ENCOPRESIS

A. Repeated passage of feces into inappropriate places (e.g., clothing of floor) whether involuntary or intentional.
B. At least one such event a month for at least 3 months.
C. Chronological age is at least 4 years (or equivalent developmental level).
D. The behavior is not due exclusively to the direct physiological effects of a substance (e.g., laxatives) or a general medical condition except through a mechanism involving constipation.

Code as follows:
With constipation and overflow incontinence
Without constipation and overflow incontinence

From American Psychiatric Association. *Diagnostic and Statistical Manual of Mental Disorders.* Text revision, 4th ed. Washington, DC: American Psychiatric Association, Copyright 2000, with permission.

TABLE 21–21
DSM-IV-TR DIAGNOSTIC CRITERIA FOR ENURESIS

A. Repeated voiding of urine into bed or clothes (whether involuntary or intentional).
B. The behavior is clinically significant as manifested by either a frequency of twice a week for at least 3 consecutive months or the presence of clinically significant distress or impairment in social academic (occupational), or other important areas of functioning.
C. Chronological age is at least 5 years (or equivalent developmental level).
D. The behavior is not due exclusively to the direct physiological effect of substance (e.g., diuretic) or a general medical condition (e.g., diabetes, spina bifida, or seizure disorder).

Specify type:
   Nocturnal only
   Diurnal only
   Nocturnal and diurnal

From American Psychiatric Association. *Diagnosis and Statistical Manual of Mental Disorders*, text revision, 4th ed. Washington, DC: American Psychiatric Association, Copyright 2000, with permission.

tracism. Behavioral techniques often are helpful. Parental guidance and family therapy often are needed. If conditions such as impaction and anal fissures are present, consultation with a pediatrician is required.

B. Enuresis (not due to a general medical condition). Prevalence: age 5, 7%; age 10, 3%; age 18, 1%. Much more common in boys. The diurnal subtype is the least prevalent and is more common in girls than in boys.

1. **Diagnosis, signs, and symptoms.** See Table 21–21.
2. **General considerations.** Enuresis tends to run in families; concordance is greater in monozygotic than in dizygotic twins. Some patients have small bladders that require frequent voiding. It does not seem to be related to a specific stage of sleep, as are sleepwalking and sleep terror disorders. Many patients have no coexisting mental disorder, and impairment reflects only conflict with caregivers, loss of self-esteem, and social ostracism, if any. Enuresis is likely to coexist with other disorders and can be precipitated by such events as birth of a sibling or parental separation. Spontaneous remissions are frequent at ages 6 to 8 and at puberty.
3. **Treatment**
   a. **Psychological.**
      (1) **Behavioral approaches**—record dry nights on a calendar and reward dry nights with a star and five to seven consecutive dry nights with a gift. A bell (or buzzer) and pad apparatus is a successful treatment but is cumbersome.
      (2) **Psychotherapy**—not recommended unless psychopathology or other problems coexist, such as reduced self-esteem. The exploration of conflicts underlying enuresis has met with little success. Parental guidance related to the management of the disorder often is necessary.
   b. **Pharmacological.** Rarely used, given the rate of spontaneous remissions, success of behavioral approaches, and development of tolerance to drugs. Imipramine often is effective in reducing or even eliminating wetting, but tolerance can develop after about 6 weeks. The mode of action is unclear; effects on bladder or sleep cycle are considered. Some success has been achieved with desmopressin (DDAVP).

X. Other disorders of infancy, childhood, or adolescence

A. Separation anxiety disorder.
Estimated prevalence is 3–4% of school age children, 10% of adolescents. The male-to-female ratio is 1:1. Onset is from preschool to adolescence.

1. **Diagnosis, signs, and symptoms.** See Table 21–22.
2. **General considerations.** The disorder clusters in families, but genetic transmission is unclear. Some data link affected children with parents who have a history of the disorder in addition to current panic disorder, agoraphobia, or depression. Anxiety disorders are likely to develop in temperamentally inhibited infants, and increased autonomic neuron system activity has been demonstrated. Social debilitation is a risk in severe cases.
3. **Treatment**
   a. **Pharmacological**—see Table 21–4.
      (1) **Anxiolytics**—little research in childhood anxiety disorders. Alprazolam (Xanax) has shown some efficacy.
      (2) **Antidepressants**—tricyclics (e.g., imipramine) can be tried.
      (3) **Antipsychotics**—not useful in anxiety disorders. The risk for side effects outweighs potential benefits.
      (4) **Antihistamines**—diphenhydramine (Benadryl) is sometimes used to relieve childhood anxiety. Its usefulness is limited, and some children can have a paradoxical reaction of excitement.

TABLE 21–22
DSM-IV-TR DIAGNOSTIC CRITERIA FOR SEPARATION ANXIETY DISORDER

A. Developmentally inappropriate and excessive anxiety concerning separation from home or from those to whom the individual is attached, as evidenced by three (or more) of the following:
   (1) recurrent excessive distress when separation from home or major attachment figures occurs or is anticipated
   (2) persistent and excessive worry about losing, or about possible harm befalling, major attachment figures
   (3) persistent and excessive worry that an untoward event will lead to separation from a major attachment figure (e.g., getting lost or being kidnapped)
   (4) persistent reluctance or refusal to go to school or elsewhere because of fear of separation
   (5) persistently and excessively fearful or reluctance to be alone or without major attachment figures at home or without significant adults in other settings
   (6) persistent reluctance or refusal to go to sleep without being near a major attachment figure or to sleep away from home
   (7) repeated nightmares involving the theme of separation
   (8) repeated complaints of physical symptoms (such as headaches, stomachaches, nausea, or vomiting) when separation from major attachment figures occurs or is anticipated
B. The duration of the disturbance is at least 4 weeks.
C. The onset is before age 18 years.
D. The disturbance causes clinically significant distress or impairment in social, academic (occupational), or other important areas of functioning.
E. The disturbance does not occur exclusively during the course of a pervasive developmental disorder, schizophrenia, or other psychotic disorder and, in adolescents and adults, is not better accounted for by panic disorder with agoraphobia.

Specify if:
Early onset: If onset occurs before age 6 years

From American Psychiatric Association. *Diagnostic and Statistical Manual of Mental Disorders*, text revision, 4th ed. Washington, DC: American Psychiatric Association, 2000, with permission.

      b. Psychological—multimodal treatment is recommended.

        (1) Individual psychotherapy—children with separation anxiety disorder exaggerate environmental dangers so that they fear for their safety and that of their parents. Their feelings and attitudes are addressed in insight-oriented or cognitive-behavioral therapy.

        (2) Family therapy or parent guidance—if parents are fostering separation anxiety.

        (3) Behavior modification—may be helpful to achieve separation from parents and a return to school.

B. Selective mutism. Rare, more common in girls. Diagnostically, a child who both speaks and comprehends refuses to talk for at least 1 month (but this period is not limited to the first month of school) in social situations. Begins between ages 4 and 8, usually resolves in weeks to months. Associated with parental overprotection, parental ambivalence, communication disorders, shyness, and oppositional behavior. Treatment can include individual psychotherapy and parent counseling. SSRIs may be helpful.

C. Reactive attachment disorder of infancy or early childhood. Prevalence and sex ratio are unknown. Often diagnosed and treated by pediatricians.

    1. Diagnosis, signs, and symptoms. Grossly inadequate care (persistent disregard of physical or emotional needs or repeated change of caretaker) results in markedly disturbed social relatedness in a child younger than 5 years. Inhibited type is characterized by a failure to initiate or respond to interactions that is accompanied by apathy, passivity, and lack of visual tracking. Disinhibited type is characterized by indiscriminate and shallow sociability. These failure-to-thrive children are apathetic and passive, and do not track visually. The disturbance is not secondary to MR or autistic disorder.

    2. General considerations. Physically, head circumference is generally normal; weight, very low; height, somewhat short. Pituitary functioning is normal. Associated with low socioeconomic status and mothers who are depressed and isolated and have experienced abuse. Course—the earlier the intervention, the more reversible the disorder. Affectionless character can develop. Death can occur.

    3. Treatment. In many cases, removal of child may be necessary. Severe malnourishment and other medical problems may require hospitalization. Some homes become adequate following parent education, the provision of a homemaker or financial aid, or treatment of mental disorders in family members.

D. Stereotypic movement disorder. Diagnostically, repetitive, seemingly nonfunctional behaviors last for at least 4 weeks (e.g., hand shaking, rocking, head banging, nail biting, nose picking, hair pulling) and markedly interfere with normal activities or cause physical injury. The disorder is common in MR. It is not diagnosed for behaviors associated with obsessive-compulsive disorder, pervasive developmental disorders, or trichotillomania. An increase in dopamine activity seems to be associated with an increase in stereotypic movements. Pervasive developmental disorder and tic disorder must be absent. Common in MR and blindness. Treatment varies. If movements increase with frustration, boredom, or tension, these conditions are addressed. Repetitive behavior may respond to an SSRI. Self-abusive behaviors may require antipsychotics or opioid antagonists (which are currently under study) (Table 21–4).

XI. Other disorders relevant to children and adolescents

A. Schizophrenia with childhood onset. Several studies confirm that some children have delusions or hallucinations (auditory or visual). Nevertheless, few children or young adolescents are schizophrenic, and delusions, hallucinations, and thought disorders are difficult to diagnose in children. Some children in whom schizophrenia is diagnosed are given a diagnosis of mood disorder when followed to adolescence. Treatment is with antipsychotic medications (although studies are few). Psychotherapy, family therapy, and special schooling may be necessary (see Chapter 8).

B. Mood disorders. Some prepubertal children meet the criteria for major depressive disorder. SSRIs may benefit some of them. Prepubertal children and adolescents with mania, hypomania, or mania-like symptoms have been successfully treated with lithium. Valproate benefits some adolescents and can be tried in prepubertal children. Risperidone appears to be effective in targeting mania-like symptoms.

C. Other disorders. Some children meet criteria for anxiety disorders, including generalized anxiety disorder, specific phobia, social phobia, obsessive-compulsive disorder, posttraumatic stress disorder, and panic disorders (see Chapter 11). Clomipramine (Anafranil) and SSRIs appear to benefit children with obsessive-compulsive disorder. Posttraumatic stress disorder can result from physical or sexual abuse.

Substance-related, gender identity, eating, somatoform, sleep, and adjustment disorders can also be diagnosed during childhood and adolescence.

XII. Other childhood issues

A. Child abuse and neglect. An estimated 1 million children are abused or neglected annually in the United States, a problem that results in 2,000 to 4,000 deaths per year. The abused are apt to be of low birth weight or born prematurely (50% of all abused children), handicapped (e.g., MR, cerebral palsy), or troubled (e.g., defiant, hyperactive). The abusing parent is usually the mother, who likely was abused herself. Abusing parents often are impulsive, substance abusers, depressed, antisocial, or narcissistic.

Each year, 150,000 to 200,000 new cases of sexual abuse are reported. Of these allegations, 2–8% appear to be false, and many other allegations cannot be substantiated. In 8 of 10 sexually abused children, the perpetrator, usually male, is known to the child. In 50%, the offender is a parent, parent surrogate, or relative.

B. Suicide.   Serious attempted and completed suicides are rare in children younger than 13 years. Suicidal ideation, threats, and less serious gestures are much more frequent and often precipitate hospitalization. Suicidal children tend to be depressed (and sometimes preoccupied with death); however, angry, impulsive children, in addition to children suffering recent emotional trauma, can be suicidal.

Suicidal behavior is increasing in adolescents and, as with children, often necessitates hospitalization. It correlates with depression, aggressive behavior, and alcohol abuse. Suicidal ideation is more common in girls, and girls make more suicidal gestures or attempts. Serious attempts and successful suicides correlate with being male and the availability of alcohol, illicit drugs, or medications, which lower impulse control and can be used to overdose.

Parents often are unaware of their children's suicidal thoughts and behavior, so that direct questioning of children and adolescents about suicide is necessary (see Chapter 20).

C. Fire setting.   Associated with other destruction of property, stealing, lying, self-destructive tendencies, and cruelty to animals. The male-to-female ratio is 9:1.

D. Violence.   Associated with conduct disorder, impulsivity, and anger. May result in homicide. Fifty percent of children in first grade who are disruptive or oppositional are at risk for teenage delinquency.

E. Obesity.   Present in 5–20% of children and adolescents. A small percentage present with an obesity-hypoventilation syndrome that is similar to adult pickwickian syndrome. These children can have dyspnea, and their sleep is characterized by snoring, stridor, perhaps apnea, and hypoxia with oxygen desaturation. Death can result. Other conditions, such as hypothyroidism or Prader-Willi syndrome, should be ruled out (see Chapter 15).

F. AIDS.   AIDS has presented child and adolescent psychiatrists with a multitude of difficult problems. For example, the care of young patients from lower socioeconomic groups, already grossly inadequate because of insufficient resources, is further burdened by HIV-related illness or the death of parents and relatives. Young psychiatric patients who have concomitant nonsymptomatic positive serology and require residential treatment are rejected for fear of transmission of the disease. In adolescence, AIDS has further complicated sexuality and the problem of substance abuse (see Chapter 5).

For more detailed discussion of this topic, see Child Psychiatry, Ch 32, p 2532; Psychiatric Examination of the Infant, Child, and Adolescent, Ch 33, p 2558; Mental Retardation, Ch 34, p 2587; Learning Disorders, Ch 35, p 2614; Motor Skills Disorder: Developmental Coordination Disorder, Ch 36, p 2629; Communication Disorders, Ch 37, p 2634; Pervasive Developmental Disorders, Ch 38, p 2659; Attention-deficit Disorders, Ch 39, p 2679; Disruptive Behavior Disorders, Ch 40, p 2693; Feeding and Eating Disorders of Infancy and Early Childhood, Ch 41, p 2704; Tic Disorders, Ch 42, p 2711; Elimination Disorders, Ch 43, p 2720; Other Disorders of Infancy, Childhood, and Adolescence, Ch 44, p 2735; Mood Disorders and Suicide in Children and Adolescents, Ch 45, p 2740; Anxiety Disorders in Children, Ch 46, p 2758; Early-onset Schizophrenia, Ch 47, p 2782; Child Psychiatry: Psychiatric Treatment, Ch 48, p 2790; and Child Psychiatry: Special Areas of Interest, Ch 49, p 2865, in CTP/VII.

22

Geriatric Psychiatry

I. Introduction

Geriatric psychiatry is the branch of medicine concerned with promoting health and preventing, diagnosing, and treating physical and mental disorders in the elderly.

II. Epidemiology

The life expectancy in the United States is approaching 80 years. For this reason, the number and relative percentage of elderly persons in the general population are markedly increased. The oldest old—people at least 85 years of age—are the fastest-growing group of the elderly population, and although the oldest old constitute only 1.2% of the total population, their numbers have increased 232% since 1960. People at least 85 years old now constitute 10% of those 65 and older.

III. Medical background

The leading five causes of death in the elderly are heart disease, cancer, stroke, Alzheimer's disease, and pneumonia. CNS changes and psychopathology are frequent causes of morbidity, as are arthritis and related symptoms. Benign prostatic hyperplasia affects three fourths of men over age 75. Urinary incontinence is believed to occur in as many as one fifth of the elderly, sometimes in association with dementia. These common disorders result in behavior modification. Arthritis, for example, may restrict activity and alter lifestyle. The elderly, like other adults, are profoundly embarrassed by urinary difficulties and will restrict activities and hide or deny their disability to maintain self-esteem.

Cardiovascular disease is a prominent cause of morbidity and mortality in the elderly. Hypertension may be present in 40% of the elderly, many of whom are receiving diuretics or antihypertensive medications. Hypertension itself can result in CNS effects ranging from headaches to stroke, and pharmacotherapy for this condition can result in mood and cognitive disorders (e.g., electrolyte disturbances due to diuretic treatment). Atherosclerosis, associated with both cardiovascular disease and hypertension, has been related to the occurrence of the major forms of dementia—not only vascular dementia but also Alzheimer's disease.

Sensory changes also accompany the aging process. One third of the aged have some degree of auditory disability. In one study, nearly one half of persons 75 to 85 years of age had lens cataracts, and more than 70% had glaucoma. Difficulties with convergence, accommodation, and macular degeneration also are sources of visual disability in the aged. These sensory changes frequently interact with psychopathological disabilities, serving to magnify psychopathological deficit and color symptoms.

IV. Clinical syndromes

A. Depression

1. **Signs and symptoms.** The frequency of depression appears to increase with age. Also, the relapse rate appears to increase as the time between depressive episodes diminishes. The frequency of suicide increases markedly with age. Nonetheless, good evidence suggests that certain features of depression, namely obsessions and phobias, decrease with age.

   Epidemiological studies of depression in the elderly are confounded by confusion between depression and dementia. Family members of patients with dementia commonly seek treatment for persons with the chief complaint of depression in the absence of any true mood disorder. The psychiatrist must recognize that paucity of speech, slowing of gait, flattening of affect, and decreased interest in and involvement with social and personal activities, which all indicate depression in a young patient, indicate early dementia in the elderly patient in the absence of clear-cut dysphoria. Cognitive assessment, which reveals deficits in the dementia patient, further clarifies the diagnosis of dementia when applicable.

   Major depressive disorder, in its classic adult form, may coexist with dementia and is a common concomitant of the early stages of Alzheimer's disease. When depressive symptoms occur in the context of Alzheimer's disease, they are commonly part of the spectrum of the behavioral and psychological symptoms of dementia (BPSD), which include characteristic sleep disturbance, suspiciousness, anxieties, and agitation. Other symptoms, reminiscent of depression in other contexts, may also occur in the BPSD syndrome of Alzheimer's disease, including tearfulness, somatic complaints, and obsessive behaviors. Pervasive dysphoria, however, is relatively rare, and patients with Alzheimer's disease and depression rarely, if ever, manifest suicidal behavior. Manneristic statements such as, "I wish I were dead," are common in Alzheimer's disease; however, such statements are not accompanied by suicidal plans, gestures, or actions.

   Depression may be the earliest manifestation of Alzheimer's disease, and the occurrence of depression in adult life is now a recognized risk factor for subsequently manifested Alzheimer's disease.

   Depression is also a common concomitant of infarction or other brain insult, with or without coexisting dementia. Disease affecting the frontal brain regions is believed to be particularly associated with affective symptoms. Depression associated with cerebral infarction is sometimes manifested as emotional incontinence (i.e., sudden episodes of tearfulness without a pervasive, consistent, or affective dysphoria).

   In addition to dementia and overt brain trauma, depression in the elderly is commonly associated with various other forms of physical disease. For example, electrolyte disturbances caused by diuretics alone or in combination with other medications can result in a mood disorder, as can vitamin B_{12} deficiency secondary to malabsorption that develops after gastrointestinal surgery.

2. **Treatment.** Primary (idiopathic) depressive disorders in the elderly are serious and, in many cases, even life-threatening conditions. Treatment

modalities that should be given primary consideration include selective serotonin reuptake inhibitors (SSRIs); tricyclic antidepressants; serotonin 5-HT$_2$ receptor antagonists such as trazodone (Desyrel); miscellaneous antidepressants, including bupropion (Wellbutrin), venlafaxine (Effexor), and mirtazapine (Remeron); electroconvulsive therapy (ECT), and monoamine oxidase inhibitors (MAOIs).

a. Antidepressants—an increasingly diverse category of compounds, all of which are potentially useful in the elderly. Considerations in selecting a particular antidepressant treatment include, prominently, the side effects and risks (if any) of the drug.

(1) SSRIs—in general, the SSRIs (e.g., fluoxetine [Prozac], sertraline [Zoloft], paroxetine [Paxil], and citalopram [Celexa]) are safe and well tolerated by elderly patients. As a group, these drugs may cause nausea and other gastrointestinal symptoms, nervousness, agitation, headache, and insomnia, most often to mild degrees. Fluoxetine is the drug most likely to cause nervousness, insomnia, and loss of appetite, particularly early in treatment. Sertraline is the drug most likely to produce nausea and diarrhea. Paroxetine causes some anticholinergic effects. SSRIs do not cause the characteristic side effects of the tricyclic agents. The absence of orthostatic hypotension is a clinically significant factor in the use of SSRIs by the elderly.

(2) Tricyclic drugs—when used by elderly patients, the secondary amine agents desipramine (Norpramin) and nortriptyline (Pamelor) are preferred because of their low propensity to cause anticholinergic, orthostatic, and sedative side effects. Nortriptyline is less likely than other tricyclic agents are to cause orthostatic hypotension in patients with congestive heart failure. Because of the quinidine-like effect of all tricyclic agents, a pretreatment electrocardiogram (ECG) may be useful to determine if the patient has a preexisting cardiac conduction defect.

(3) Trazodone—pharmacologically affects the serotonergic neurotransmitter system. The sedative side effect can be useful when sleep disturbance is a problem. Conversely, orthostatic hypotension can pose a problem for the elderly. Arrhythmias are another side effect that must be given serious consideration.

(4) Bupropion—generally well tolerated; it is nonsedating and does not produce orthostasis; it should be given in three divided doses with the immediate-release formulation or two divided doses with the sustained-release formulation.

(5) MAOIs—useful in treating depression because MAO levels decrease in the aging brain and may account for diminished catecholamines and a resultant depression. MAOIs should be used with caution in elderly patients. Orthostatic hypotension is common and severe with MAOIs. Patients need to adhere to a tyramine-free diet to avoid hypertensive crises. The potential for serious drug interactions involving certain analgesics, such as meperidine (Demerol), and sympathomimetics also requires that patients understand what food and drugs they may use. Tranylcypromine (Parnate) and phenelzine (Nardil) should be used cautiously in patients prone to hypertension.

(6) **ECT**—may be the treatment of choice for depression in the elderly, particularly if cardiac factors limit or preclude the use of antidepressant medications or if refusal to eat presents an immediate, perhaps even life-threatening, problem. The risk of ECT is very low and is often less than that of pharmacotherapy. Any risks of treatment must be weighed against the risks of depression, including the patient's mental status and any suicidal risk.

B. **Bipolar disorders.**   The relapse rate of patients with mania and bipolar disorders increases with age. The mean length of morbid episodes is at least as long in aged patients as in younger adults. The great majority of cases of bipolar disorders begin before age 50; onset after age 65 is considered unusual. When a manic episode occurs for the first time after the age of 65, an overt pathophysiological (organic) cause should be strongly suspected. Possible causes include medication side effects.

The use of lithium in elderly patients is more hazardous than in young patients because age-related morbidity and physiologic changes are common. Lithium is excreted by the kidneys, and decreased renal clearance or renal disease can increase the risk for toxicity. Thiazide diuretics decrease the renal clearance of lithium; consequently, the concomitant use of these medications can necessitate adjustment in lithium dosage. Other medications may also interfere with lithium clearance. Lithium may cause CNS effects, to which the elderly are more sensitive. Because of these factors, more frequent serum monitoring of lithium concentrations is recommended in the elderly. Drugs used to treat elderly patients with bipolar disorders are listed in Table 22–1.

C. **Schizophrenia, paranoid states, and other late-life psychoses**

1. **Signs and symptoms.** Initial admissions to psychiatric hospitals for schizophrenia peak between 25 and 34 years of age and are relatively uncommon after age 65. Paranoid psychoses of diverse causes, however, are common in aged persons, including many elderly patients without any premorbid history of significant psychopathology. Sensory deficits appear to predispose to paranoid psychoses in some elderly patients. In others, cerebrovascular events and dementia are associated with the onset of paranoid symptoms. Medications or pathophysiologic causes should be carefully explored in all cases. Paranoid and delusional psychoses sometimes precede the onset of dementia of the Alzheimer's type. In other instances, these states may be associated with cerebrovascular factors that are not always evidenced by clinical or neuroimaging findings. Neurotransmitter changes associated with aging may also predispose the elderly to psychosis. More specifically, decrements in various

TABLE 22–1
GERIATRIC DOSAGES OF DRUGS COMMONLY USED TO TREAT BIPOLAR DISORDER

Generic Name	Trade Name	Geriatric Dosage Range (mg/d)
Lithium carbonate	Eskalith, Lithotabs, Lithonate, Lithobid	75–900
Carbamazepine	Tegretol	200–1,200
Valproate (valproic acid, divalproex)	Depakene, Depakote	250–1,000

neurotransmitter systems have been convincingly demonstrated in the elderly. For example, decrements in dopaminergic functioning are associated with age-related cell loss in the substantia nigra, with or without overt parkinsonian symptoms. Age-related changes in noradrenergic functioning are associated with physical evidence of cellular loss in the locus ceruleus. Similarly, age-related cholinergic neurotransmitter system changes are associated with decreased choline acetyltransferase enzyme activity. Collectively, these and other CNS neurochemical changes result in a resetting of the CNS neurotransmitter balance; these changes often predispose to psychosis in the elderly.

2. **Treatment.** The changes in neurotransmitter systems in the elderly appear to be important to both the causes and the treatment of psychosis. In general, psychosis in the elderly frequently responds to much lower doses of medication than psychosis in younger patients. The elderly also are more sensitive to many of the adverse effects of antipsychotic medications than younger adults are.

Specifically, the elderly are very sensitive to extrapyramidal side effects. Elderly patients have been known to stop speaking, ambulating, and swallowing after doses of medication that would be unlikely to produce significant problems in younger patients. Partly as a result of age-related autonomic changes, the elderly also are highly susceptible to the orthostatic side effects of antipsychotics. Falling may be associated with extrapyramidal side effects, orthostatic side effects, and sedating effects of antipsychotics. These side effects frequently act in conjunction with the side effects of other medications and with arthritis, peripheral vascular disease, arrhythmias, transient ischemic attacks, idiopathic parkinsonism, and other age-associated diseases to increase further the risk for falling. Hip fractures resulting from falls that are partly associated with the side effects of medication are a major cause of morbidity in the elderly and can be an immediate or more remote cause of death. Consequently, the potentially deleterious, and even life-threatening, side effects of antipsychotics in the elderly must be minimized.

Changes in cholinergic neurotransmitters predispose the elderly to anticholinergic side effects. It should be noted, however, that the antipsychotic with the highest anticholinergic potency, thioridazine (Mellaril), is roughly equivalent in anticholinergic potency to desipramine, the least anticholinergic antidepressant of the commonly used tricyclic antidepressants and their derivatives. Furthermore, dosages of antipsychotics prescribed in elderly patients are frequently much lower than those used in the treatment of younger adult patients. Consequently, in practice, anticholinergic side effects of antipsychotics in elderly patients are not as serious a concern as extrapyramidal, orthostatic, and sedating effects.

Clinical experience also indicates that the therapeutic effects of antipsychotic medications in the elderly may not become evident on a given dosage of medication for 4 weeks or longer. Because of these therapeutic factors and risks, the dictum in treating psychosis in the elderly is, "Start low and go slow." As in younger patients, side effect profiles should help determine the choice of medication; however, no consensus has been reached regarding the antipsychotic of choice for the elderly or even whether high-potency or low-potency typical antipsychotics or the atypical antipsychotics are more desirable. Among the low-potency typical antipsychotics, mesoridazine (Serentil) is frequently prescribed for the elderly, and a typical starting dosage is 10 mg/day; among the high-potency antipsychotics, haloperidol (Haldol) is frequently prescribed, and a typical starting dosage is 0.25 mg or 0.5 mg taken one to three times daily. In recent years, the atypical, newer antipsychotics have come to be preferred over traditional antipsychotics in treating the elderly. These include risperidone (Risperdal), with a typical starting dosage of 0.25 mg/day, and olanzapine (Zyprexa), with a typical starting dosage of 2.5 or 5 mg/day.

D. Age-associated memory impairment, mild cognitive impairment, Alzheimer's disease, and other dementing disorders. Changes in cognition are among the most frequent and most important (in terms of morbidity, mortality, and impact on family members and society in general) age-related medical conditions.

1. Cognitive changes in normal aging and in progressive Alzheimer's disease occur on a continuum. Barry Reisberg and associates describe seven major clinically distinguishable stages, from normality to most severe Alzheimer's disease, in the Global Deterioration Scale. These stages and their implications are summarized below.

Stage 1: Normal—no objective or subjective evidence of cognitive decrement. Current epidemiologic data indicate that only a minority of elderly persons fall within this category, perhaps 20–40% of persons over age 65.

Stage 2: Normal for age—subjective complaints of cognitive decrement.

Most persons over age 65 have subjective symptoms of not remembering people's names and the location of objects as well as they did in the previous 5 to 10 years.

Elderly persons commonly take preparations containing lecithin and choline, vitamins (including vitamin E) and multivitamins, and various herbal preparations or nostrums for these complaints.

Present prognostic data do not indicate that symptoms of age-associated memory impairment are the precursor of further decline in most elderly persons. Although medications and nostrums are frequently taken, convincing evidence of their efficacy is lacking.

Stage 3: Mild cognitive impairment—subtle evidence of objective decrement in cognition or executive functioning.

Subtle deficits may become evident in various ways. For example, the patient may become hopelessly lost when traveling to an unfamiliar location; decreased performance in a demanding occupation may be noted by coworkers; patients may display overt word- and name-finding deficits; concentration deficits may be evident on clinical testing; and an overt tendency to forget what has just been said and to repeat oneself may be manifest.

The prognosis associated with these subtle but identifiable symptoms varies. In some cases, the symptoms are the result of brain insults, such as small strokes, that may not be evident from the clinical history, neurological examination, or neuroimaging findings. In many cases, symptoms are secondary to subtle, and perhaps not clearly identifiable, psychiatric, medical, and neurological disorders of diverse causes. In many cases, the symptoms represent the earliest manifestations of Alzheimer's disease and may last as long as 7 years. The diagnosis of Alzheimer's disease at this stage, however, can be made with confidence only in retrospect. Accordingly, a separate diagnosis, *mild cognitive impairment,* is currently applied for persons in this stage.

Anxiety is a frequent psychiatric concomitant of the cognitive losses in subjects with mild cognitive impairment. Given the frequently benign prognosis, the inability to diagnose a degenerative dementing disorder with confidence at this stage, and the prolonged duration of these symptoms when they do represent the earliest signs of Alzheimer's disease, the most effective treatment for such anxiety is that the patient withdraw from anxiety-provoking activities. For example, withdrawal from a job that is beyond the patient's cognitive capacities can eliminate daily stress and humiliation. It can also eliminate, at least temporarily, the patient's problems because patients at this stage do not have difficulty with the routine tasks of daily living.

Because many patients with stage 3 symptoms of mild cognitive impairment do manifest overt Alzheimer's disease in subsequent years, the efficacy and utility of cholinesterase inhibitors such as donepezil are being investigated in this population.

Stage 4: Mild Alzheimer's disease—clearly manifested deficits on a careful clinical interview.

Deficits are apparent in concentration, memory, orientation, or functional capacity. The concentration deficit may be large enough that the patient not only displays a deficit on the standard subtraction of serial 7s task, but also has difficulty subtracting serial 4s from 40. Recent memory may suffer such that some major events of the previous week are not recalled. Detailed questioning may reveal that the spouse's knowledge of the patient's past is superior to the patient's own recall of his or her personal history. The patient may mistake the date by 10 days or more. The spouse (or other family members) may note that the patient no longer is able to balance a checkbook, no longer remembers to pay the rent or other bills properly, has difficulty preparing meals, or displays similar deficits in the ability to manage complex occupational and social tasks.

Alzheimer's disease can be diagnosed with confidence in this stage. It is possible to follow patients through the course of this stage, the mean duration of which has been estimated to be 2 years. Symptoms may plateau in this stage, and some patients may not manifest a further overt decline for 4 years or longer.

The most prominent psychiatric features of stage 4 are the patient's decreased interest in personal and social activities, accompanied by a flattening of affect. Depressive symptoms also may be noted but are generally mild enough that no specific treatment is indicated. Depressive symptoms sometimes are severe enough to warrant treatment, frequently with a low dosage of an antidepressant. Patients are still capable of living alone if assistance or guidance is provided with such complex activities as paying the rent and managing a bank account.

Cholinesterase inhibitors such as donepezil (Aricept) and rivastigmine (Exelon) have been found to be useful in relieving some of the cognitive deficits in this stage. Experience with donepezil indicates that it is well tolerated, although cholinergic side effects can occur. The therapeutic effects are modest.

Stage 5: Moderate Alzheimer's disease—deficits large enough to prevent patients from surviving independently in the community without assistance.

Patients at this stage often can no longer recall major relevant aspects of their lives (e.g., they may not recall the name of the President, their correct current address, or the names of the schools they attended). Patients at this stage frequently do not recall the current year and have enough difficulty in concentration and calculation that they err in subtracting serial 2s from 20. In addition to their inability to manage complex activities of daily living, patients generally have difficulty choosing the proper clothing to wear for the season and the occasion.

The duration of this stage is approximately a year and a half, although, as in the previous stage, the symptoms may plateau in some patients for many years.

Although generally more overt, the psychiatric symptoms at stage 5 are in many ways similar to those noted in stage 4. Consequently, the patient's denial and flattening of affect tend to be more evident. Depressive symptoms may occur. Anger and some of the more overt behavioral symptoms of Alzheimer's disease also are common. Depending on the nature and magnitude of the psychiatric symptoms, treatment with an antidepressant or an antipsychotic medication may be indicated. When the latter is used, the dictum previously stated for the treatment of psychosis in the elderly, "Start low and go slow," applies.

Patients who are living alone at this stage require at least part-time assistance for continued community survival. When additional community assistance is not feasible or available, institutionalization may be required. Patients who are residing with a spouse frequently resist additional assistance as an invasion of their home.

Cholinesterase inhibitors have been found to be useful in providing modest relief of cognitive symptoms in this stage.

Stage 6: Moderately severe Alzheimer's disease—deficits large enough to necessitate assistance with basic activities of daily living.

Patients at this stage may occasionally forget the name of the spouse on whom they depend for survival. They frequently do not know their address but can generally recall some important aspects of their domicile, such as the street or town. Patients have generally forgotten the schools they attended but recall some aspects of their early lives, such as their birthplace, former occupation, or one or both of their parents' names. Patients generally still can state their correct personal name. They may have difficulty counting backward from 10 by 1s.

During the course of stage 6, which lasts approximately $2\frac{1}{2}$ years, deficits in dressing and bathing increase progressively. In the latter part of this stage, toileting and continence become compromised.

Emotional and behavioral problems become most apparent and disturbing in this stage. Agitation, anger, sleep disturbances, physical violence, and negativity are examples of symptoms that commonly require treatment at this point in the illness. Low doses of antipsychotics may be useful. The atypical antipsychotics with a low extrapyramidal side effect profile are generally preferred. For example, risperidone in a dosage of 1.0 mg/day has been found to be useful, although clinicians may find that a quarter of a 1-mg tablet daily treats symptoms with minimal adverse effects, if any.

Patients require full-time assistance in community settings. If the patient lives with his or her spouse, the spouse will generally require at least part-time additional management assistance.

Cholinesterase inhibitors have not been shown to be useful in patients at this stage or in those with more severe dementia.

Stage 7: Severe Alzheimer's disease—deficits that necessitate continuous assistance with activities of daily living.

The capacity for speech is severely circumscribed early in this stage and is eventually lost. Ambulation and other motor capacities are also lost during the progression of this stage. Most patients survive until this stage. Studies indicate that patients commonly die at all points in this stage. The median point at which patients succumb is approximately the time ambulatory ability is lost. Although some patients survive in this stage for 7 years or longer, most die approximately 2 to 3 years after stage 7 begins. Pneumonia appears to be the most common immediate cause of death.

Although agitation is a problem for some patients, psychotropic medication can frequently be tapered gradually from the onset of this stage and eventually discontinued. Nursing homes may be better equipped than spouses to manage these patients. Many devoted spouses, however, prefer to continue to care for their partner, in which case round-the-clock home health care assistance may be a necessary adjunct as management of incontinence and other basic life activities, such as bathing and feeding, become major concerns. Psychiatrists should be prepared to counsel family members regarding such issues as institutionalization and the continued meaning of life.

2. **Vascular dementia**—the second major cause of dementia in the elderly. It occurs most frequently in conjunction with Alzheimer's disease. Classic pathological studies have indicated that approximately 50% of cases of dementia coming to autopsy are associated with Alzheimer's disease alone, 25% with Alzheimer's disease plus cerebrovascular factors, and 15% with vascular factors in the absence of neuropathological evidence of Alzheimer's disease.

Vascular dementia is believed to be the result of cerebral infarctions of varying size in multiple regions of the brain. Conditions associated with cerebral infarction (e.g., cardiac arrhythmias and hypertension) predispose to vascular dementia.

The course of vascular dementia was formerly believed to be more stepwise than the relatively gradual course of Alzheimer's disease. However, a stepwise course is rarely observed in the absence of strokes. The time course of decline in vascular dementia is at least as rapid as that in Alzheimer's disease. In mixed cases, the presence of cerebral infarction appears to increase morbidity. Consequently, the rate of progression of dementia and the time to death are relatively rapid in vascular dementia and mixed dementia in comparison with the rate of decline and time to death in Alzheimer's disease.

The clinical presentation of vascular dementia is more diverse than that of Alzheimer's disease. Speech disturbance or gait disturbance, for example, may occur at varying points in the evolution of vascular dementia, whereas in Alzheimer's disease, these deficits tend to occur at a specific point in the evolution of the dementia process.

The psychiatric disturbances occurring in vascular dementia include general dementia-related psychiatric conditions, such as the affective and psychotic disturbances and agitation described at each stage of Alzheimer's disease. The emotional changes characteristic of stroke-related dementia also occur (e.g., emotional incontinence and other sudden, labile mood changes). Emotional incontinence generally is not treated with medication. The guidelines for the treatment of dementia-related psychiatric disturbances, previously outlined for Alzheimer's disease, also apply in the treatment of affective, psychiatric, and other behavioral disturbances in vascular dementia.

Management of the underlying cause of vascular dementia includes steps to prevent strokes, such as the treatment of hypertension and cardiac arrhythmias and the use of platelet-deaggregating agents. Among the latter, salicylates (e.g., aspirin) are perhaps the most effective.

3. **Other dementing disorders and differential diagnosis of dementia**—other causes of dementia include Lewy body dementia; frontotemporal dementias, of which a prominent example is Pick's disease; Creutzfeldt-Jakob disease; Huntington's disease; alcohol abuse; normal-pressure hydrocephalus; and dementias due to diverse physiological disturbances.

   a. **Lewy body dementia**—Lewy bodies occur in approximately 15–25% of all cases of dementing disorder. In the great majority of dementia patients with Lewy bodies, coexisting Alzheimer's or cerebrovascular disease is found. In cases with mixed Alzheimer's or vascular dementia and Lewy body pathology, the clinical picture is not distinctively altered by the presence of a Lewy body condition. However, Lewy bodies occur in the absence of concomitant dementia pathology in approximately 4% of all cases of dementia. The terminology *Lewy body dementia* should probably be applied only to these pure Lewy body cases, for which a distinctive clinical picture has been described. This is marked by prominent parkinsonian features, a relatively fluctuating clinical course, vivid and well-focused visual hallucinations, and relatively rapid progression of dementia. Patients with Lewy body dementia may be very sensitive to neuroleptic medications, and the frequent development of "sensitivity reactions," marked by parkinsonism, cognitive decline, drowsiness, and features of the neuroleptic malignant syndrome with increased mortality, has been noted. Accordingly, neuroleptic medications should be used with great caution in patients with Lewy body dementia. Many clinicians avoid neuroleptics with any potential parkinsonian side effects. Consequently, the antipsychotics that are sometimes utilized to treat uncontrollable agitation in Lewy body dementia include quetiapine (Seroquel) and other agents that cause either minimal or no extrapyramidal side effects. Another distinct aspect of the psychopharmacological treatment of Lewy body dementia is a favorable and more marked therapeutic response to cholinesterase inhibitor treatment with donepezil or similar medications, which appear to ameliorate both cognitive and behavioral symptomatology.

b. **Frontotemporal dementias**—a diverse group of dementing disorders marked by disproportionate degeneration in the frontal and temporal regions of the brain, generally demonstrable on neuroimaging. Many of these conditions, of which a prominent example is Pick's disease, are characterized pathologically by the presence of an abnormally phosphorylated tau within neurons, as neurofibrillary structures. However, unlike Alzheimer's disease, in which abnormally phosphorylated tau is also present, the frontotemporal dementias are not marked by the abnormal deposition and accumulation of amyloid β-protein in senile plaques.

   In general, the frontotemporal dementias occur at a younger age than Alzheimer's disease or vascular dementia. Disorders of insight and judgment indicative of frontal lobe-type disturbance are particularly marked clinical features. No treatments are available for these disorders at present.

c. **Creutzfeldt-Jakob disease**—a rare condition, occurring in approximately one person per million under ordinary circumstances. This condition is now believed to be caused by a change in the conformation of a normal brain protein into a pathological form, known as a *prion*. It can be contracted by eating meat from infected animals or by coming in contact with infected tissues. The onset and course are variable and acute, but subacute and chronic forms have been described. Frequently, Creutzfeldt-Jakob disease is distinguished from Alzheimer's disease by its course, which may be more rapid, or by the occurrence of focal and localized neural disease. The latter is manifested by cranial nerve signs, such as auditory deficits associated with eighth nerve involvement, and gait disturbance, associated with cerebellar involvement. Occasionally, Creutzfeldt-Jakob disease closely mimics the course of Alzheimer's disease.

d. **Huntington's disease**—may present with a dementia disturbance before the appearance of choreiform disease and should be considered in the differential diagnosis of dementia.

e. **Alcohol-induced persisting dementia or amnestic disorder**—frequently distinguished from Alzheimer's disease by the presence of confabulation and by a memory deficit out of proportion to cognitive and functional disturbances in other areas.

f. **Normal-pressure hydrocephalus**—marked by gait disturbance, urinary incontinence, and dilated cerebral ventricles out of proportion to the magnitude of cortical atrophy and dementia. Urinary incontinence, neuroradiological findings, and the relatively early appearance of gait disturbance assist in distinguishing this condition from Alzheimer's disease.

g. **Dementias due to diverse physiological disturbances**—the diagnosis of dementia, which may be a consequence of more than 50 possible primary conditions, and the differentiation of these conditions from the major cause of dementia, Alzheimer's disease, is based on laboratory investigations and knowledge of the clinical course of Alzheimer's disease. The basic laboratory workup for dementia includes a complete blood cell count and differential, serum electrolyte and serum enzyme studies, serum B_{12} and serum folate levels, thyroid levels, a urinalysis, and a cerebral neuroimaging study. Positive findings on any of these studies must be interpreted by the clinician. They may indicate a primary cause of dementia, which may be treatable; they may indicate added insult in the context of degenerative dementia; or they may be incidental. Knowledge of the clinical course of Alzheimer's disease can help the clinician to distinguish between these possibilities. Premature deficits should alert the clinician to possible increased morbidity or a possibly remediable underlying process.

V. Psychotherapy in the elderly

Fundamental psychological processes in the elderly do not differ from those of younger adults. However, the aging process and associated pathological changes do result in psychological issues that are relatively particular to this age group. Common issues in therapy include evolving and changing relationships of the elderly with their adult children. For example, in the presence of disease, the elderly may have both a desire for independence and, in the present social context, unrealistic expectations with regard to their adult children. Adult chil-

TABLE 22–2
FUNCTIONAL STAGES IN NORMAL HUMAN DEVELOPMENT AND ALZHEIMER'S DISEASE

Approximate Age	Acquired Abilities	Lost Abilities		Alzheimer's Stage
12+ years	Hold a job	Hold a job	3	INCIPIENT
8–12 years	Handle simple finances	Handle simple finances	4	MILD
5–7 years	Select proper clothing	Select proper clothing	5	MODERATE
5 years	Put on clothes unaided	Put on clothes unaided	6a	MODERATELY SEVERE
4 years	Shower unaided	Shower unaided	b	
4 years	Toilet unaided	Toilet unaided	c	
3–4½ years	Control urine	Control urine	d	
2–3 years	Control bowels	Control bowels	e	
15 months	Speak five or six words	Speak five or six words	7a	SEVERE
1 year	Speak one word	Speak one word	b	
1 year	Walk	Walk	c	
6–10 months	Sit up	Sit up	d	
2–4 months	Smile	Smile	e	
1–3 months	Hold up head	Hold up head	f	

From Reisberg B: Dementia: a systematic approach to identifying reversible causes. *Geriatrics* 1986;41(4):30–46; Reisberg B: Functional assessment staging (FAST). *Psychopharmacol Bull* 1988;24:653–659; and Reisberg B, Franssen EH, Souren LEM, Auer S, Kenowsky S: Progression of Alzheimer's disease: variability and consistency; ontogenic models, their applicability and relevance. *J Neural Transm Suppl* 1998;54:9–20, with permission.

TABLE 22–3
MANAGEMENT NEEDS IN NORMAL DEVELOPMENT AND OF THE ALZHEIMER'S PATIENT AT THE CORRESPONDING DEVELOPMENTAL AGE

Global Deterioration and Functional Stage of Aging and Alzheimer's Disease	Development Age	Management Needs of Aged and Alzheimer's Patients
1	Adult	None.
2	Adult	None.
3	12+ years	None.
4	8–12 years	Independent survival still attainable.
5	5–7 years	Patient can no longer survive in the community without part-time assistance.
6	2–5 years	Patient requires full-time supervision.
7	0–2 years	Patient requires continuous care.

Adapted from Reisberg B, Franssen EH, Souren LEM, Auer S, Kenowsky S: Progession of Alzheimer's disease: variability and consistency; ontogenic models, their applicability and relevance. *J Neural Transm Suppl* 1998;54:9–20, with permission.

dren, in turn, may harbor resentments toward their parents continued from childhood, or, conversely, they may experience unrealistic feelings of guilt in regard to what they should be doing for their parents in the event of illness or other traumatic events.

Family therapy, consequently, can be of particular value in the elderly, sometimes in conjunction with group or individual psychotherapy. Other goals of individual therapy particular to the elderly include the maintenance of self-esteem despite physical, marital, and social change; the meaningful use of unaccustomed leisure time; and clarification of options in the context of more or less overwhelming physical and social change. In general, psychotherapy in the elderly is relatively situation- and problem-oriented and seeks solutions within the established personality framework, rather than overwhelming personality change. Many elderly persons, however, respond remarkably well to seemingly overwhelming changes and personal tragedies (e.g., loss of health, loss of a spouse) and display hitherto unseen social strengths and adaptive capacities.

Dementia poses special psychotherapeutic challenges. In a phenomenon termed *retrogenesis,* which occurs in Alzheimer's dementia and to a variable extent in other dementing conditions, the patient's cognitive, functional, and physiologic changes reverse the patterns of normal human development. This is illustrated for the functional changes in Alzheimer's disease in Table 22–2. Consequently, each functional stage of Alzheimer's disease can be formulated as a corresponding developmental age of childhood. The developmental age of the Alzheimer's patient provides a rapid appreciation of his or her overall management and care needs (Table 22–3). Thus, a stage 7 patient with severe Alzheimer's disease requires approximately the same amount of care as an infant. Similarly, one can leave a stage 4 patient with mild Alzheimer's disease alone to a large extent, just as an 8- to 12-year-old child may require only limited supervision. The developmental age of the Alzheimer's patient is also useful in understanding his or her emotional needs, behavioral disturbances, and physical needs. As noted, these principles are also to some extent applicable to dementing disorders other than Alzheimer's disease.

For more detailed discussion of this topic, see Geriatric Psychiatry, Ch 51, p 2980, in CTP/VII.

23

End-of-Life Care, Death, Dying, and Bereavement

I. End-of-life care

End-of-life care involves complex issues such as euthanasia, physician-assisted suicide, and palliative care.

A. Euthanasia. Defined as a physician's deliberate act to cause a patient's death by directly administering a lethal dose of medication or other agent (sometimes called *mercy killing*).

B. Physician-assisted suicide. Defined as a physician's imparting information or providing means that enable a person to take his or her own life deliberately.

C. Ethical issues. Euthanasia and physician-assisted suicide are opposed by the American Medical Association and the American Psychiatric Association. In Oregon, physicians are legally permitted to prescribe lethal medication for patients who are terminally ill (1994 Oregon Death with Dignity Law [Table 23–1]).

D. Palliative care. Defined as treatment geared to alleviate the pain and suffering of patients who are dying. Such care provides pain relief and emotional, social, and spiritual support, including psychiatric treatment if indicated.

Palliative care differs from euthanasia and physician-assisted suicide in important ways: (1) The intent of palliative care is to treat the patient, not to cause death, as in euthanasia. (2) If patients are prescribed medicine, it is intended to reduce pain and suffering, not to enable them to commit suicide. (3) Palliative care always includes a psychiatric examination for patients who are thinking about suicide. (4) Patients may die as a result of palliative treatment to relieve suffering, but death associated with palliative care is not intentional and is not the goal of treatment.

E. End-of-life decisions. The principle of patient autonomy requires that physicians respect the decision of a patient to forego life-sustaining treatment. Life-sustaining treatment is defined as any medical treatment that serves to prolong life without reversing the underlying medical condition. It includes, but is not limited to, mechanical ventilation, renal dialysis, blood transfusions, chemotherapy, antibiotics, and artificial nutrition and hydration. Patients *in extremis* should never be forced to endure intolerable, prolonged suffering in an effort to prolong life.

II. Grief, mourning, and bereavement

Generally synonymous terms that describe a syndrome precipitated by the loss of a loved one. Attempts have been made to characterize the stages of grief,

TABLE 23–1
OREGON'S ASSISTED SUICIDE LAW

- Oregon residents whose physicians determine they have less than 6 months to live are eligible to ask for suicide medication.
- A second doctor must determine if the patient is mentally competent to make the decision and is not suffering from mental illness such as depression.
- The law does not compel doctors to comply with patients' requests for suicide medication.
- Doctors who agree to provide medication must receive a request in writing from the patient, signed by two witnesses. The written request must be made 48 hours before the doctor delivers the prescription. A second oral request is made just before the doctor writes the prescription.
- Pharmacists who are opposed to suicide may refuse to fill the prescriptions.
- The law does not specify which medication may be used. Supporters of the law say an overdose of barbiturates combined with antinausea medication would probably be used.

which are listed in Table 23–2. Characteristics of bereavement in parents and children are listed in Table 23–3.

Grief can occur for reasons other than the death of a loved one: (1) loss of a loved one through separation, divorce, or incarceration; (2) loss of an emotionally charged object or circumstance (e.g., a prized possession or valued job or position); (3) loss of a fantasized love object (e.g., death of an intrauterine fetus, birth of a malformed infant); and (4) loss resulting from narcissistic injury (e.g., amputation, mastectomy).

Grief differs from depression in a number of ways, which are described in Table 23–4. Risk factors for a major depressive episode after the death of a

TABLE 23–2
GRIEF AND BEREAVEMENT

Stage	John Bowlby	Stage	C.M. Parkes
1	**Numbness or protest.** Characterized by distress, fear, and anger. Shock may last moments, days, or months.	1	**Alarm.** A stressful state characterized by physiological changes (e.g., rise in blood pressure and heart rate); similar to Bowlby's first stage.
2	**Yearning and searching for the lost figure.** World seems empty and meaningless, but self-esteem remains intact. Characterized by preoccupation with lost person, physical restlessness, weeping, and anger. May last several months or even years.	2	**Numbness.** Person appears superficially affected by loss but is actually protecting himself or herself from acute distress.
3	**Disorganization and despair.** Restlessness and aimlessness. Increase in somatic preoccupation, withdrawal, introversion, and irritability. Repeated reliving of memories.	3	**Pining (searching).** Person looks for or is reminded of the lost person. Similar to Bowlby's second stage.
		4	**Depression.** Person feels hopeless about future, cannot go on living, and withdraws from family and friends.
4	**Reorganization.** With establishment of new patterns, objects, and goods, grief recedes and is replace by cherished memories. Healthy identification with deceased occurs.	5	**Recovery and reorganization.** Person realizes that his or her life will continue with new adjustments and different goods.

TABLE 23–3
BEREAVEMENT IN PATIENTS AND CHILDREN

Loss of a Parent	Loss of a Child
Protest phase. Child has strong desire for the deceased parent.	May be a more intense experience than the death of an adult.
Despair phase. Child experiences hopelessness, withdrawal, and apathy.	Feelings of guilt and helplessness may be overwhelming.
Detachment phase. Child relinquishes emotional attachment to dead parent.	Stages of shock, denial, anger, bargaining, and acceptance occur.
Child may transfer need for a parent to one or more adults.	Manifestations of grief may last a lifetime.
	Up to 50% of marriages in which a child dies end in divorce.

spouse are listed in Table 23–5. Complications of bereavement are listed in Table 23–6.

III. Dos and don'ts of grief management and therapy

A. *Do* encourage the ventilation of feelings. Allow the patient to talk about loved ones. Reminiscing about positive experiences can be helpful.

B. *Don't* tell a bereaved person not to cry or get angry.

C. *Do* try to have a small group of people who knew the deceased talk about him or her in the presence of the grieving person.

D. *Don't* prescribe antianxiety or antidepressant medication on a regular basis. If the person becomes acutely agitated, it is better to offer verbal comfort than a pill. However, small doses of medications (5 mg of diazepam [Valium]) may help in the short-term.

E. *Do* note that frequent short visits are better than a few long visits.

F. *Do* be aware of delayed grief reaction, which occurs some time after a death and may be marked by behavioral changes, agitation, lability of mood, and substance abuse. Such reactions may occur close to the anniversary of a death (*anniversary reaction*).

TABLE 23–4
GRIEF VERSUS DEPRESSION

Grief	Depression
Normal identification with deceased. Little ambivalence toward deceased.	Abnormal overidentification with deceased. Increased ambivalence and unconscious anger toward deceased.
Crying, weight loss, decreased libido, withdrawal, insomnia, irritability, decreased concentration and attention.	Similar.
Suicidal ideas rare.	Suicidal ideas common.
Self-blame relates to how deceased was treated. No global feelings of worthlessness.	Self-blame is global. Person thinks he or she is generally bad or worthless.
Evokes empathy and sympathy.	Usually evokes interpersonal annoyance or irritation.
Symptoms abate with time. Self-limited. Usually clears within 6 months to 1 year.	Symptoms do not abate and may worsen. May still be present after years.
Vulnerable to physical illness.	Vulnerable to physical illness.
Responds to reassurance and social contacts.	Does not respond to reassurance and pushes away social contacts.
Not helped by antidepressant medication.	Helped by antidepressant medication.

TABLE 23–5
RISK FACTORS FOR MAJOR DEPRESSIVE EPISODE AFTER DEATH OF A SPOUSE

History of depression; major depressive disorder, dysthymic disorder, depressive personality disorder, bipolar disorder
Under 30 years of age
Poor general health
Limited social support system
Unemployment
Poor adaptation to the loss

G. *Do* note that an anticipatory grief reaction occurs in advance of loss and can mitigate acute grief reaction at the actual time of loss. This can be a useful process if it is recognized when occurring.

H. *Do* be aware that the person grieving for a family member who died by suicide may not want to talk about his or her feelings of being stigmatized.

IV. Death and dying

The reactions of patients to being told by a physician that they have a terminal illness vary. The reactions are described as a series of stages by thanatologist Elisabeth Kübler-Ross (Table 23–7).

Be aware that stages do not always occur in sequence. Shifts from one stage to another may occur. Moreover, children under 5 years of age do not appreciate death; they see it as a separation, similar to sleep. Between 5 and 10 years of age, they become increasing aware of death as something that happens to others, particularly parents. After 10 years of age, children conceptualize death as something that can happen to them.

V. Dos and don'ts with the dying patient

A. *Don't* have a rigid attitude (e.g., "I always tell the patient"); let the patient be your guide. Many patients will want to know the diagnosis, whereas others will not. Determine what the patient already knows and understands about the prognosis. Do not stifle hope or break through a patient's denial if that is the major defense, so long as the patient can obtain and accept necessary help. If the patient refuses to obtain help as a result of denial, gently and gradually help the patient to understand that help is necessary and available. Reassure the patient that he or she will be taken care of regardless of behavior.

TABLE 23–6
COMPLICATIONS OF BEREAVEMENT

Disturbance in the process of grief
  Absent or delayed grief
  Exaggerated grief
  Prolonged grief
Increased vulnerability to adverse affects
  General medical morbidity
  Mortality
  Psychiatric disorders
    Anxiety disorders
    Substance use disorders
    Depressive disorders

Adapted from and courtesy of Sidney Zisook, M.D.

TABLE 23–7
DEATH AND DYING (REACTIONS OF DYING PATIENTS)

	Elisabeth Kübler-Ross
Stage 1	**Shock and denial.** Patient's initial reaction is shock, followed by denial that anything is wrong. Some patients never pass beyond this state and may go doctor shopping until they find one who supports their position.
Stage 2	**Anger.** Patients became frustrated, irritable, and angry that they are ill; they ask, "Why me?" Patients in this stage are difficult to manage because their anger is displaced onto doctors, hospital staff, and family. Sometimes anger is directed at themselves in the belief that illness has occurred as punishment for wrongdoing.
Stage 3	**Bargaining.** Patient may attempt to negotiate with physicians, friends, or even God, that in return for a cure, he or she will fulfill one or many promises (e.g., give to charity, attend church regularly).
Stage 4	**Depression.** Patient shows clinical signs of depression; withdrawal, psychomotor retardation, sleep disturbances, hopelessness, and possibly suicidal ideation. The depression may be a reaction to the effects of illness on his or her life (e.g., loss of job, economic hardship, isolation from friends and family), or it may be in anticipation of the actual loss of life that will occur shortly.
Stage 5	**Acceptance.** Person realizes that death is inevitable and accepts its universality.

B. *Do* stay with the patient for a period of time after informing him or her of the condition or diagnosis. A period of shock may ensue. Encourage the patient to ask questions and provide truthful answers. Indicate that you will return to answer any questions that the patient or family may have.

C. *Do* make a return visit after a few hours, if possible, to check on the patient's reaction. If the patient exhibits anxiety, 5 mg of diazepam can be prescribed as needed for 24 to 48 hours.

D. *Do* advise family members of the medical facts. Encourage them to visit and allow the patient to talk of his or her fears. Family members not only have to deal with the loss of a loved one but also must face their own personal mortality, which causes anxiety.

E. *Do* always check for the presence of living will or do not resuscitate (DNR) wishes of the patient or family. Try to anticipate their wishes regarding life-sustaining procedures.

F. *Do* alleviate pain and suffering. There is no reason for withholding narcotics for fear of dependence in a dying patient. Pain management should be vigorous.

For more detailed discussion of this topic, see Zisook S, Downs NS: Death, Dying, and Bereavement, Section 28.5, p 1963, in CTP/VII.

24

Psychotherapy

I. General introduction

The primary aim of psychiatric treatments is to alter pathological behavior. Although the dynamics of human behavior are not completely understood, it is clear that all behaviors, whether normal or pathological, are the result of highly complex interactions involving biological, psychological, and environmental factors. Thus, the physiology of a person's brain, the person's developmental history, store of cognitive information, interpersonal relations, sensory input, and affective experience, and the characteristics of the environment with which the person interacts are all among the variables that determine his or her ultimate personality and behavior.

II. Psychoanalysis and psychoanalytic psychotherapy

These two forms of treatment are based on Sigmund Freud's theories of a dynamic unconscious and psychological conflict. The major goal of these forms of therapy is to help the patient develop insight into unconscious conflicts, based on unresolved childhood wishes and manifested as symptoms, and develop more adult patterns of interacting and behaving.

A. Psychoanalysis. The most intensive and rigorous of this type of therapy. The patient is seen three to five times a week, generally for a minimum of several hundred hours over a number of years. The patient lies on a couch with the analyst seated behind, out of the patient's visual range. The patient attempts to say freely and without censure whatever comes to mind, to associate freely, so as to follow as deeply as possible the train of thoughts to their earliest roots. The patient also associates to dream material and to transference feelings that are evoked in the process. The analyst uses interpretation and clarification to help the patient work through and resolve conflicts that have been affecting the patient's life, often unconsciously. Psychoanalysis requires that the patient be stable, highly motivated, verbal, and psychologically minded. The patient also must be able to tolerate the stress generated by analysis without becoming overly regressed, distraught, or impulsive.

B. Psychoanalytically oriented psychotherapy. Based on the same principles and techniques as classic psychoanalysis, but less intense. The two types are insight-oriented or expressive psychotherapy and supportive or relationship psychotherapy. Patients are seen one to two times a week and sit up facing the psychiatrist. The goal of resolution of unconscious psychological conflict is similar to that of psychoanalysis, but a greater emphasis is placed on day-to-day reality issues and a lesser emphasis on the development of transference issues. Patients suitable for psychoanalysis are suitable for this therapy, as are patients with a wider range of symptomatic and characterologic problems. Patients with personality disorders are also suitable for this therapy. A comparison of psychoanalysis and psychoanalytically oriented psychotherapy is presented in Table 24–1.

TABLE 24–1
SCOPE OF PSYCHOANALYTIC PRACTICE: A CLINICAL CONTINUUM[a]

Feature	Psychoanalysis	Psychoanalytic Psychotherapy	
		Expressive Mode	Supportive Mode
Frequency	Regular, four to five times a week, 30–50 minute session.	Regular, one to three times a week, half to full hour.	Flexible, once a week or less or as needed, half to full hour.
Duration	Long-term, usually 3 to 5+ years.	Short-term or long-term, several sessions to months of years.	Short-term or intermittent long-term; single session to lifetime.
Setting	Patient primarily on couch with analyst out of view.	Patient and therapist face to face; occasional use of couch.	Patient and therapist face to face; couch contraindicated.
Modus operandi	Systematic analysis of all (positive and negative) transference and resistance; primary focus on analyst and intrasession events; transference neurosis facilitated; regression encouraged.	Partial analysis of dynamics and defenses; focus on current interpersonal events and transference to others outside sessions; analysis of negative transference; positive transference left unexplored unless it impedes progress; limited regression encouraged.	Formation of therapeutic alliance and real object relationship; analysis of transference contraindicated with rare exceptions; focus on conscious external events; regression discouraged.
Analyst–therapist role	Absolute neutrality; frustration of patient; reflector-minor role.	Modified neutrality; implicit gratification of patient and great activity.	Neutrality suspended; limited explicit gratification, direction, and disclosure.
Putative change agents	Insight predominates within relatively deprived environment.	Insight within empathic environment; identification with benevolent object.	Auxiliary or surrogate ego as temporary substitute; holding environment; insight to degree possible.
Patient population	Neuroses; mild character psychopathology.	Neuroses; mild to moderate character psychopathology, especially narcissistic and borderline personality disorders.	Severe character disorders; latent or manifest psychoses; acute crises; physical illness.
Patient requisites	High motivation; psychological-mindedness; good previous object relationships; ability to maintain transference neurosis; good frustration tolerance.	High to moderate motivation and psychological-mindedness; ability to form therapeutic alliance; some frustration tolerance.	Some degree of motivation and ability to form therapeutic alliance.

TABLE 24-1—*continued*

| Feature | Psychoanalysis | Psychoanalytic Psychotherapy | |
		Expressive Mode	Supportive Mode
Basic goals	Structural reorganization of personality; resolution of unconscious conflicts; insight into intrapsychic events; symptom relief an indirect result.	Partial reorganization of personality and defenses; resolution of preconscious and conscious derivatives of conflicts; insight into current interpersonal events; improved object relations; symptom relief a goal or prelude to further exploration.	Reintegration of self and ability to cope; stabilization or restoration of preexisting equilibrium; strengthening of defenses; better adjustment or acceptance of pathology; symptom relief and environmental restructuring as primary goals.
Major techniques	Free association method predominates; fully dynamic interpretation (including confrontation, clarification, and working through), with emphasis on genetic reconstruction.	Limited free association; confrontation, clarification, and partial interpretation predominate, with emphasis on here-and-now interpretation and limited genetic interpretation.	Free association method contraindicated; suggestion (advice) predominates; abreaction useful; confrontation, clarification, and interpretation in the here and now secondary; genetic interpretation contraindicated.
Adjunct treatment	Primarily avoided; if applied, all negative and positive meanings and implications thoroughly analyzed.	May be necessary (e.g., psychotropic drugs as temporary measure); if applied, negative implications explored and diffused.	Often necessary (e.g., psychotrophic drugs, family therapy, rehabilitative therapy, or hospitalization); if applied, positive implications are emphasized.

^aThis division is not categoric; all practice resides on a clinical continuum.
Table by Toksoz Byram Karasu, M.D.

In supportive psychotherapy, the essential element is support rather than the development of insight. This type of therapy often is the treatment of choice for patients with serious ego vulnerabilities, particularly psychotic patients. Patients in a crisis situation, such as acute grief, also are suitable. This therapy can be continued on a long-term basis and last many years, especially in the case of patients with chronic problems. Support can take the form of limit setting, increasing reality testing, reassurance, advice, and help with developing social skills.

C. **Brief dynamic psychotherapy.**   A short-term treatment, generally consisting of 10 to 40 sessions during a period of less than 1 year. The goal, based on psychodynamic theory, is to develop insight into underlying conflicts; such insight leads to psychological and behavioral changes.

This therapy is more confrontational than the other insight-oriented therapies in that the therapist is very active in repeatedly directing the patient's associations and thoughts to conflictual areas. The number of hours is explicitly agreed on by the therapist and patient before to the beginning of therapy, and a specific, circumscribed area of conflict is chosen to be the focus of treatment. More extensive change is not attempted. Patients suitable for this therapy must be able to define a specific central problem to be addressed and must be highly motivated, psychologically minded, and able to tolerate the temporary increase in anxiety or sadness that this type of therapy can evoke. Patients who are not suitable include those with fragile ego structures (e.g., suicidal or psychotic patients) and those with poor impulse control (e.g., borderline patients, substance abusers, and antisocial personalities).

III. Behavior therapy

The basic assumption of this therapy is that maladaptive behavior can be changed without insight into its underlying causes. Behavioral symptoms are taken at face value and not as symptoms of a deeper problem. Behavior therapy is based on the principles of learning theory, including operant and classical conditioning. Operant conditioning is based on the premise that behavior is shaped by its consequences; if behavior is positively reinforced, it will increase; if it is punished, it will decrease; and if it elicits no response, it will be extinguished. Classical conditioning is based on the premise that behavior is shaped by being coupled with or uncoupled from anxiety-provoking stimuli. Just as Ivan Pavlov's dogs were conditioned to salivate at the sound of a bell once the bell had become associated with meat, a person can be conditioned to feel fear in neutral situations that have come to be associated with anxiety. Uncouple the anxiety from the situation, and the avoidant and anxious behavior will decrease.

Behavior therapy is believed to be most effective for clearly delineated, circumscribed maladaptive behaviors (e.g., phobias, compulsions, overeating, cigarette smoking, stuttering, and sexual dysfunctions). In the treatment of conditions that can be strongly affected by psychological factors (e.g., hypertension, asthma, pain, and insomnia), behavioral techniques can be used to induce relaxation and decrease aggravating stresses (Table 24–2).

A. Token economy.   A form of **positive reinforcement** used with inpatients. A patient is rewarded with various tokens (e.g., food, passes) for performing desired behaviors (e.g., dressing in street clothes, attending group therapy). Has been used to treat schizophrenia, especially in inpatient settings.

B. Aversion therapy.   A form of conditioning in which an aversive stimulus (e.g., a shock or unpleasant smell) is paired with an undesired behavior. In a less controversial form of aversion therapy, the patient couples imagining something unpleasant with the undesired behavior. Has been used to treat substance abuse.

C. Systematic desensitization.   A technique in which a patient engaging in avoidant behavior linked to a specific stimulus (e.g., heights or airplane travel) is asked to construct a hierarchy of anxiety-provoking

TABLE 24–2
SOME COMMON CLINICAL APPLICATIONS OF BEHAVIOR THERAPY

Disorder	Comments
Agoraphobia	Graded exposure and flooding can reduce the fear of being in crowded places. About 60% of patients so treated are improved. In some cases, the spouse can serve as the model while accompanying the patient into the fear situation; however, the patient cannot get a secondary gain by keeping the spouse nearby and displaying symptoms.
Alcohol dependence	Aversion therapy, in which the alcohol-dependent patient is made to vomit (by adding an emetic to the alcohol) every time a drink is ingested, is effective in treating alcohol dependence. Disulfiram (Antabuse) can be given to alcohol-dependent patients when they are alcohol-free. Such patients are warned of the severe physiological consequences of drinking (e.g., nausea, vomiting, hypotension, collapse) with disulfiram in the system.
Anorexia nervosa	Observe eating behavior; contingency management; record weight.
Bulimia nervosa	Record bulimic episodes; log moods.
Hyperventilation	Hyperventilation test; controlled breathing; direct observation.
Other phobias	Systematic desensitization has been effective in treating phobias, such as fears of heights, animals, and flying. Social skills training has also been used for shyness and fear of other people.
Paraphilias	Electric shocks or other noxious stimuli can be applied at the time of a paraphilic impulse, and eventually the impulse subsides. Shocks can be administered by either the therapist or the patient. The results are satisfactory but must be reinforced at regular intervals.
Schizophrenia	The token economy procedure, in which tokens are awarded for desirable behavior and can be used to buy ward privileges, has been useful in treating schizophrenic inpatients. Social skills training teaches schizophrenic patients how to interact with others in a socially acceptable way so that negative feedback is eliminated. In addition, the aggressive behavior of some schizophrenic patients can be diminished through those methods.
Sexual dysfunctions	Sex therapy, developed by William Masters and Virginia Johnson, is a behavior therapy technique used for various sexual dysfunctions, especially male erectile disorder, orgasm disorders, and premature ejaculation. It uses relaxation, desensitization, and graded exposure as the primary techniques.
Shy bladder	Inability to void in a public bathroom; relaxation exercises.
Type A behavior	Physiological assessment muscle relaxation, biofeedback (on electromyogram).

images, from least to most fearful, and to remain at each level of the imaginary hierarchy until the anxiety diminishes. When this procedure is performed in real life rather in the imagination, it is called *graded exposure*. The efficacy of the technique is based on positive reinforcement for confronting anxiety-provoking stimuli; in addition, maladaptive behavior is extinguished by the realization of an absence of negative consequences. Hierarchy construction often is associated with relaxation techniques because it is felt that anxiety and relaxation are incompatible, so that the imagined images become uncoupled from anxiety (reciprocal inhibition).

D. Flooding.   A technique in which the patient is exposed immediately to the most anxiety-provoking stimulus (e.g., the top of a tall building if he or she is afraid of heights) instead of being exposed gradually or systematically to a hierarchy of feared situations. If this technique is carried out in the imagination rather than in real life, it is called *implosion*. Flooding is thought to be an effective behavioral treatment of such disorders as phobias, provided the patient can tolerate the associated anxiety.

IV. Cognitive-behavioral therapy

This therapy is based on the theory that behavior is determined by the way in which persons think about themselves and their roles in the world. Maladaptive behavior is secondary to ingrained, stereotyped thoughts, which can lead to cognitive distortions or errors in thinking. The theory is aimed at correcting cognitive distortions and the self-defeating behaviors that result from them. Therapy is on a short-term basis, generally lasting for 15 to 20 sessions during a period of 12 weeks. Patients are made aware of their own distorted cognitions and the assumptions on which they are based. Homework is assigned; patients are asked to record what they are thinking in certain stressful situations (e.g., "I'm no good" or "No one cares about me") and to ascertain the underlying, often relatively unconscious, assumptions that fuel the negative cognitions. This process has been referred to as "recognizing and correcting automatic thoughts." The cognitive model of depression includes the cognitive triad, which is a description of the thought distortions that occur when a person is depressed. The triad includes (1) a negative view of the self, (2) a negative interpretation of present and past experience, and (3) a negative expectation of the future (Table 24–3).

Cognitive therapy has been most successfully applied to the treatment of mild to moderate, nonpsychotic depressions. It also has been effective as an adjunctive treatment in substance abuse and in increasing compliance with medication. It has been used recently to treat schizophrenia.

V. Family therapy

Family therapy is based on the theory that a family is a system that attempts to maintain homeostasis, regardless of how maladaptive the system may be. This theory has been referred to as a "family systems orientation," and the techniques include focusing on the family rather than on the identified patient. The family therefore becomes the patient, rather than the individual family member who has been identified as sick. One of the major goals of a family therapist is to determine what homeostatic role, however pathological, the identified patient is serving in the particular family system. One example is the triangulated child—the child who is identified by the family as the patient is actually serving to maintain the family system by becoming involved in a marital conflict as a scapegoat, referee, or even surrogate spouse. The therapist's

TABLE 24–3
GENERAL ASSUMPTIONS OF COGNITIVE THERAPY

Perception and experiencing in general are active processes that involve both inspective and introspective data.

The patient's cognitions represent a synthesis of internal and external stimuli.

How persons appraise a situation is generally evident in their cognitions (thoughts and visual images).

Those cognitions constitute their stream of consciousness or phenomenal field, which reflects their configuration of themselves, their world, their past and future.

Alterations in the content of their underlying cognitive structures affect their affective state and behavioral pattern.

Through psychological therapy, patients can become aware of their cognitive distortions.

Correction of those faulty dysfunctional constructs can lead to clinical improvement.

Adapted from Beck AT, Rush AJ. Shaw BF, Emery G: *Cognitive Therapy of Depression*. New York: Guilford, 1979:47, with permission.

job is to help the family understand the triangulation process and address the deeper conflict that underlies the child's apparent disruptive behavior. Techniques include reframing and positive connotation (a relabeling of all negatively expressed feelings or behaviors as positive); for example, "This child is impossible" becomes "This child is desperately trying to distract and protect you from what he or she perceives is an unhappy marriage."

Other goals of family therapy include changing maladaptive rules that govern a family, increasing awareness of cross-generational dynamics, balancing individuation and cohesiveness, increasing one-on-one direct communication, and decreasing blaming and scapegoating.

VI. Interpersonal therapy

This is a short-term psychotherapy, lasting 12 to 16 weeks, developed specifically for the treatment of nonbipolar, nonpsychotic depression. Intrapsychic conflicts are not addressed. Emphasis is on current interpersonal relationships and on strategies to improve the patient's interpersonal life. Antidepressant medication is often used as an adjunct to interpersonal therapy. The therapist is very active in helping to formulate the patient's predominant interpersonal problem areas, which define the treatment focus (Table 24–4).

VII. Group therapy

Group therapies are based on as many theories as are individual therapies. Groups range from those that emphasize support and an increase in social skills, to those that emphasize specific symptomatic relief, to those that work through unresolved intrapsychic conflicts. The focus may be on a person within the context of a group, on interactions that occur among persons in the group, or on the group as a whole. Both individual and interpersonal issues can be resolved. Groups provide a forum in which imagined fears and transference distortions can be immediately subjected to exploration and correction. Therapeutic factors in group therapy are listed in Table 24–5.

Groups tend to meet one to two times a week, usually for $1\frac{1}{2}$ hours. They may be homogeneous or heterogeneous, depending on the diagnosis. Examples of homogeneous groups include those for patients attempting to lose weight or stop smoking, and groups whose members share the same medical or psychiatric problem (e.g., AIDS, posttraumatic stress disorder, substance

TABLE 24–4
INTERPERSONAL PSYCHOTHERAPY

Goal	Improvement in current interpersonal skills
Selection criteria	Outpatient, nonbipolar disorder, nonpsychotic depressive disorder
Duration	12–16 weeks, usually once-weekly meetings
Technique	Reassurance
	Clarification of feeling states
	Improvement of interpersonal communication
	Testing perceptions
	Development of interpersonal skills
	Medication

From Ursano RJ, Silberman EK: Individual psychotherapies. In: Talbott JA, Hales RE, Yudofsky SC, eds. *The American Psyciatric Press Textbook of Psychiatry.* Washington, DC: American Psychiatric Press, 1988:868, with permission.

TABLE 24-5
TWENTY THERAPEUTIC FACTORS IN GROUP PSYCHOTHERAPY

Factor	Definition
Abreaction	A process by which repressed material, particularly a painful experience or conflict, is brought back to consciousness. In the process, the person not only recalls but relives the material, which is accompanied by the appropriate emotional response; insight usually results from the experience.
Acceptance	The feeling of being accepted by other members of the group; differences of opinion are tolerated, there is an absence of censure.
Altruism	The act of one member's being of help to another; putting another person's need before one's own and learning that there is value in giving to others. The term was originated by Auguste Cornte (1738-1857), and Sigmund Freud believed it was a major factor in establishing group cohesion and community feeling.
Catharsis	The expression of ideas, thoughts, and suppressed material that is accompanied by an emotional response that produces a state of relief in the patient.
Cohesion	The sense that the group is working together toward a common goal; also referred to as a sense of "we-ness"; believed to be the most important factor related to positive therapeutic effects.
Consensual validation	Confirmation of reality by comparing one's own conceptualizations with those of other group members; interpersonal distortions are thereby corrected. The term was introduced by Harry Stack Sullivan. Trigant Burrow had used the phrase *consensual observation* to refer to the same phenomenon.
Contagion	The process in which the expression of emotion by one member stimulates the awareness of a similar emotion in another member.
Corrective familial experience	The group re-creates the family of origin for some members who can work through original conflicts psychologically through group interaction (e.g., sibling rivalry, anger toward parents).
Empathy	The capacity of a group member to put himself or herself into the psychological frame of reference of another group member and thereby understand his or her thinking, feeling or behavior.
Identification	An unconscious defense mechanism in which the person incorporates the characteristics and the qualities of another person or object into his or her ego system.
Imitation	The conscious emulation or modeling of one's behavior after that of another (also called *role modeling*); also known *as spectator therapy*, as one patient learns from another.
Insight	Conscious awareness and understanding of one's own psychodynamics and symptoms of maladapting behavior. Most therapists distinguish two types: (1) intellectual insight—knowledge and awareness without any changes in maladaptive behavior; (2) emotional insight—awareness and understading leading to positive changes in personality and behavior.
Inspiration	The process of imparting a sense of optimism to group members; the ability to recognize that one has the capacity to overcome problems; also known as *instillation of hope*.
Interaction	The free and open exchange of ideas and feeings among group members; effective interaction is emotionally charged.
Interpretation	The process during which the group leader formulates the meaning or significance of a patient's resistance, defenses, and symbols; the result is that the patient has a cognitive framework within which to understand his or her behavior.
Learning	Patients acquire knowledge about new areas, such as social skills and sexual behavior; they receive advice, obtain guidance, and attempt to influence and are influenced by other group members.
Reality testing	Ability of the person to evaluate objectively the world outside the self; includes the capacity to perceive oneself and other group members accurately. *See also* consensual validation.
Transference	Projection of feelings, thoughts, and wishes onto the therapist, who has come to represent an object from the patient's past. Such reactions, while perhaps appropriate for the condition prevailing in the patient's earlier life, are inappropriate and anachronistic when applied to the therapist in the present. Patients in the group may also direct such feelings toward one another, a process called *multiple transferences*.
Universalization	The awareness of the patient that he or she is not alone in having problems; others share similar complaints or difficulties in learning; the patient is not unique.
Ventilation	The expression of suppressed feelings, ideas, or events to other group members; the sharing of personal secrets that ameliorate a sense of sin or guilt (also referred to as *self-disclosure*).

use disorders). Certain types of patients do not do well in certain types of groups. Psychotic patients, who require structure and clear direction, do not do well in insight-oriented groups. Paranoid patients, antisocial personalities, and substance abusers can benefit from group therapy but do not do well in heterogeneous, insight-oriented groups. In general, acutely psychotic or suicidal patients do not do well in groups.

A. Alcoholics Anonymous (AA). An example of a large, highly structured, peer-run group that is organized around persons with a similar central problem. AA emphasizes sharing experiences, role models, ventilation of feelings, and a strong sense of community and mutual support. Similar groups include Narcotics Anonymous (NA) and Sex Addicts Anonymous (SAA).

B. Milieu therapy. The multidisciplinary therapeutic approach used on inpatient psychiatric wards. The term *milieu therapy* reflects the idea that all activities on a ward are oriented toward increasing a patient's ability to cope in the world and relate appropriately to others. Milieu therapy generally involves groups and may include art therapy, occupational therapy, activities of daily living, community meetings, group passes, and social events.

C. Multiple family groups. Composed of families of schizophrenic patients. The groups discuss issues and problems related to having a schizophrenic person in the family and share suggestions and means of coping. Multiple family groups are an important factor in decreasing relapse rates among the schizophrenic patients whose families participate in the groups.

VIII. Couple and marital therapy

As many as 50% of patients are estimated to enter psychotherapy primarily because of marital problems; another 25% experience marital problems along with their other presenting problems. Marital or couples therapy is an effective tool for helping each partner to achieve self-knowledge while working on his or her problems. Couple and marital therapy encompasses a wide range of treatment techniques with the goal of increasing marital satisfaction or addressing marital impairment. As in family therapy, the relationship rather than either of the individuals is viewed as the patient.

IX. Dialectical behavior therapy

This form of therapy has been used successfully in patients with borderline personality disorder and parasuicidal behavior. It is eclectic, drawing on methods from supportive, cognitive, and behavioral therapies. Some elements are derived from Franz Alexander's view of therapy as a corrective emotional experience, and also from certain Eastern philosophical schools (e.g., Zen). Patients are seen weekly, with the goal of improving interpersonal skills and decreasing self-destructive behavior by means of techniques involving advice, use of metaphor, storytelling, and confrontation, among many others. Borderline patients especially are helped to deal with the ambivalent feelings that are characteristic of the disorder.

X. Hypnosis

Hypnosis is a complex mental state in which consciousness is altered in such a way that the subject is amenable to suggestion and receptive to direction by the therapist. When hypnotized, the patient is in a trance state, during which memories can be recalled and events experienced. The material can be used to gain insight into the makeup of a personality. Hypnosis is used to treat

TABLE 24–6
BIOFEEDBACK APPLICATIONS

Condition	Effects
Asthma	Both frontal EMG and airway resistance biofeedback have been reported as producing relaxtion from the panic associated with asthma, as well as improving air flow rate.
Cardiac arrhythmias	Specific biofeedback of the ECG has permitted patients to lower the frequency of premature ventricular contractions.
Fecal incontinence and enuresis	The timing sequence of internal and external anal sphincters has been measured with triple-lumen rectal catheters providing feedback to incontinent patients for them to reestablish normal bowel habits in a relatively small number of biofeedback sessions. An actual precursor of biofeedback dating to 1938 was the sounding of a buzzer for sleeping enuretic children at the first sign of moisture (the pad and bell).
Grand mal epilepsy	A number of EEG biofeedback procedures have been used experimentally to suppress seizure activity prophylactically in patients not responsive to anticonvulsant medication. The procedures permit patient to enhance the sensorimotor brain wave rhythm or to normalize brain activity as computed in real-time power spectrum displays.
Hyperactivity	EEG biofeedback procedures have been used on children with attention-deficit/hyperactivity disorder to train them to reduce their motor reslessness.
Idiopathic hypertension and orthostatic hypotension	A variety of specific (direct) and nonspecific biofeedback procedures—including blood pressure feedback, galvanic skin response, and foot-hand thermal feedback combined with relaxation procedures—have been used to teach patients to increase or decrease their blood pressure. Some follow-up data indicate that the changes may persist for years and often permit the reduction or elimination of antihypertensive medications.
Migraine	The most common biofeedback strategy with classic or common vascular headaches has been thermal biofeedback from a digit accompanied by autogenic self-suggestive phrases encouraging hand warming and head cooling. The mechanism is thought to help prevent excessive cerebral artery vasoconstriction, often accompanied by an ischemic prodromal symptom, such as scintillating scotomata, followed by rebound engorgement of arteries and stretching of vessel wall pain receptors.
Myofacial and temparomandibular joint pain	High levels of EMG activity over the powerful muscles associated with bilateral temporomandibular joints have been decreased by means of biofeedback in patients who are jaw clenchers or have bruxism.
Neuromuscular rehabilitation	Mechanical devises or an EMG measurement of muscle activity displayed to a patient increases the effectiveness of traditional therapies, as documented by relatively long clinical histories in peripheral nerve–muscle damage, spasmodic torticollis, selected cases of tardive dyskinesia, cerebral palsy, and upper motor neuron hemiplegias.
Raynaud's syndrome	Cold hands and cold feet are frequent concomitants of anxiety and also occur in Raynaud's syndrome, caused by vasospasm of arterial smooth muscle. A number of studies report that thermal feedback from the hand, an inexpensive and benign procedure compared with surgical sympathectomy, is effective in about 70% of cases of Raynaud's syndrome.
Tension headaches	Muscle contraction headaches are most frequently treated with two large active electrodes spaced on the forehead to provide visual or auditory information about the levels of muscle tension. The frontal electrode placement is sensitive to EMG activity in the frontalis and occipital muscles, which the patient learns to relax.

EMG, electromyogram.

many disorders, including obesity, substance-related disorders (especially nicotine dependence), sexual disorders, and dissociative states.

XI. Guided imagery

Used alone or with hypnosis. The patient is instructed to imagine scenes with associated colors, sounds, smells, and feelings. The scene may be pleasant (used to decrease anxiety) or unpleasant (used to master anxiety). Imagery has been used to treat patients with generalized anxiety disorders, posttraumatic stress disorder, and phobias, and as an adjunct therapy for medical or surgical disease.

XII. Biofeedback

Biofeedback provides information to a person about his or her physiological functions, usually related to the autonomic nervous system (e.g., blood pressure), with the goal of producing a relaxed, euthymic mental state. It is based on the idea that the autonomic nervous system can be brought under voluntary control through operant conditioning. It is used in the management of tension states associated with medical illness (e.g., to increase hand temperature in patients with Raynaud's syndrome and to treat headaches and hypertension) (Table 24–6).

XIII. Paradoxical therapy

In this approach, the therapist suggests that the patient intentionally engage in an unwanted or undesirable behavior (called *paradoxical injunction*)—for example, avoiding a phobic object or performing a compulsive ritual. This approach can create new insights for some patients.

XIV. Sex therapy

In sex therapy, the therapist discusses the psychological and physiologic aspects of sexual functioning in great detail. Therapists adopt an educative attitude, and aids such as models of the genitalia and videotapes may be used. Treatment is on a short-term basis and behaviorally oriented. Specific exercises are prescribed, depending on the disorder being treated (e.g., graduated dilators for vaginismus). Usually, the couple is treated, but individual sex therapy is also effective.

For more detailed discussion of this topic, see Psychotherapies, Ch 30, p 2056, in CTP/VII.

25

Psychopharmacology and Other Biological Therapies

I. Introduction

Psychotherapeutic drugs are the mainstay of treatment for a broad range of mental disorders, such as psychotic disorders, mood disorders, anxiety, and attention-deficit/hyperactivity disorders, among others. A recent explosion of research and development has filled today's psychopharmacological armamentarium with many safe and well-tolerated drugs.

In current practice, a specific agent may be used to treat a wide range of disorders. Moreover, the diversity of drug treatment options has been further expanded by the favorable adverse effect profiles of newer drugs, which permit many new combination treatments. At present, for example, polypharmacy is common in the treatment of psychotic and bipolar disorders.

This chapter reviews the current principles of psychopharmacology and discusses currently available psychotropic medications. The drugs are grouped in an outline format according to their primary therapeutic indications: anxiolytics and hypnotics, antipsychotics, antidepressants, antimanics and mood stabilizers, stimulants, cholinesterase inhibitors (cognitive enhancers), and other drugs. Electroconvulsive therapy (ECT) and other biological modalities used in psychiatric practice are also discussed.

II. Basic principles of psychopharmacology

A. Pharmacological actions. Pharmacological actions are divided into two categories, pharmacokinetic and pharmacodynamic. In simple terms, *pharmacokinetics* describes *what the body does to the drug,* and *pharmacodynamics* describes *what the drug does to the body*. Pharmacokinetic data trace the absorption, distribution, metabolism, and excretion of a drug in the body. Pharmacodynamic data measure the effects of a drug on cells in the brain and other tissues of the body.

1. Pharmacokinetics

a. Absorption. Orally administered drugs dissolve in the fluid of the gastrointestinal tract and then reach the brain through the bloodstream. Some drugs are available in *depot* preparations, which are injected intramuscularly once every 1 to 4 weeks. Intravenous administration is the quickest route for achieving therapeutic blood concentrations, but it also carries the highest risk for sudden and life-threatening adverse effects.

b. Distribution and bioavailability. Drugs that circulate bound to plasma proteins are *protein-bound,* and those that circulate unbound are said to be *free*. Only the free fraction can pass through the blood–brain barrier. The *distribution* of a drug to the brain is promoted by high rates of cerebral blood flow, lipid solubility, and receptor affinity.

Bioavailability refers to the fraction of administered drug that can eventually be recovered from the bloodstream. Bioavailability is an important variable because FDA regulations specify that the bioavailability of a generic formulation can differ from that of the brand name formulation by no more than 30%.

c. **Metabolism and excretion.** The four metabolic routes—*oxidation, reduction, hydrolysis,* and *conjugation*—usually produce metabolites that are relatively more polar and therefore more readily excreted. However, metabolic processes may also transform inactive prodrugs into therapeutically active metabolites. The liver is the principal site of *metabolism,* and bile, feces, and urine are the major routes of *excretion.* Psychotherapeutic drugs are also excreted in sweat, saliva, tears, and breast milk, an important fact to be considered for mothers who want to nurse their children.

The *half-life* of a drug is the amount of time it takes for its plasma concentration to be reduced by half during metabolism and excretion. A greater number of daily doses are required for drugs with shorter half-lives than for drugs with longer half-lives. Drug interactions or disease states that inhibit the metabolism of continuously administered psychoactive drugs can produce toxicity.

2. **Pharmacodynamics.** The major pharmacodynamic considerations include the *molecular site of action, dose–response curve, therapeutic index,* and the development of *tolerance, dependence, and withdrawal symptoms.*

   a. **Molecular site of action.** The *molecular site of action* is determined in laboratory assays and may or may not correctly identify the drug–receptor interactions responsible for a drug's clinical effects, which are identified empirically in clinical trials.

   b. **Dose–response curve.** The *dose–response curve* plots the effects of a drug against its plasma concentration. *Potency* refers to the ratio of drug dosage to clinical effect. For example, risperidone (Risperdal) is more potent than olanzapine (Zyprexa) because about 4 mg of risperidone is required to achieve the comparable therapeutic effect of 20 mg of olanzapine. However, because both are capable of eliciting a similar beneficial response at their respective optimal dosages, the *clinical efficacies* of risperidone and olanzapine are equivalent.

   c. **Therapeutic index.** The *therapeutic index* is the ratio of a drug's toxic dosage to its maximally effective dosage. Drugs such as lithium, for example, have a low therapeutic index, so that close monitoring of plasma concentrations is required to avoid toxicity.

   d. **Tolerance, dependence, and withdrawal symptoms.** When a person becomes less responsive to a particular drug with time, *tolerance* to the effects of the drug has developed. The development of tolerance can be associated with the appearance of physical *dependence,* which is the need to continue taking a drug to prevent the appearance of *withdrawal symptoms.*

III. Clinical guidelines

Optimizing the results of psychotropic drug therapy involves consideration of the five *D*s: diagnosis, drug selection, dosage, duration, and dialogue.

A. The five *D*s.

1. **Diagnosis.** A careful diagnostic investigation should identify specific target symptoms with which the drug response can be objectively assessed.

2. **Drug selection.** Factors that determine drug selection include diagnosis, past personal and family history of response to a particular agent, and the overall medical status of the patient. Certain drugs will be excluded because concurrent drug treatment of medical and other psychiatric disorders creates a risk for drug–drug interactions. Other drugs will be excluded because they have unfavorable adverse effect profiles. A choice of the ideal drug should emerge based on a review of the clinician's experience and preferences.

    The Drug Enforcement Administration (DEA) has classified drugs according to their potential for abuse (Table 25–1), and clinicians are advised to use caution when prescribing controlled substances.

3. **Dosage.** The two most common causes of failure of psychotropic drug treatment are inadequate dosing and an incomplete therapeutic trial of a drug. Once the decision has been made to treat a person with medication, efforts should be directed toward achieving therapeutic dosages for an adequate trial period to permit a valid assessment of efficacy.

4. **Duration.** For antipsychotic, antidepressant, and mood-stabilizing drugs, a therapeutic trial should continue for 4 to 6 weeks. In the treatment of these conditions, drug efficacy tends to improve with time, whereas drug discontinuation is frequently associated with relapses. In contrast, for most anxiolytic and stimulant drugs, the maximum therapeutic benefit is usually evident within an hour of administration.

5. **Dialogue.** Persons will generally be less upset by adverse effects if they have been told to expect them. Clinicians should distinguish between probable or expected adverse effects and rare or unexpected adverse effects.

    People often feel that taking a psychotherapeutic drug means that they are really sick or not in control of their lives, or that they may become addicted to the drug and have to take it forever. A simplified approach to these concerns is to explain that the psychiatric disorder for which the patient is being treated causes a chemical imbalance of the brain, analogous to the chemical imbalances in the blood caused by diabetes. Clinicians should explain the difference between how psychotropic drugs of abuse affect the normal brain and how approved psychiatric drugs help correct emotional disorders.

TABLE 25-1
CHARACTERISTICS OF DRUGS AT EACH DRUG ENFORCEMENT AGENCY LEVEL

DEA Control Level (Schedule)	Characteristics of Drug at Each Control Level	Examples of Drugs at Each Control Level
I	High abuse potential No accepted use in medical treatment in the United States at the present time and, therefore, not for prescription use Can be used for research	Lysergic acid diethylamide (LSD), heroin, marijuana, peyote, 3,4-methylenedioxymethamphetamine (MDMA), methcathinone, gamma hydroxybutyrate (GHB), phencyclidine (PCP), mescaline, psilocybin, nicocodeine, nicomorphine
II	High abuse potential Severe physical dependence liability Severe psychological dependence liability No refills; no telephone prescriptions	Amphetamine, opium, morphine, codeine, hydromorphone, phenmetrazine, amobarbital, secobarbital, pentobarbital, methylphenidate, ketamine
III	Abuse potential less than levels I and II Moderate or low physical dependence liability High psychological liability Prescriptions must be rewritten after 6 months or five refills	Glutethimide, methyprylon, nalorphine, sulfonmethane, benzphetamine, phendimetrazine, chlorphentermine; compounds containing codeine, morphine, opium, hydrocodone, dihydrocodeine, naltrexone, diethylpropion, dronabinol
IV	Low abuse potential Limited physical dependence liability Limited psychological dependence liability Prescriptions must be rewritten after 6 months or five refills	Phenobarbital, benzodiazepines,[a] chloral hydrate, ethchlorvynol, ethinamate, meprobamate, paraldehyde, phentermine
V	Lowest abuse potential of all controlled substances	Narcotic preparations containing limited amounts of nonnarcotic active medicinal ingredients

[a]In New York State benzodiazepines are treated as schedule II substances, which require a triplicate prescription for a maximum of 1 month's supply.

B. Special considerations

1. **Children.** It is best to begin with a small dosage and increase it until clinical effects are observed. However, the clinician should not hesitate to use adult dosages in children if the dosage is effective and no adverse effects develop.

2. **The elderly.** Clinicians should begin treating elderly patients with a small dosage, usually approximately one-half the usual dosage. The dosage should be increased in small amounts, until either a clinical benefit is achieved or unacceptable adverse effects appear. Although many elderly patients require only a small dosage of medication, others require the usual adult dosage.

3. **Pregnant and nursing women.** Clinicians are best advised to avoid administering any drug to a woman who is pregnant (particularly during the first trimester) or nursing a child. This rule, however, occasionally needs to be broken when the mother's psychiatric disorder is severe. The risk to mother and fetus of the untreated psychiatric disorder must be weighed against the risk of psychotropic drug use during pregnancy. It has been suggested that withdrawing a drug during pregnancy could cause a discontinuation syndrome in both mother and fetus.

4. **Medically ill persons.** Like children and the elderly, medically ill persons should be treated according to the most conservative clinical practice, which is to begin with a small dosage, increase it slowly, and watch for both clinical and adverse effects. If applicable, plasma drug concentrations may be particularly helpful during the treatment of these persons.

IV. Anxiolytics and hypnotics
A. Treatment recommendations
1. **Treatment of acute anxiety.** Acute anxiety responds best to either oral or parenteral administration of benzodiazepines. Dopamine receptor antagonists (typical antipsychotics) are sometimes used to control acutely anxious persons who also exhibit agitated and violent behavior.
2. **Treatment of chronic anxiety**
   a. **Antidepressants.** The selective serotonin reuptake inhibitors (SSRIs), venlafaxine (Effexor), and nefazodone (Serzone) are antidepressants that also are first-line agents for the control of chronic anxiety disorders, including generalized anxiety disorder, panic disorder, obsessive-compulsive disorder, social anxiety disorder, and posttraumatic stress disorder; phobias; and agitation associated with bipolar I disorder. It appears that an antidepressant drug must have inherent serotonergic activity to be effective in the treatment of obsessive-compulsive symptoms.
   b. **Benzodiazepines.** Benzodiazepines, which lack serotonergic activity, are used on a long-term basis for the treatment of generalized anxiety symptoms and panic disorder, but not obsessive-compulsive disorder.
   c. **Buspirone (BuSpar).** Buspirone is approved by the FDA for the treatment of anxiety disorders, specifically generalized anxiety disorder. However, many experts view it as a second-line agent because of its limited efficacy.
   d. **Bupropion (Wellbutrin).** Bupropion is a nonserotonergic antidepressant that is not generally as effective for the treatment of anxiety symptoms as are serotonergic agents.
   e. **Mirtazapine (Remeron).** Mirtazapine is effective for the treatment of anxiety symptoms, but its utility is limited by its marked sedative qualities.
   f. **Third-line treatments.** The older agents—monoamine oxidase inhibitors (MAOIs) and tricyclic and tetracyclic drugs—are efficacious, but they may cause serious adverse effects.
3. **Treatment of insomnia**
   a. **Nonbenzodiazepines.** The nonbenzodiazepine agents zolpidem (Ambien) and zaleplon (Sonata) have certain advantages over benzodiazepines for the treatment of insomnia. They have a rapid onset of action, specifically target insomnia, lack muscle relaxant and anticonvulsant properties, are completely metabolized within 4 or 5 hours, and rarely cause withdrawal symptoms or rebound insomnia. The usual bedtime dose of each is 10 mg. Zolpidem is said to be ef-

TABLE 25–2
HALF-LIVES, DOSES, AND PREPARATIONS OF BENZODIAZEPINE RECEPTOR AGONISTS AND ANTAGONISTS

Drug	Dose Equivalents	Half-life (h)	Rate of Absorption	Usual Adult Dosage	Dose Preparations
Agonists					
Clonazepam	0.5	Long (metabolite, >20)	Rapid	1–6 mg bid	0.5-mg, 1.0-mg, and 2.0-mg tablets
Diazepam	5	Long (>20) (nordiazepam—long, >20)	Rapid	4–40 mg bid to qid	2-mg, 5-mg, and 10-mg tablets (slow release 15-mg capsules)
Alprazolam	0.25	Intermediate (6–20)	Medium	0.5–10 mg bid to qid	0.25-mg, 0.5-mg, 1.0 mg, and 2.0-mg tablets
Lorazepam	1	Intermediate (6–20)	Medium	1–6 mg tid	0.5-mg, 1.0-mg, and 2.0-mg tablets, 2 mg/mL, 4 mg/mL parenteral
Oxazepam	15	Intermediate (6–20)	Slow	30–120 mg tid or qid	10-mg, 15-mg, and 30-mg capsules (15-mg tablets)
Temazepam	5	Intermediate (6–20)	Medium	7.5–30 mg hs	7.5-mg, 15-mg, and 30-mg capsules
Chlordiazepoxide	10	Intermediate (6–20) (demethylchlordiazepoxide— intermediate, 6–20) (demoxapam—long, >20) (nordiazepam—long, >20)	Medium	10–150 mg tid or qid	5-mg, 10-mg, and 25-mg tablets and capsules
Flurazepam	5	Short (<6) (N-hydroxyethylflurazepam—short, <6) (N-desalkylflurazepam—long, >20)	Rapid	15–30 mg hs	15-mg and 30-mg capsules
Triazolam	0.1–0.03	Short (<6)	Rapid	0.125 mg or 0.250 mg hs	0.125-mg or 0.250-mg tablets
Clorazepate	7.5	Short (<6) (nordiazepam—long, >20)	Rapid	15–60 mg bid or qid	3.75-mg, 7.5-mg, and 15-mg tablets (slow release 11.25-mg and 22.5-mg tablets)
Halazepam	20	Short (<6) (nordiazepam—long, >20)	Medium	60–160 mg tid or qid	20-mg and 40-mg tablets
Prazepam	10	Short (<6) (nordiazepam—long, >20)	Slow	30 mg (20–60 mg) qid or tid	5-mg, 10-mg, or 20-mg capsules
Estazolam	0.33	Intermediate (6–20) (4-hydroxyestazolam— intermediate, 6–20)	Rapid	1.0 or 2.0 hs	1-mg and 2-mg tablets
Quazepam	5	Long (>20) (2-oxoquazepam-N-desalkylflurazepam—long, >20)	Rapid	7.5 or 15 mg hs	7.5-mg and 15-mg tablets
Midazolam	1.25–1.3	Short (<6)	Rapid	5 to 50 mg parenteral	5 mg/mL parenteral, 1-mL, 2-mL, 5-mL, and 10-mL vials
Zolpidem	2.5	Short (<6)	Rapid	5 mg or 10 mg hs	5-mg and 10-mg tablets
Zaleplon	?	Short (1)	Rapid	10 mg hs	5-mg and 10-mg capsules
Antagonist					
Flumazenil	0.06	Short (<6)	Rapid	0.2–0.5 mg/min injection over 3–10 min (total, 1–5 mg)	0.1 mg/mL (5 mL and 10-mL vials)

fective for 5 hours and zaleplon for 4 hours. Adverse events may include dizziness, nausea, and somnolence.

b. **Benzodiazepines.** The five benzodiazepines used primarily as hypnotics are flurazepam (Dalmane), temazepam (Restoril), quazepam (Doral), estazolam (ProSom), and triazolam (Halcion). Benzodiazepines shorten sleep latency and increase sleep continuity, so that they are useful for the treatment of insomnia.

Benzodiazepines also curtail sleep stages III and IV (deep or slow-wave sleep) and so are good treatments for sleepwalking and night terrors, which occur in the deep stages of sleep. Benzodiazepines suppress disorders related to rapid eye movement (REM) sleep, most notably violent behavior during REM sleep (REM behavior disorder).

c. **Trazodone (Desyrel).** Low dose trazodone, 25 to 100 mg at bedtime, is widely used to treat insomnia. It has a favorable effect on sleep architecture.

B. **Benzodiazepine agonists and antagonists.** Fifteen benzodiazepines are available for clinical use in the United States (Table 25–2). They are widely prescribed, with at least 10% of the population using one of these drugs each year. They are safe, effective, and well tolerated in both short-term and long-term use. The pharmacological effects of the benzodiazepines are listed in Table 25–3.

1. **Indications.** Benzodiazepines are often used to augment the effects of antidepressant drugs during the first month of use, before the antidepressant drug has begun to exert its anxiolytic effects; they are then tapered once the antidepressant becomes effective. High-potency benzodiazepines are used as maintenance therapy for persons with panic symptoms.

2. **Choice of drug.** The most important differences among the benzodiazepines relate to potency and elimination half-life.

a. **Potency.** High-potency benzodiazepines, such as alprazolam (Xanax) and clonazepam (Klonopin), appear to be effective in suppressing panic attacks. Low-potency benzodiazepines cause sedation.

TABLE 25–3
PHARMACOLOGIC EFFECTS OF BENZODIAPINES

Effects	Clinical Application/Consequences
Therapeutic effects	
Sedative	Insomnia, conscious sedation, alcohol withdrawal
Anxiolytic	Panic attacks, generalized anxiety
Anticonvulsant	Seizures
Muscle relaxant	Muscle tension, muscle spasm
Amnestic	Adjunct to chemotherapy or anesthesia
Antistress	Mild hypertension, irritable bowel syndrome, angina
Adverse effects	
Sedative	Daytime sleepiness, impaired concentration
Amnestic	Mild forgetfulness, anterograde memory impairment
Psychomotor	Accidents, falls
Behavioral	Depression, agitation
Decreased CO_2 response	Worsening of sleep apnea and other obstructive pulmonary disorders
Withdrawal syndrome	Dependence—anxiety, insomnia, excess sensitivity to light, excess sensitivity to sound, tachycardia, mild systolic hypertension, tremor, headache, sweating, abdominal distress, craving, seizures

b. Duration of action. Diazepam (Valium) and triazolam are readily absorbed and have a rapid onset; chlordiazepoxide (Librium) and oxazepam (Serax) work more slowly.

Compounds with a long half-life tend to accumulate with repeated dosing, so that the risk for excessive daytime sedation, difficulties with concentration and memory, and falls is increased. Rates of hip fractures resulting from falls are higher in elderly persons taking long-acting drugs than in those taking more rapidly eliminated compounds. Benzodiazepines with short half-lives also have the advantage of causing less impairment with regular use. However, they appear to produce a more severe withdrawal syndrome. Drugs affecting the rate of elimination of benzodiazepines are listed in Table 25–4.

c. Dependence and withdrawal symptoms. A major concern with long-term benzodiazepine use is the development of dependence, particularly with high-potency agents. Not only can discontinuation of benzodiazepines result in symptom recurrence and rebound, but it can also precipitate withdrawal symptoms. Several factors contribute to the development of benzodiazepine withdrawal symptoms (Table 25–5). Drug type and duration of use are the most significant factors, but other considerations are also important.

Concerns about dependence should lead to caution in prescribing but should not preclude the use of benzodiazepines when indi-

TABLE 25–4
DRUGS AFFECTING THE RATE OF ELIMINATION OF OXIDIZED BENZODIAZEPINES

Increase Elimination Half-life	Decrease Elimination Half-life
Cimetidine	Chronic ethyl alcohol use
Propranolol	Rifampin
Oral contraceptives (estrogens)	
Chloramphenicol	
Propoxyphene	
Isoniazid	
Disulfiram	
Allopurinol	
Tricyclic antidepressants	
Acute ethyl alcohol use	

TABLE 25–5
KEY FACTORS IN THE DEVELOPMENT OF BENZODIAZEPINE WITHDRAWAL SYMPTOMS

Factor	Explanation
Drug type	High-potency, short half-life compounds (e.g., alprazolam, triazolam, lorazepam)
Duration of use	Risk increases with time
Dose level	Higher doses increase risk
Rate of discontinuation	Abrupt withdrawal instead of taper increases risk for severe symptoms, including seizures
Diagnosis	Panic disorder patients more prone to withdrawal symptoms
Personality	Patients with passive-dependent, histrionic, somatizing, or asthenic traits more likely to experience withdrawal.

cated. In some persons who take benzodiazepines for years, withdrawal reactions never develop, whereas others have difficulties after only a few weeks of use.

Apart from being subjectively distressing, withdrawal symptoms can be misconstrued as part of the underlying disorder and thus prompt unnecessary continuation of drug use.

3. **Benzodiazepine antagonist.** Flumazenil (Romazicon) is a benzodiazepine antagonist used to reverse the effects of benzodiazepine receptor agonists in overdose and in clinical situations such as sedation or anesthesia. It has also been used to reverse benzodiazepine effects immediately before the administration of ECT. Adverse effects include nausea, vomiting, and agitation. Flumazenil can precipitate seizures, particularly in persons who have seizure disorders, are dependent on benzodiazepines, or have taken large overdoses. The usual regimen is to give 0.2 mg intravenously over 30 seconds. If consciousness is not regained, an additional 0.3 mg can be given intravenously over 30 seconds. Most persons respond to a total of 1 to 3 mg. Doses larger than 3 mg are unlikely to add benefit.

V. Antipsychotics

Antipsychotic drugs are effective in both the short-term and the long-term management of schizophrenia, schizophreniform disorder, schizoaffective disorder, delusional disorder, brief psychotic disorder, manic episodes, and major depressive disorder with psychotic features.

A. **Serotonin-dopamine antagonists (SDAs, atypical antipsychotic drugs).** The SDAs include risperidone, olanzapine, quetiapine (Seroquel), ziprasidone (Geodon), and clozapine (Clozaril). These drugs improve three classes of disability typical of schizophrenia: positive symptoms (hallucinations, delusions, disordered thoughts, agitation); negative symptoms (withdrawal, flat affect, anhedonia, catatonia); and cognitive impairment (perceptual distortions, memory deficits, inattentiveness). The SDAs, except clozapine, are first-line agents for the treatment of schizophrenia and psychotic symptoms of any cause. They have largely replaced the typical antipsychotics (dopamine receptor antagonists) for all indications except acute control of violent or agitated behavior. Unlike dopamine receptor agonists, SDAs are associated with a relatively small risk for extrapyramidal symptoms. Thus, they eliminate the need for anticholinergic drugs that tend to blunt memory. SDAs are also effective for the treatment of mood disorders with psychotic or manic features. Olanzapine is FDA-approved for the treatment of bipolar I disorder.

1. **Pharmacological actions**
   a. **Risperidone.** Between 70% and 85% of risperidone is absorbed from the gastrointestinal tract, and the combined half-life of risperidone and its active metabolite 9-hydroxyrisperidone averages 20 hours, so that it is effective in once-daily dosing.
   b. **Olanzapine.** Approximately 85% of olanzapine is absorbed from the gastrointestinal tract, and its half-life averages 30 hours. Therefore, it is also effective in once-daily dosing.

      c. Quetiapine. Quetiapine is rapidly absorbed from the gastrointestinal tract. Its half life is about 6 hours, so that dosing two or three times per day is necessary.

      d. Ziprasidone. Ziprasidone is well absorbed. Its half life is 5 to 10 hours, so that twice-daily dosing is optimal.

      e. Clozapine. Clozapine is variably absorbed from the gastrointestinal tract. Its half-life is 10 to 16 hours, so that it is taken twice daily.

  2. Therapeutic indications. SDAs are effective for initial and maintenance treatment of psychosis in schizophrenia and schizoaffective disorders in both adults and adolescents. They are also effective for psychotic depression, psychosis secondary to head trauma, psychosis and aggressiveness secondary to dementia, and drug-induced psychosis (e.g., psychosis resulting from treatment with sympathomimetics or from levodopa or dopamine agonist treatment in people with Parkinson's disease). SDAs are effective in acutely ill and treatment-refractory persons, and they prevent relapses, even at low doses. In comparison with persons treated with dopamine receptor agonists, persons treated with SDAs require less frequent hospitalization, fewer emergency room visits, less phone contact with mental health professionals, and less treatment in day programs.

      Clozapine was the first atypical drug, and it remains one of the most efficacious antipsychotic drugs. However, because clozapine causes potentially life-threatening adverse effects, it is now considered appropriate for use only in persons with schizophrenia resistant to all other dopamine receptor agonists and SDAs. Clozapine provides a therapeutic niche for patients with severe tardive dyskinesias, unmanageable extrapyramidal symptoms, and psychosis secondary to antiparkinsonian drugs.

  3. Clinical guidelines

      a. Risperidone. Risperidone is available in 1-, 2-, 3-, and 4-mg tablets, and as an oral solution with a concentration of 1 mg/mL. The initial dosage is usually 1 to 2 mg/day, taken at night. It can then be raised gradually (by 1 mg every 2 or 3 days) to 4 to 6 mg at night. Dosages higher than 6 mg/day are associated with increased adverse effects. Dosages below 6 mg/day have generally not been associated with extrapyramidal symptoms, but dystonic and dyskinetic reactions have been seen at dosages of 4 to 16 mg/day.

      b. Olanzapine. Olanzapine is available in 2.5-, 5-, 7.5-, 10-, and 15-mg tablets. The initial dosage is usually 5 or 10 mg once daily. A starting dosage of 5 mg/day is recommended for elderly and medically ill persons, and for persons with hepatic impairment or hypotension. After 1 week, the dosage can be raised to 10 mg/day. Dosages in clinical use range from 5 to 20 mg/day, but benefit in both schizophrenia and bipolar mania is noted in most people at dosages of 10 to 15 mg/day. The higher dosages are occasionally associated with increased extrapyramidal and other adverse effects. The manufacturer recommends "periodic" assessment of transaminases during treatment with olanzapine.

c. **Quetiapine.** Quetiapine is available in 25-, 100-, and 200-mg tablets. The dosage should begin at 25 mg twice daily and can be raised by 25 to 50 mg per dose every 2 to 3 days up to a target dosage of 300 to 400 mg/day, divided into two or three daily doses. Studies have shown efficacy in the range of 300 to 800 mg/day, with most people receiving maximum benefit at 300 to 500 mg/day.

d. **Ziprasidone.** Ziprasidone is available in 20-, 40-, 60-, and 80-mg capsules. Dosing should be initiated at 40 mg/day, divided into two daily doses. Studies have shown efficacy in the range of 40 to 200 mg, divided into two daily doses.

e. **Clozapine.** Clozapine is available in 25- and 100-mg tablets. The initial dosage is usually 25 mg one or two times daily, although a conservative initial dosage is 12.5 mg twice daily. The dosage can then be raised gradually (by 25 mg every 2 or 3 days) to 300 mg/day, usually divided into two or three daily doses. Dosages of up to 900 mg/day can be used.

(1) **Pretreatment evaluation.** Before the initiation of treatment with clozapine, an informed consent procedure should be documented. The patient's history should include information about blood disorders, epilepsy, cardiovascular disease, hepatic and renal diseases, and drug abuse. The presence of a hepatic or renal disease necessitates the use of low starting dosages. The physical examination should include supine and standing blood pressure measurements to screen for orthostatic hypotension. The laboratory examination should include an electrocardiogram (ECG); several complete blood cell counts including white blood cell counts, which can then be averaged; and tests of hepatic and renal function.

(2) **Monitoring during treatment.** During treatment with clozapine, weekly white blood cell counts are indicated for the first 6 months to monitor for the development of agranulocytosis; they should be obtained thereafter every 2 weeks. Although monitoring is expensive, early detection of agranulocytosis can prevent a fatal outcome. Probably more important than screening blood cell counts is educating persons to seek immediate medical evaluation if fever or any signs of infection develop. If the white cell count is less than 2,000/mm^3 or the granulocyte count is less than 1,000/mm^3, clozapine should be discontinued, a hematologic consultation should be obtained, and a bone marrow biopsy should be considered. Persons with agranulocytosis should not be reexposed to the drug. Clinicians can monitor the white blood cell count through any laboratory. Proof of monitoring must be presented to the pharmacist to obtain the medication.

f. **Switching from and to another antipsychotic drug.** Clozapine and olanzapine both have anticholinergic effects, and the transition from one to the other can be accomplished with little risk for cholinergic rebound. The transition from risperidone to olanzapine is best accomplished by tapering the risperidone during 3 weeks while simultaneously beginning olanzapine directly at a dosage of 10 mg/day.

Risperidone, quetiapine, and ziprasidone lack anticholinergic effects, and the abrupt transition from a dopamine receptor agonist, olanzapine, or clozapine to one of these agents may cause cholinergic rebound, which consists of excessive salivation, nausea, vomiting, and diarrhea. The risk for cholinergic rebound can be mitigated by initially augmenting risperidone, quetiapine, or ziprasidone with an anticholinergic drug, which is then tapered slowly.

With depot formulations of a dopamine receptor agonist, the first dose of the SDA is given on the day the next injection is due. At present, SDAs are available only in oral formulations. If it is approved by the FDA, ziprasidone will likely be available in a depot formulation.

4. **Adverse effects**
   a. **All SDAs**
      (1) **Neuroleptic malignant syndrome.** The development of neuroleptic malignant syndrome is considerably rarer with SDAs than with dopamine receptor agonists. This syndrome consists of muscular rigidity, fever, dystonia, akinesia, mutism, oscillation between obtundation and agitation, diaphoresis, dysphagia, tremor, incontinence, labile blood pressure, leukocytosis, and elevated creatine phosphokinase. Clozapine, especially if combined with lithium, and risperidone have been associated with neuroleptic malignant syndrome.
      (2) **Tardive dyskinesias.** SDAs are significantly less likely than dopamine receptor agonists to be associated with treatment-emergent tardive dyskinesias. Moreover, SDAs relieve the symptoms of tardive dyskinesias and are especially indicated for psychotic persons with preexisting tardive dyskinesias. For this reason, long-term maintenance treatment with dopamine receptor agonists has become a questionable practice.
   b. **Risperidone.** Risperidone causes few adverse effects at the usual therapeutic dosages of 6 mg/day or less. The most common adverse effects include anxiety, insomnia, somnolence, dizziness, constipation, nausea, dyspepsia, rhinitis, rash, and tachycardia. At the rarely used higher dosages, it causes dosage-dependent extrapyramidal effects, hyperprolactinemia, sedation, orthostatic hypotension, palpitations, weight gain, decreased libido, and erectile dysfunction. Rare adverse effects associated with long-term use include neuroleptic malignant syndrome, priapism, thrombocytopenic purpura, and seizures in persons with hyponatremia.
   c. **Olanzapine.** Olanzapine is generally well tolerated except for moderate somnolence and weight gain of 10 to 25 lb in up to 50% of persons on long-term therapy. Infrequent adverse effects include anticholinergic effects, hyperglycemia, orthostatic hypotension,

transaminase elevations, and rarely extrapyramidal symptoms. Diabetes mellitus and acute-onset diabetic ketoacidosis have been reported in patients using olanzapine.

d. **Quetiapine.** The most common adverse effects of quetiapine are somnolence, postural hypotension, and dizziness, which are usually transient and are best managed with initial gradual upward titration of the dose. Quetiapine appears no more likely than placebo to cause extrapyramidal symptoms. Quetiapine is associated with modest transient weight gain, transient rises in liver transaminases, small increases in heart rate, and constipation.

e. **Ziprasidone.** Adverse effects are unusual with ziprasidone. In particular, it is the only SDA not associated with weight gain. The most common adverse effects are somnolence, dizziness, nausea, and light-headedness. Ziprasidone causes almost no significant effects outside the CNS.

f. **Clozapine.** Significant potential for the development of serious adverse effects is the reason that clozapine is reserved for use in only the most treatment-refractory persons. The most common adverse effects are sedation, seizures, dizziness, syncope, tachycardia, hypotension, ECG changes, nausea, vomiting, leukopenia, granulocytopenia, agranulocytosis, and fever. Weight gain can be marked. Diabetes mellitus has been linked to clozapine, regardless of any weight gain. Other common adverse effects include fatigue, sialorrhea, various gastrointestinal symptoms (most commonly constipation), anticholinergic effects, and subjective muscle weakness. Clozapine is best used in a structured setting.

Because of additive risks of agranulocytosis, clozapine should not be combined with carbamazepine (Tegretol), or other drugs known to cause bone marrow suppression.

5. **Drug interactions**

a. **All SDAs.** CNS depressants, alcohol, or tricyclic drugs coadministered with SDAs may increase the risk for seizures, sedation, and cardiac effects. Antihypertensive medications may exacerbate the orthostatic hypotension caused by SDAs. The coadministration of benzodiazepines and SDAs may be associated with an increased incidence of orthostasis, syncope, and respiratory depression. Risperidone, olanzapine, quetiapine, and ziprasidone can antagonize the effects of levodopa and dopamine agonists. Long-term use of SDAs together with drugs that induce hepatic cytochrome P450 (CYP) metabolic enzymes (e.g., carbamazepine, barbiturates, omeprazole [Prilosec], rifampin [Rifadin, Rifamate], glucocorticoids) may increase the clearance of SDAs by 50% or more.

b. **Risperidone.** The concurrent use of risperidone and phenytoin or SSRIs may produce extrapyramidal symptoms. The use of risperidone by persons with opioid dependence may precipitate opioid withdrawal symptoms. The addition of risperidone to the regimen of a person taking clozapine can raise clozapine plasma concentrations by 75%. Otherwise, risperidone has little effect on other drugs.

   c. **Olanzapine.** Cimetidine (Tagamet) and warfarin (Coumadin) do not influence olanzapine metabolism. Olanzapine does not affect the metabolism of imipramine (Tofranil), desipramine (Norpramin), warfarin, diazepam, lithium, or biperiden (Akineton). Fluvoxamine (Luvox) increases the serum concentrations of olanzapine.

   d. **Quetiapine.** Phenytoin increases quetiapine clearance fivefold, and thioridazine (Mellaril) increases quetiapine clearance by 65%. Cimetidine reduces quetiapine clearance by 20%. Fluoxetine (Prozac), imipramine, haloperidol (Haldol), and risperidone do not influence quetiapine metabolism. Quetiapine reduces lorazepam (Ativan) clearance by 20% and does not affect lithium clearance.

   e. **Ziprasidone.** Ziprasidone has a low potential for causing clinically significant drug interactions.

   f. **Clozapine.** Clozapine should not be used with any other drug that can cause bone marrow suppression. Such drugs include carbamazepine, phenytoin, propylthiouracil, sulfonamides, and captopril (Capoten). The addition of paroxetine (Paxil) may precipitate clozapine-associated neutropenia. Lithium combined with clozapine may increase the risk for seizures, confusion, and movement disorders. Lithium should not be used in combination with clozapine by persons who have experienced an episode of neuroleptic malignant syndrome. Risperidone, fluoxetine, paroxetine, and fluvoxamine increase serum concentrations of clozapine. When initiated carefully, risperidone augmentation can increase the antipsychotic efficacy of clozapine.

B. **Dopamine receptor antagonists.** The dopamine receptor antagonists are presently second-line agents for the treatment of schizophrenia and other psychotic disorders. Because of their immediate calming effects, however, dopamine receptor antagonists are first-line agents for the management of acute psychotic episodes.

   The therapeutic effects and the neurological and endocrinologic adverse effects of these drugs result from their blockade of dopamine receptors. In addition, various dopamine receptor antagonists also block noradrenergic, cholinergic, and histaminergic receptors. Dopamine receptor agonists range from high-potency drugs, which are more likely to cause parkinsonian adverse effects, to low-potency drugs, which are more likely to interact with nondopaminergic receptors and thus cause cardiotoxic, epileptogenic, and anticholinergic adverse effects.

   Dopamine receptor antagonists effectively control positive symptoms (hallucinations, delusions, disordered thoughts, agitation) but have little effect on negative symptoms (withdrawal, flat affect, anhedonia, catatonia), and they cause adverse effects that may actually appear to worsen negative symptoms. Dopamine receptor antagonists are also ineffective for the treatment of cognitive impairment (perceptual distortions, memory deficits, inattentiveness).

   Dopamine receptor antagonists are commonly used to treat persons who are severely agitated and violent, although other drugs, such as benzodiazepines and barbiturates, are also usually effective for the immediate control of agitated and violent behavior. Symptoms such as extreme irritability, lack of impulse control, severe hostility, gross hyperactivity, and agitation are responsive to short-term treatment with dopamine receptor agonists.

1. **Choice of drug.** Although dopamine receptor antagonists potency varies widely (Table 25–6), all available typical dopamine receptor agonists are equally efficacious in the treatment of schizophrenia. The dopamine receptor agonists are available in a wide range of formulations and doses (Table 25–7).

   a. **Short-term treatment.** The equivalent of 5 to 10 mg of haloperidol is a reasonable dose for an adult person in an acute state. An elderly person may benefit from as little as 1 mg of haloperidol. The administration of more than 50 mg of chlorpromazine in one injection may result in serious hypotension. Intramuscular administration of the dopamine receptor agonist results in peak plasma concentrations in about 30 minutes, versus 90 minutes with the oral route. Doses of dopamine receptor antagonists for intramuscular administration are about half the doses given by the oral route. In a short-term treatment setting, the patient should be observed for 1 hour after the first dose of dopamine receptor agonist medication. After that time, most clinicians administer a second dose of a dopamine receptor agonist or a sedative agent (e.g., a benzodiazepine) to achieve effective behavioral control. Possible sedatives include 2 mg of lorazepam intramuscularly and 50 to 250 mg of amobarbital (Amytal) intramuscularly.

   b. **Long-acting depot medications.** Because some persons with schizophrenia do not comply with oral dopamine receptor agonist regimens, long-acting depot preparations may be needed. A clinician usually administers the intramuscular preparations once every 1 to 4 weeks. Therefore, the clinician immediately knows whether a person has missed a dose of medication. Depot dopamine receptor agonists may be associated with an increase in adverse effects, including tardive dyskinesia.

TABLE 25–6
DOPAMINE RECEPTOR ANTAGONISTS: TYPICAL THERAPEUTIC DOSES

Drug	Chlorpromazine Equivalent (mg)	Relative Potency	Therapeutic Dose (mg/day)[a]
Chlorpromazine (Thorazine)	100	Low	150–2000
Triflupromazine (Vesprin)	30	Medium	20–150
Thioridazine (Mellaril)	100	Low	100–800
Perphenazine (Trillafon)	10	Medium	8–64
Trifluoperazine (Stelazine)	3–5	High	5–60
Fluphenazine (Prolixin)	3–5	High	5–60
Acetophenazine (Tindal)	15	Medium	20–100
Chlorprothixene (Taractan)	75	Low	100–600
Thiothixene (Navane)	3–5	High	5–60
Loxapine (Loxitane)	10–15	Medium	30–250
Haloperidol (Haldol)	2–5	High	2–100
Pimozide (Orap)	1–2	High	2–20

[a] Extreme range.

TABLE 25–7
DOPAMINE RECEPTOR ANTAGONIST PREPARATIONS

	Tablets	Capsules	Solution	Parenteral	Rectal Suppositories
Acetophenazine	20 mg	—	—	—	—
Chlorpromazine	10, 25, 50, 100, 200 mg	30, 75, 150, 200, 300 mg	10 mg/5 mL, 30 mg/mL, 100 mg/mL	25 mg/mL	25, 100 mg
Droperidol	—	—	—	2.5 mg/mL	—
Fluphenazine	1, 2.5, 5, 10 mg	—	2.5 mg/5 mL, 6 mg/mL	2.5 mg/mL (IM only)	—
Fluphenazine deconoate	—	—	—	25 mg/mL	—
Fluphenazine enanthate	—	—	—	25 mg/mL	—
Haloperidol	0.5, 1, 2, 10, 20 mg	—	2 mg/mL	5 mg/mL (IM only)	—
Haloperidol decanoate	—	—	—	50 mg/mL, 100 mg/mL (IM only)	—
Loxapine	—	5, 10, 25, 50 mg	25 mg/mL	50 mg/mL	—
Mesoridazine	10, 25, 50, 100 mg	—	25 mg/mL	25 mg/mL	—
Molindone	5, 10, 25, 50, 100 mg	—	20 mg/mL	—	—
Perphenazine	2, 4, 8, 16 mg	—	16 mg/5 mL	5 mg/mL	—
Pimozide	2 mg	—	—	—	—
Prochlorperazine	5, 10, 25 mg	10, 15, 30 mg (SR)	5 mg/5 mL	5 mg/mL	2.5, 5, 25 mg
Promazine	25, 50, 100 mg	—	25 mg/5 mL, 100 mg/5 mL	25 mg/mL, 50 mg/mL	—
Thioridazine	10, 15, 25, 50, 100, 150, 200 mg	—	30 mg/mL, 100 mg/mL	—	—
Thiothixene	—	1, 2, 5, 10, 20 mg	5 mg/mL	10 mg (IM only), 2 mg/mL (IM only)	—
Trifluoperazine	1, 2, 5, 10 mg	—	10 mg/mL	2 mg/mL	—
Triflupromazine	—	—	—	10 mg/mL, 20 mg/mL	—

TABLE 25–8
POTENCIES AND ADVERSE EFFECT PROFILES OF DOPAMINE RECEPTOR ANTAGONISTS

Drug	Potency	Sedative Effect	Hypotensive Effect	Anticholinergic Effect	Extrapyramidal Effect
Phenothiazines					
Aliphatic					
Chlorpromazine (Thorazine)	Low	High	High	Medium	Low
Piperidines					
Mesoridazine (Serentil)	Low	Medium	Medium	Medium	Medium
Thioridazine (Mellaril)	Low	High	High	High	Low
Piperazines					
Fluphenazine (Prolixin, Permitil)	High	Medium	Low	Low	High
Perphenazine (Trilafon)	Medium	Low	Low	Low	High
Trifluoperazine (Stelazine)	High	Medium	Low	Low	High
Thioxanthene					
Thiothixene (Navane)	High	Low	Low	Low	High
Dibenzodiazepines					
Loxapine (Loxitane)	Medium	Medium	Medium	Medium	High
Butyrophenones					
Droperidol (Inapsine) injection only	Medium	Low	Low	Low	High
Haloperidol (Haldol)	High	Low	Low	Low	High
Indolone					
Molindone (Moban)	Medium	Medium	Low	Medium	High
Diphenylbutylpiperidine					
Pimozide (Orap)	High	Low	Low	Low	High

From Hyman SE, Arana GW, Rosenbaum JF. *Handbook of Psychiatric Drug Therapy*, 3rd ed. Boston: Little, Brown and Company, 1996, with permission.

2. **Precautions and adverse reactions.** Low-potency dopamine receptor agonists are most likely to cause non-neurological adverse effects, and high-potency dopamine receptor agonists are most likely to cause neurological (i.e., extrapyramidal) adverse effects (Table 25–8).

3. **Drug interactions.** Because they produce numerous receptor effects and are for the most part metabolized in the liver, the dopamine receptor agonists are associated with many pharmacokinetic and pharmacodynamic drug interactions (Table 25–9).

VI. Antidepressants

A. **SSRIs.** Four SSRIs are first-line agents for the treatment of depression. Fluoxetine was introduced in 1988, and it has since become the single most widely prescribed antidepressant in the world. During the subsequent decade, sertraline (Zoloft) and paroxetine became nearly as widely prescribed as fluoxetine. Citalopram (Celexa) was introduced in the United States in 1998. A fifth SSRI, fluvoxamine, is generally not used as an antidepressant but as a treatment for obsessive-compulsive disorder.

1. **Pharmacological actions**
   a. **Pharmacokinetics.** All SSRIs are well absorbed after oral administration and reach their peak concentrations in 4 to 8 hours. Fluoxetine has the longest half-life, 2 to 3 days; its active metabolite nor-

TABLE 25–9
ANTIPSYCHOTIC DRUG INTERACTIONS

Drug	Consequences
Tricyclic antidepressants	Increased concentration of both
Anticholinergics	Anticholinergic toxicity, decreased absorption of antipsychotics
Antacids	Decreased absorption of antipsychotics
Cimetidine	Decreased absorption of antipsychotics
Food	Decreased absorption of antipsychotics
Buspirone	Elevation of haloperidol levels
Barbiturates	Increased metabolism of antipsychotics, excessive sedation
Phenytoin	Decreased phenytoin metabolism
Guanethidine	Reduced hypotensive effect
Clonidine	Reduced hypotensive effect
α-Methyldopa	Reduced hypotensive effect
Levodopa	Decreased effects of both
Succinylcholine	Prolonged muscle paralysis
Monoamine oxidase inhibitors	Hypotension
Halothane	Hypotension
Alcohol	Potentiation of CNS depression
Cigarettes	Decreased plasma levels of antipsychotics
Epinephrine	Hypotension
Propranolol	Increased plasma concentration of both
Warfarin	Decreased plasma concentrations of warfarin

fluoxetine has a half-life of 7 to 9 days. The half-life of sertraline is 26 hours, and its significantly less active metabolite has a half-life of 3 to 5 days. The half-lives of the other three SSRIs, which do not have metabolites with significant pharmacological activity, are 35 hours for citalopram, 21 hours for paroxetine, and 15 hours for fluvoxamine.

The administration of the SSRIs with food has little effect on absorption and may reduce the incidence of nausea and diarrhea.

b. Pharmacodynamics. The clinical benefits of SSRIs are attributed to the relatively selective inhibition of serotonin reuptake, with little effect on the reuptake of norepinephrine and dopamine. The same degree of clinical benefit can usually be achieved through either steady use of a low dosage or more rapid escalation of the dosage. However, the clinical response varies considerably from person to person.

2. Therapeutic indications

a. Depression. Fluoxetine, sertraline, paroxetine, and citalopram are indicated for the treatment of depression, based on several multicenter, double-blinded, placebo-controlled studies. SSRIs are first-line agents for the treatment of depression in the general population, the elderly, the medically ill, and pregnant women. SSRIs are as effective as any other class of antidepressants for mild and moderate depression. For severe depression and melancholia, several studies have found that the maximum efficacy of serotonin-norepinephrine reuptake inhibitors, such as venlafaxine or tricyclic drugs, often exceeds that of SSRIs. However, recent evidence suggests that sertraline is more effective than the other SSRIs for severe depression with melancholia. It is appropriate to initiate antidepressant therapy with SSRIs for all degrees of depression.

(1) **Choice of drug.** Direct comparisons of the benefits of specific SSRIs have not shown any one to be generally superior to the others. However, responses to the various SSRIs can vary considerably within a given patient. A number of reports indicate that more than 50% of people who respond poorly to one SSRI will respond favorably to another. Thus, it is most reasonable for patients who do not respond to their first SSRI to try other agents in the SSRI class before shifting to non-SSRI antidepressants.

(2) **Comparison with tricyclic antidepressants.** Several controlled studies have shown that the efficacy of the SSRIs is similar to that of the tricyclic antidepressants, but that their adverse effect profile is markedly better. These studies have also consistently shown that some degree of nervousness or agitation, sleep disturbances, gastrointestinal symptoms, and perhaps sexual adverse effects are more common in persons treated with SSRIs than in those treated with tricyclic drugs.

b. **Suicide.** In the overwhelming majority of people at risk for suicide, SSRIs reduce the risk. In the late 1980s, a widely publicized report suggested an association between fluoxetine use and violent acts, including suicide, but many subsequent reviews have clearly refuted this association. A few persons, however, become especially anxious and agitated when given fluoxetine. The appearance of these symptoms in a suicidal person could conceivably aggravate the seriousness of their suicidal ideation. An additional caveat is the observation that suicidal persons often act out their suicidal thoughts more effectively as they recover from their depression. Thus, potentially suicidal persons should be closely monitored during the first few weeks of SSRI therapy.

c. **Depression during and after pregnancy.** The use of fluoxetine during pregnancy is not associated with increases in perinatal complications, congenital fetal anomalies, learning disabilities, language delays, or specific behavioral problems. Emerging data for sertraline, paroxetine, and fluvoxamine indicate that these agents are probably similarly safe when taken during pregnancy.

Prospective studies have found that the risk for relapse into depression when a newly pregnant mother discontinues SSRI treatment is several times greater than the risk to the fetus caused by exposure to SSRIs. Because maternal depression is a independent risk factor for fetal morbidity, the data clearly indicate that SSRI use before pregnancy should be continued without interruption during pregnancy. SSRIs very rarely produce transient neonatal jitteriness and mild tachypnea.

Highly sensitive laboratory techniques generally do not detect any evidence of SSRIs in the plasma of babies being breast-fed by mothers taking SSRIs. However, at least one breast-fed infant is reported to have had a plasma concentration of sertraline equal to one half of the maternal concentration. Nevertheless, this infant showed no abnormal behaviors. Therefore, the use of these drugs probably does not expose most nursing infants to any more risk than does exposure in utero.

d. Depression in the elderly and medically ill. The ideal antidepressant in this population would cause no cognitive, cardiotoxic, anticholinergic, antihistaminergic, or α-adrenergic adverse effects. Of the SSRIs, only paroxetine has some anticholinergic activity, although this is clinically relevant only at higher doses. All SSRIs are useful for elderly, medically frail persons. Fluoxetine has been approved by the FDA for the treatment of geriatric depression.

e. Chronic depression. SSRI treatment combined with monthly interpersonal psychotherapy markedly reduces the rate of relapse of patients with depression during a 3-year period. Because discontinuation of SSRIs within 6 months after a depressive episode is associated with a high rate of relapse, a person with chronic depression should remain on SSRI therapy for several years. SSRIs are well tolerated in long-term use.

f. Depression in children. SSRIs are increasingly prescribed to treat childhood depression and to forestall efforts by children and adolescents to self-medicate their depressed feelings with alcohol or illicit drugs. The adverse effect profile of SSRIs in children includes gastrointestinal symptoms, insomnia, motor restlessness, social disinhibition, mania, hypomania, and psychosis.

g. Premenstrual dysphoric disorder. SSRIs reduce the debilitating mood and behavioral changes that occur in the week preceding menstruation in women with premenstrual dysphoric disorder. Scheduled administration of SSRIs either throughout the cycle or only during the luteal phase (the 2-week period between ovulation and menstruation) is equally effective for this purpose.

The use of fluoxetine has been associated with both increases and decreases in the duration of the menstrual period of more than 4 days. The significance of SSRI effects on the length of the menstrual cycle is mostly unknown and warrants further study.

3. Clinical guidelines

a. Dosage and administration.

(1) Fluoxetine. Fluoxetine is available in 10- and 20-mg capsules, a scored 10-mg tablet, and as a liquid (20 mg/5 mL). For the treatment of depression, the initial dosage is usually 10 or 20 mg/day orally. The drug is generally taken in the morning because insomnia is a potential adverse effect. Fluoxetine may be taken with food to minimize possible nausea. Because of the long half-lives of the drug and its metabolite, a 4-week period is required to reach steady-state concentrations. As with all available antidepressants, the antidepressant effects of fluoxetine may be seen in the first 1 to 3 weeks, but the clinician should wait until the patient has been taking the drug for 4 to 6 weeks before definitively evaluating its antidepressant activity.

Several studies indicate that 20 mg may be as effective as higher doses for the treatment of depression. The maximum daily dosage recommended by the manufacturer is 80 mg/day, and higher dosages may cause seizures. A reasonable strategy is to maintain a patient on 20 mg/day for 3 weeks. If the patient shows no signs of clinical improvement at that time, an increase to 40 mg/day may be warranted.

To minimize the early adverse effects of anxiety and restlessness, some clinicians initiate fluoxetine at 5 to 10 mg/day, with use of the scored 10-mg tablets. Alternatively, because of the long half-life of fluoxetine, the drug can be initiated with an every-other-day administration schedule.

At least 2 weeks should elapse between the discontinuation of MAOIs and the initiation of fluoxetine. Fluoxetine must be discontinued for at least 5 weeks before the initiation of MAOI treatment.

(2) Sertraline. Sertraline is available in scored 25-mg, 50-mg, and 100-mg tablets. For the initial treatment of depression, sertraline should be initiated at a dosage of 50 mg taken once daily. To limit the gastrointestinal effects, some clinicians begin at 25 mg/day and increase the dosage to 50 mg/day after 3 weeks. Persons who do not respond after 1 to 3 weeks may benefit from increases of 50 mg every week up to a maximum dosage of 200 mg taken once daily. Sertraline generally is given in the evening because it is somewhat more likely to cause sedation than insomnia. Persons who experience gastrointestinal symptoms may benefit by taking the drug with food.

The guidelines for dosage increases of sertraline are similar to those for fluoxetine. Several studies suggest that maintaining a dosage of 50 mg/day for many weeks may be nearly as beneficial as rapidly increasing the dosage. Nevertheless, many clinicians tend to use maintenance dosages of 100 to 200 mg/day.

(3) Paroxetine. Paroxetine is available in scored 20-mg tablets, unscored 10-mg, 30-mg, and 40-mg tablets, and an orange-flavored oral suspension with a concentration of 10 mg/5 mL. Paroxetine is usually initiated for the treatment of depression at a dosage of 10 or 20 mg/day. An increase should be considered when an adequate response is not seen in 1 to 3 weeks. At that point, the clinician can initiate upward titration in 10-mg increments at weekly intervals to a maximum dosage of 50 mg/day. Dosages of up to 80 mg/day may be tolerated. Persons who experience gastrointestinal symptoms may benefit by taking the drug with food.

Paroxetine should be taken initially as a single daily dose in the evening. Higher dosages may be divided into two doses per day. Persons with melancholic features may require dosages greater than 20 mg/day. The suggested therapeutic dosage range for elderly persons is 10 to 20 mg/day.

Paroxetine is the SSRI most likely to produce a discontinuation syndrome because its plasma concentrations drop rapidly in the absence of continuous dosing. To limit the development of symptoms of abrupt discontinuation, the dosage of paroxetine should be reduced by 10 mg each week until it is 10 mg/day, at which point it may be stopped either directly or after an additional decrease to 5 mg/day.

(4) **Citalopram.** Citalopram is available in scored 20- and 40-mg tablets. The usual starting dosage is 20 mg/day for the first week, after which it is generally increased to 40 mg/day. Some persons may require 60 mg/day, but no controlled trials are available to support this dosage. For elderly persons or persons with hepatic impairment, a dosage of 20 mg/day is recommended, with an increase to 40 mg/day only if no response is noted at 20 mg/day. Tablets should be taken once daily, either in the morning or evening, with or without food.

b. **Strategies for limiting adverse effects.** Three fourths of people experience no adverse effects at low starting dosages of SSRIs, and dosages may be increased relatively rapidly (i.e., on the order of an increase every 1 to 2 weeks) in this group. In the remaining fourth of persons, most of the adverse effects of the SSRIs appear within the first 1 to 2 weeks, and they generally subside or resolve spontaneously if the drugs are continued at the same dosage. However, 10–15% of people are not able to tolerate the lowest dosage of a particular SSRI and may discontinue the drug after taking only a few doses. One approach for such persons is to fractionate the dose over a week, with one dose taken every 2, 3, or 4 days. Some people may tolerate a different SSRI or another class of antidepressant, such as a tricyclic drug or one of the other newer agents. However, some people appear unable to tolerate even tiny doses of any antidepressant drug.

Because SSRI adverse effects generally come and go before the desired effect is noted, many experts begin with a very low dosage for the first 3 to 6 weeks, then increase gradually once a therapeutic benefit is seen. Because of the long half-lives of the SSRIs, especially fluoxetine, and the even longer time it may take for the full benefit of a particular dosage to be appreciated, steep increases in dosage are to be avoided. For example, the lowest dosage may provide more than 90% of the benefit of the highest dosage if enough time is allowed. On the other hand, adverse effects are much more predictably dosage-dependent, and too rapid an increase in dosage may provoke an adverse response in a sensitive person.

c. **Augmentation strategies.** In depressed people with a partial response to SSRIs, augmentation strategies have generally not proved superior to increases in the SSRI dosage. However, one such drug combination, SSRIs plus bupropion, has demonstrated marked added benefits. Some persons have also responded favorably to the addition of lithium, levothyroxine (Levoxine, Levothroid, Synthroid), or amphetamines.

  d. **Loss of efficacy.** Potential methods to manage attenuation of the response to an SSRI include increasing or decreasing the dosage; tapering the drug, then rechallenging with the same medication; switching to another SSRI or non-SSRI antidepressant; and augmenting with bupropion, thyroid hormone, lithium, sympathomimetics, buspirone, anticonvulsants, naltrexone (ReVia), or another non-SSRI antidepressant. A change in response to an SSRI should be explored in psychotherapy, which may reveal the underlying conflicts causing an increase in depressive symptoms.

4. Precautions and adverse reactions

  a. **Sexual dysfunction.** Sexual inhibition is the most common adverse effect of SSRIs. Rates of sexual dysfunction are reported in premarketing trials at less than 10%, but this is a consequence of considerable undersampling. As clinicians have become more active in questioning persons about their sexual functioning, the true incidence appears to be closer to 80%. Most of the sexual dysfunction is mild, and the SSRIs all appear to be equally likely to cause it. The most common complaints are inhibited orgasm and decreased libido, which are dosage-dependent. Unlike most of the other adverse effects of SSRIs, sexual inhibition does not resolve within the first few weeks of use but usually continues as long as the drug is taken.

  Treatment for SSRI-induced sexual dysfunction includes decreasing the dosage; switching to bupropion or nefazodone, which causes less sexual dysfunction; adding 150 mg of the sustained-release preparation of bupropion once or twice per day; and adding sildenafil (Viagra), yohimbine (Yocon), cyproheptadine (Periactin), or dopamine agonists. The combination of an SSRI with bupropion is effective both in producing an antidepressant effect and in reducing sexual inhibition.

  b. **Gastrointestinal adverse effects.** Sertraline, citalopram, and fluvoxamine have the highest rates of gastrointestinal adverse effects, but these are also caused by fluoxetine and paroxetine. The most common gastrointestinal complaints are nausea, diarrhea, anorexia, vomiting, and dyspepsia. The nausea and loose stools are dosage-related and transient, usually resolving within a few weeks. Anorexia is most common with fluoxetine, but some people gain weight while taking fluoxetine. Fluoxetine-induced loss of appetite and loss of weight begin as soon as the drug is taken and peak at 20 weeks, after which weight often returns to baseline.

  c. **Weight gain.** Up to one third of people taking SSRIs gain weight, sometimes more than 20 pounds. Among those who gained weight in clinical trials, the mean weight gain was 21 lb with fluoxetine, 15 lb with sertraline, and 16 lb with citalopram. Paroxetine has anticholinergic activity and is the SSRI most often associated with weight gain. Weight usually returns to baseline by the end of the first year of treatment.

d. Headaches. The incidence of headache in SSRI trials was 18–20%, only one percentage point higher than the placebo rate. Fluoxetine is the most likely to cause headache. On the other hand, all SSRIs are effective prophylaxis against both migraine and tension-type headaches in many people.

e. CNS adverse effects

   (1) Anxiety. Fluoxetine is the most likely to cause anxiety, agitation, and restlessness, particularly in the first few weeks. These initial effects usually give way to an overall reduction in anxiety after the first month of use. Five percent of people discontinue taking fluoxetine because of increased nervousness. An increase in anxiety is caused considerably less frequently by the other SSRIs.

   (2) Insomnia and sedation. The major effect in this area attributable to SSRIs is improved sleep resulting from the treatment of depression and anxiety. However, as many as one fourth of people taking SSRIs note either trouble sleeping or excessive somnolence. Fluoxetine is the most likely to cause insomnia, for which reason it is often taken in the morning. Sertraline is about equally likely to cause insomnia or somnolence; citalopram and especially paroxetine are more likely to cause somnolence than insomnia. With the latter agents, people usually report that taking the dose before retiring helps them sleep better and does not cause residual daytime somnolence.

   SSRI-induced insomnia can be treated with benzodiazepines, trazodone (clinicians must explain the risk for priapism), or other sedating medicines. The presence of significant SSRI-induced somnolence often requires switching to another SSRI or to bupropion.

   (3) Vivid dreams and nightmares. A minority of people taking SSRIs report recalling extremely vivid dreams or nightmares. A patient experiencing such dreams with one SSRI may derive the same therapeutic benefit without disturbing dream images by switching to another SSRI. This adverse effect often resolves spontaneously during several weeks.

   (4) Seizures. Seizures have been reported in 0.1–0.2% of all persons treated with SSRIs. This incidence is comparable with the incidence reported with other antidepressants and is not significantly different from that noted with placebo. Seizures are more frequent at the highest dosages of SSRIs (100 mg or more of fluoxetine per day).

   (5) Extrapyramidal symptoms. Tremor is seen in 5–10% of people taking SSRIs, a frequency two to four times that seen with placebo. SSRIs may rarely cause akathisia, dystonia, tremor, cogwheel rigidity, torticollis, opisthotonos, gait disorders, and bradykinesia. People with well-controlled Parkinson's disease may experience acute worsening of their motor symptoms when they take SSRIs. Extrapyramidal adverse effects are most closely associated with the use of fluoxetine; they are particularly noted at dosages in excess of 40 mg/day but may occur at any time during the course of therapy.

f. Anticholinergic effects. Paroxetine has mild anticholinergic activity that causes dry mouth, constipation, and sedation in a dosage-dependent fashion. However, the anticholinergic activity of paroxetine is perhaps only one-fifth that of nortriptyline, and most persons taking paroxetine do not experience cholinergic adverse effects. Although not considered to have anticholinergic activity, the other SSRIs are associated with dry mouth in 14–20% of people, a rate one and one-half to two times that of placebo.

g. Hematologic adverse effects. SSRIs affect platelet function but are rarely associated with increased bruisability. Paroxetine and fluoxetine are rarely associated with the development of reversible neutropenia, particularly if administered concurrently with clozapine.

h. Electrolyte and glucose disturbances. SSRIs are rarely associated with a decrease in glucose concentrations; therefore, persons with diabetes should be carefully monitored and the dosage of their hypoglycemic drug decreased as necessary. Rare cases of SSRI-associated hyponatremia and the secretion of inappropriate antidiuretic hormone (SIADH) have been seen in persons treated with diuretics who are also water-deprived.

i. Rash and allergic reactions. Various types of rashes may appear in about 4% of all persons; in a small subset, generalization of the allergic reaction and involvement of the pulmonary system result rarely in fibrotic damage and dyspnea. SSRI treatment may have to be discontinued in persons with drug-related rashes.

j. Galactorrhea. SSRIs may cause reversible galactorrhea, presumably a consequence of interference with dopaminergic regulation of prolactin secretion.

k. Serotonin syndrome. Concurrent administration of an SSRI with an MAOI can raise plasma serotonin concentrations to toxic levels and produce a constellation of symptoms called *serotonin syndrome*. This serious and possibly fatal syndrome of serotonin overstimulation comprises, in order of appearance as the condition worsens, (1) diarrhea; (2) restlessness; (3) extreme agitation, hyperreflexia, and autonomic instability with possible rapid fluctuations of vital signs; (4) myoclonus, seizures, hyperthermia, uncontrollable shivering, and rigidity; and (5) delirium, coma, status epilepticus, cardiovascular collapse, and death.

Treatment of the serotonin syndrome consists of removing the offending agents and promptly instituting comprehensive supportive care with nitroglycerine, cyproheptadine, methysergide (Sansert), cooling blankets, chlorpromazine (Thorazine), dantrolene (Dantrium), benzodiazepines, anticonvulsants, mechanical ventilation, and paralyzing agents.

l. **SSRI discontinuation syndrome.** The abrupt discontinuance of an SSRI, especially one with a relatively short half-life, such as paroxetine, has been associated with a syndrome that may include dizziness, weakness, nausea, headache, rebound depression, anxiety, insomnia, poor concentration, upper respiratory symptoms, paresthesias, and migraine-like symptoms. It usually does not appear until after at least 6 weeks of treatment and generally resolves spontaneously in 3 weeks. Persons who experience transient adverse effects in the first weeks of SSRI therapy are more likely to experience discontinuation symptoms. Fluoxetine is the least likely to be associated with this syndrome because the half-life of its metabolite is more than 1 week and it effectively tapers itself. Fluoxetine has therefore been used in some cases to treat the discontinuation syndrome associated with the termination of therapy with other SSRIs, although the syndrome itself is self-limited.

5. **Drug interactions.** See Table 25–10. SSRIs do not interfere with most other drugs. A serotonin syndrome can develop with concurrent administration of MAOIs, L-tryptophan, lithium, or other antidepressants that inhibit the reuptake of serotonin. Fluoxetine, sertraline, and paroxetine can raise the plasma concentrations of tricyclic antidepressants to levels that can cause clinical toxicity. A number of potential pharmacokinetic interactions have been described based on in vitro analyses of the CYP enzymes, but clinically relevant interactions are rare.

The combination of lithium and all serotonergic drugs should be used with caution because of the possibility of precipitating seizures. SSRIs may increase the duration and severity of zolpidem-induced hallucinations.

a. **Fluoxetine.** Fluoxetine can be administered with low dosages of tricyclic drugs. Because it is metabolized by the hepatic CYP 2D6 isoenzyme, fluoxetine may interfere with the metabolism of other drugs in the 7% of the population that has an inefficient isoform of this enzyme, the so-called poor metabolizers. Fluoxetine may slow the metabolism of carbamazepine, antineoplastic agents, diazepam, and phenytoin. Possibly significant drug interactions have been described for fluoxetine with benzodiazepines, antipsychotics, and lithium. Fluoxetine does not interact with warfarin, tolbutamide (Orinase), or chlorothiazide (Diuril).

b. **Sertraline.** Sertraline may displace warfarin from plasma proteins and may increase the prothrombin time. The drug interaction data on sertraline support a generally similar profile to that of fluoxetine, although sertraline does not interact as strongly with the CYP 2D6 enzyme.

c. **Paroxetine.** Paroxetine is associated with a higher risk for drug interactions than either fluoxetine or sertraline because it is a more potent inhibitor of the CYP 2D6 enzyme. Cimetidine can increase

TABLE 25–10
INTERACTIONS OF DRUGS WITH THE SSRI's

SSRI	Other Drugs	Effect	Clinical Importance
Fluoxetine	Desipramine	Inhibits metabolism	Possible
	Carbamazepine	Inhibits metabolism	Possible
	Diazepam	Inhibits metabolism	Not important
	Haloperidol	Inhibits metabolism	Possible
	Warfarin	No interaction	
	Tolbutamide	No interaction	
Fluvoxamine	Antipyrine	Inhibits metabolism	Not important
	Propranolol	Inhibits metabolism	Unlikely
	Tricyclics	Inhibits metabolism	Unlikely
	Warfarin	Inhibits metabolism	Possible
	Atenolol	No interaction	
	Digoxin	No interaction	
Paroxetine	Phenytoin	AUC increases by 12%	Possible
	Procyclidine	AUC increases by 39%	Possible
	Cimetidine	Paroxetine AUC increases by 50%	Possible
	Antipyrine	No interaction	
	Digoxin	No interaction	
	Propranolol	No interaction	
	Tranylcypromine	No interaction	Caution with combined treatment
	Warfarin	No interaction	Not important
Sertraline	Antipyrine	Increased clearance	
	Diazepam	Clearance decreased by 13%	Not important
	Tolbutamide	Clearance decreased by 16%	Not important
	Digoxin	No interaction	
	Lithium	No pharmacokinetic interaction	Caution with combined treatment
	Desipramine	No interaction	
	Atenolol	No pharmacokinetic interaction	
Citalopram	Cimetidine	Citalopram AUC increases	
	Metoprolol	May double blood concentration	

Adapted from Warrington SJ: Clinical implications of the pharmacology of serotonin reuptake inhibitors. *Int Clin Psychopharmacol* 1987; 7(Suppl 2):13, with permission.
AUC, area under curve.

the concentrations of sertraline and paroxetine, and phenobarbital (Solfoton, Luminal) and phenytoin can decrease the concentrations of paroxetine. Because of the potential for interference with the CYP 2D6 enzyme, the coadministration of paroxetine with other antidepressants, phenothiazine, and antiarrhythmic drugs should be undertaken with caution. Paroxetine may increase the anticoagulant effect of warfarin. Coadministration of paroxetine and tramadol (Ultram) may precipitate a serotonin syndrome in elderly persons.

d. **Citalopram.** Citalopram is not a potent inhibitor of any CYP enzymes. Concurrent administration of cimetidine increases concentrations of citalopram by about 40%. Citalopram does not significantly affect the metabolism of, nor is its metabolism significantly affected by, digoxin (Lanoxicaps, Lanoxin), lithium, warfarin, carbamazepine, or imipramine. Citalopram increases plasma concentrations of metoprolol (Toprol XL, Lopressor) twofold, but this usually has no effect on blood pressure or heart rate. Data on the coadministration of citalopram and potent inhibitors of CYP 3A4 or CYP 2D6 are not available.

B. Venlafaxine. Venlafaxine is an effective antidepressant drug with a rapid onset of action. Venlafaxine is among the most efficacious drugs for the treatment of severe depression with melancholic features.

1. **Pharmacological actions.** Venlafaxine is well absorbed from the gastrointestinal tract and reaches peak plasma concentrations within 2.5 hours. It has a half-life of about 3.5 hours, and its one active metabolite, O-desmethylvenlafaxine, has a half-life of 9 hours. Therefore, venlafaxine must be taken 2 to 3 times daily.

   Venlafaxine is a nonselective inhibitor of the reuptake of three biogenic amines—serotonin, norepinephrine, and, to a lesser extent, dopamine. Venlafaxine does not have activity at muscarinic, nicotinic, histaminergic, opioid, or adrenergic receptors, and it is not active as an MAOI.

2. **Therapeutic efficacy.** Venlafaxine is approved for the treatment of major depressive disorder and generalized anxiety disorder. Many severely depressed persons respond to venlafaxine at a dosage of 200 mg/day within 2 weeks, a period of time somewhat shorter than the 2 to 4 weeks usually required for the SSRIs to take effect. Therefore, venlafaxine at high dosages may become a preferred drug for seriously ill persons in whom a rapid response is desired. However, sympathomimetics (e.g., amphetamines) and ECT appear to have the most rapid onset of antidepressant action, usually taking effect within 1 week. In direct comparison with fluoxetine for the treatment of seriously depressed persons with melancholic features, venlafaxine is considered superior. A direct comparison of venlafaxine and sertraline, the most effective SSRI for the treatment of severe depression with melancholia, has not yet been reported.

3. **Clinical guidelines.** Venlafaxine is available in 25-, 37.5-, 50-, 75-, and 100-mg immediate-release tablets and in 37.5-, 75-, and 150-mg extended-release capsules (Effexor XR). The immediate-release tablets should be given in two or three daily doses, and the extended-release capsules are taken in a single dose before sleep up to a maximum dosage of 225 mg/day. The tablets and the extended-release capsules are equally potent, and persons stabilized with one can switch to an equivalent dosage of the other.

   The usual starting dosage in depressed persons is 75 mg/day, given as tablets in two to three divided doses or as extended-release capsules in a single dose before sleep. Some persons require a starting dosage of 37.5 mg/day for 4 to 7 days to minimize adverse effects, particularly nausea, before titration up to 75 mg/day. In persons with depression, the dosage can be raised to 150 mg/day, given as tablets in two or three divided doses or as extended-release capsules once at night, after an appropriate period of clinical assessment at the lower dosage (usually 2 to 3 weeks). The dosage can be raised in increments of 75 mg/day every 4 days or more. Moderately depressed persons probably do not require dosages in excess of 225 mg/day, whereas severely depressed persons may require dosages of 300 to 375 mg/day for a satisfactory response.

A rapid antidepressant response—within 1 to 2 weeks—may result from the administration of a dosage of 200 mg/day from the beginning. The maximum dosage of venlafaxine is 375 mg/day. The dosage of venlafaxine should be halved in persons with significant diminished hepatic or renal function. If discontinued, venlafaxine should be gradually tapered during 2 to 4 weeks.

4. **Precautions and adverse reactions.** Venlafaxine is generally well tolerated. The following were the most common adverse reactions, occurring significantly more frequently with venlafaxine than with placebo in controlled studies: nausea (37% of all persons treated), somnolence (23%), dry mouth (22%), dizziness (19%), nervousness (13%), constipation (15%), asthenia (12%), anxiety (6%), anorexia (11%), blurred vision (6%), abnormal ejaculation or orgasm (12%), and impotence (6%). The incidence of nausea is reduced somewhat with use of the extended-release capsules. The sexual adverse effects of venlafaxine can be treated like those of the SSRIs. Because of its rapid metabolism and relative lack of protein binding, abrupt discontinuation of venlafaxine may produce a discontinuation syndrome consisting of nausea, somnolence, and insomnia. Therefore, venlafaxine should be tapered gradually during 2 to 4 weeks.

The most potentially worrisome adverse effect associated with venlafaxine is an increase in blood pressure in some persons, particularly those treated with more than 300 mg/day. In clinical trials, a mean increase in diastolic blood pressure of 7.2 mm Hg was observed in persons receiving 375 mg of venlafaxine per day, in contrast to no significant change in persons receiving 75 or 225 mg/day and a mean decrease of 2.2 mm Hg in persons receiving placebo. In one study, sustained elevations of blood pressure to levels higher than 140/90 were noted in 2% of persons who received placebo, 3% of persons who received less than 100 mg of venlafaxine per day, 5% of persons who received 101 to 200 mg/day, 7% of persons who received 201 to 300 mg/day, and 13% of persons who received more than 300 mg/day. Thus, the drug should be used cautiously by persons with preexisting hypertension, and then only at lower dosages.

Information about the use of venlafaxine by pregnant and nursing women is not available at this time. However, clinicians should avoid prescribing all newly introduced drugs to pregnant and nursing women until more clinical experience has been acquired.

5. **Drug interactions.** Cimetidine appears to inhibit the first-pass hepatic metabolism of venlafaxine and raise concentrations of the unmetabolized drug. However, because the metabolite is mainly responsible for the therapeutic effect, this interaction is of concern only in persons with preexisting hypertension or hepatic disease, in whom the combination should be avoided. Venlafaxine may raise plasma concentrations of concurrently administered haloperidol. Like all antidepressant medications, venlafaxine should not be used within 14 days of the use

of MAOIs, and it may potentiate the sedative effects of other drugs that act on the CNS.

C. Bupropion. Bupropion is a first-line agent for the treatment of depression and for smoking cessation. It generally is more effective against symptoms of depression than of anxiety, and it is quite effective in combination with SSRIs. Despite early warnings that it could cause seizures, clinical experience now shows that when used at recommended dosages, bupropion is no more likely to cause seizures than any other antidepressant drug. Smoking cessation is most successful when bupropion (called Zyban for this indication) is used in combination with behavioral modification techniques.

Bupropion is a unique antidepressant in the available armamentarium of drugs, with a highly favorable profile of adverse effects. Of particular note among antidepressants, inhibition of sexual function is minor with this drug. It has some dopaminergic effects and may serve as a mild psychostimulant as well as an antidepressant.

1. **Pharmacological actions.** Bupropion is well absorbed from the gastrointestinal tract. Peak plasma concentrations of the immediate-release formulation of bupropion are usually reached within 2 hours of oral administration, and peak concentrations of the sustained-release formulation are seen after 3 hours. The half-life of the compound ranges from 8 to 40 hours (mean, 12 hours).

2. **Therapeutic efficacy.** The therapeutic efficacy of bupropion in depression is well established in both outpatient and inpatient settings. Bupropion is a good choice for depressed persons who do not respond to serotonergic drugs. Improvement in sleep early in the course of treatment is seen less often with bupropion than with most other antidepressants.

3. **Dosage and administration.** Immediate-release bupropion is available in 75- and 100-mg tablets, and sustained-release bupropion (Wellbutrin SR) is available in 100- and 150-mg tablets. Treatment in the average adult person should be initiated at 100 mg of the immediate-release version orally twice a day, or 150 mg of the sustained-release version once a day. On the fourth day of treatment, the dosage can be raised to 100 mg of the immediate release preparation orally three times a day, or 150 mg of the sustained-release preparation orally twice a day. Alternatively, 300 mg of the sustained-release version can be taken once each morning. The dosage of 300 mg/day should be maintained for several weeks before it is increased further. Because of the risk for seizures, increases in dosage should never exceed 100 mg in a 3-day period; a single dose of immediate-release bupropion should never exceed 150 mg, and a single dose of sustained-release bupropion should never exceed 300 mg; the total daily dose should not exceed 450 mg (immediate-release) or 400 mg (sustained-release).

4. **Precautions and adverse reactions.** The most common adverse effects associated with the use of bupropion are headache, insomnia, upper respiratory complaints, and nausea. Restlessness, agitation, and irritability may also occur. Most likely because of its potentiating effects on dopaminergic neurotransmission, bupropion has rarely been

associated with psychotic symptoms (e.g., hallucinations, delusions, and catatonia) and delirium. Most notable about bupropion is the absence of significant drug-induced orthostatic hypotension, weight gain, daytime drowsiness, and anticholinergic effects. Some persons, however, may experience dry mouth or constipation, and weight loss may occur in about 25% of persons. Bupropion causes no significant cardiovascular or clinical laboratory changes.

A major advantage of bupropion over SSRIs is that bupropion is virtually devoid of any adverse effects on sexual functioning, whereas the SSRIs are associated with such effects in up to 80% of all persons. Some people taking bupropion experience an increase in sexual responsiveness and even spontaneous orgasm.

At dosages of 300 mg/day or less, the incidence of seizures is about 0.1%, which is no worse, and in some cases superior, to the incidence of seizures with other antidepressants. The risk for seizures increases to about 5% in dosages between 450 and 600 mg/day. Risk factors for seizures, such as a past history of seizures, use of alcohol, recent benzodiazepine withdrawal, organic brain disease, head trauma, or epileptiform discharges on EEG, warrant critical examination of the decision to use bupropion.

Care should be used in anyone with a history of head trauma, brain tumor, or other organic brain disease because bupropion may reduce the patient's seizure threshold. The presence of EEG abnormalities and recent withdrawal from alcohol or a sedative-hypnotic may also increase the risk for a bupropion-induced seizure. Because high dosages (> 450 mg/day) of bupropion may be associated with a euphoric feeling, bupropion may be relatively contraindicated in persons with a history of substance abuse. The use of bupropion by pregnant women has not been studied and is not recommended. Because bupropion is secreted in breast milk, its use in nursing women is not recommended.

Overdoses of bupropion are associated with a generally favorable outcome, except in cases of huge doses and overdoses of mixed drugs. Seizures occur in about a third of all cases of overdose, and fatalities may result from uncontrollable seizures, bradycardia, and cardiac arrest. In general, however, overdoses of bupropion are less harmful than overdoses of other antidepressants, except perhaps the SSRIs.

5. **Drug interactions.** Bupropion should not be used concurrently with MAOIs because of the possibility of inducing a hypertensive crisis, and at least 14 days should pass after an MAOI is discontinued before treatment with bupropion is initiated. Delirium, psychotic symptoms, and dyskinetic movements may be associated with the coadministration of bupropion and dopaminergic agents (e.g., levodopa [Laradopa], pergolide [Permax], ropinirole [Requip], pramipexole [Mirapex], amantadine [Symmetrel], and bromocriptine [Parlodel]). Bupropion in combination with lithium is effective and well tolerated in some persons with refractory depression, but this combination may rarely cause CNS toxicity, including seizures.

The combination of bupropion and fluoxetine is one of the most effective and well-tolerated treatments for all types of depression, but a few case reports indicate that panic, delirium, or seizures may be associated with this combination. Carbamazepine may decrease plasma concentrations of bupropion, and bupropion may increase plasma concentrations of valproic acid (Depakene).

D. Nefazodone. Nefazodone has antidepressant effects comparable with those of SSRIs, yet unlike SSRIs, nefazodone improves sleep continuity and has little effect on sexual functioning. Nefazodone is generally well tolerated. It is chemically related to trazodone but causes less sedation. However, some experts believe that nefazodone is generally a less effective antidepressant than the SSRIs.

1. **Clinical guidelines.** Nefazodone is available in 50-, 200-, and 250-mg unscored and 100- and 150-mg scored tablets. The recommended starting dosage of nefazodone is 100 mg twice daily, but 50 mg twice daily may be better tolerated, especially in elderly persons. To limit the development of adverse effects, the daily dose should be slowly increased in increments of 100 to 200 mg, with intervals of no less than 1 week between each increase. Elderly patients should receive about two-thirds the usual nongeriatric dosages, with a maximum of 400 mg/day. The clinical benefits of nefazodone, like those of other antidepressants, usually become apparent after 2 to 4 weeks of treatment.

2. **Precautions and adverse reactions.** In preclinical trials, 16% of persons discontinued nefazodone because of an adverse event. The most common reasons for discontinuance were nausea (3.5%), dizziness (1.9%), insomnia (1.5%), weakness (1.3%), and agitation (1.2%). The adverse reactions reported with nefazodone are listed in Table 25–11. The adverse events were dosage-dependent and tended to appear at significant concentrations (dosages >300 mg/day).

E. Mirtazapine. Mirtazapine is as effective as amitriptyline in lifting mood, yet it lacks the anticholinergic effects of the tricyclic antidepressants and the gastrointestinal and anxiogenic effects of the SSRIs. It is little used because it is no more efficacious than other antidepressants and causes as much somnolence as tricyclic drugs.

TABLE 25–11
ADVERSE REACTIONS REPORTED WITH NEFAZODONE (300–600 mg/d) AND PLACEBO

Reaction	Nefazodone (%)	Placebo (%)
Headache	36	33
Dry mouth	25	13
Somnolence	25	14
Nausea	22	12
Dizziness	17	5
Constipation	14	8
Insomnia	11	9
Weakness	11	5
Lightheadedness	10	3
Blurred vision	9	3
Dyspepsia	9	7
Confusion	7	2

F. **Reboxetine (Vestra).** Reboxetine is not yet approved for sale in the United States. It selectively inhibits norepinephrine reuptake and has little effect on serotonin reuptake. It is thus a mirror image of the SSRIs, which inhibit the reuptake of serotonin but not of norepinephrine. In direct clinical comparison with fluoxetine, reboxetine was a more effective treatment for persons with severe depression, poor self-image, and little motivation.

1. **Therapeutic efficacy.** Reboxetine is effective for the treatment of acute and chronic depressive disorders, such as major depressive disorder and dysthymia. Reboxetine can also produce a relatively rapid decrease in the symptoms of social phobia. Reboxetine is as effective as imipramine and may be more effective than fluoxetine for the treatment of persons with severe depression. Early clinical evaluation of reboxetine has focused on social adaptation, motivation to interact socially, and other aspects of the relationship between the self and the environment. Social impairments, particularly those revolving around negative self-perception and a low level of social activity, appear to respond more rapidly to reboxetine than to fluoxetine. Thus, reboxetine may facilitate a more satisfactory social adjustment by increasing drive and facilitating a person's sense of control over his or her life. It may be a particularly effective agent for the treatment of melancholic persons whose ability to cope with stress is poor. Reboxetine increases sleep efficiency, unlike fluoxetine, yet is not associated with daytime somnolence.

   Because reboxetine and SSRIs directly act on nonoverlapping neurotransmitter systems, it would be logical to combine them to treat persons whose depression is not responsive to either agent alone. No clinical data yet support the use of this combination.

2. **Clinical guidelines.** Most persons respond at 4 mg twice a day; the maximum dosage is 10 mg/day. The dosage of reboxetine should be lowered for elderly persons and those with severe renal impairment.

3. **Precautions and adverse reactions.** The most common adverse effects are urinary hesitancy, headache, constipation, nasal congestion, diaphoresis, dizziness, dry mouth, decreased libido, and insomnia. In long-term use, persons taking reboxetine experience no more adverse effects than those taking a placebo.

G. **Tricyclic and tetracyclic drugs.** The tricyclic and tetracyclic antidepressants (Table 25–12) are little used because of their adverse effects (Chapter 10).

H. **MAOIs.** The MAOIs (Table 25–13) are highly effective antidepressants, but they are little used because of the dietary precautions that must be followed to avoid tyramine-induced hypertensive crises and because of harmful drug interactions (see Table 10–11 in Chapter 10).

VII. **Antimanic drugs**

A. **Lithium.** Lithium is used for the short-term and prophylactic treatment of bipolar I disorder.

1. **Pharmacological actions.** After ingestion, lithium is completely absorbed by the gastrointestinal tract. Serum concentrations peak in 1 to $1^1/_2$ hours for standard preparations and in 4 to $4^1/_2$ hours for controlled-released preparations. Lithium does not bind to plasma proteins, is not metabolized, and is excreted through the kidneys. The plasma half-life is initially 1.3 days and is 2.4 days after administration for more than 1 year. The blood–brain barrier permits only slow passage of lithium, which is why a single overdose does not necessarily cause toxicity and why long-term lithium intoxication is slow to resolve. The half-life of lithium is about 20 hours, and equilibrium is reached after 5 to 7 days of regular intake. The renal clearance of lithium is decreased in persons with renal insufficiency (common in the elderly). The excretion of lithium is increased during pregnancy but decreased after delivery. Lithium is excreted in breast milk and in insignificant amounts in feces and sweat.

2. **Therapeutic efficacy**

   a. **Manic episodes.** Lithium controls acute mania. It prevents relapse in about 80% of persons with bipolar I disorder and in a somewhat smaller percentage of persons with mixed or dysphoric mania, rapid cycling bipolar disorder, comorbid substance abuse, or encephalopathy. Lithium alone at therapeutic concentrations exerts its antimanic effects in 1 to 3 weeks. To control mania acutely, therefore, a benzodiazepine (e.g., clonazepam or lorazepam) or a dopamine receptor agonist (e.g., haloperidol or chlorpromazine) should also be administered for the first few weeks.

   Lithium is effective as long-term prophylaxis for both manic and depressive episodes in about 70–80% of persons with bipolar I disorder.

   b. **Depressive episodes.** Lithium is effective in the treatment of major depressive disorder and depression associated with bipolar I disorder. Lithium exerts a partial or complete antidepressant effect in about 80% of persons with bipolar I disorder. Many persons take lithium and an antidepressant together as long-term maintenance for their bipolar disease. Augmentation of lithium therapy with valproate or carbamazepine is usually well tolerated, with little risk for the precipitation of mania.

   When a depressive episode occurs in a person taking maintenance lithium, the differential diagnosis should include lithium-induced hypothyroidism, substance abuse, and lack of compliance with the lithium therapy. Possible treatment approaches include increasing the lithium concentration (up to 1 to 1.2 mEq/L); adding supplemental thyroid hormone (e.g., 25 mg of liothyronine [Cytomel] per day), even in the presence of normal findings on thyroid function tests; augmenting lithium with valproate or carbamazepine; judiciously using antidepressants; ECT; and psychotherapy. Some experts report that administering ECT to a person taking lithium increases the risk for cognitive dysfunction, but this point is controversial. Once the acute depressive episode resolves, other therapies should be tapered in favor of lithium monotherapy, if clinically tolerated.

c. Maintenance. Maintenance treatment with lithium markedly decreases the frequency, severity, and duration of manic and depressive episodes in persons with bipolar I disorder. During placebo treatment, about 80% of persons with bipolar I disorder relapse, whereas only about 35% of persons treated with lithium relapse. Lithium provides relatively more effective prophylaxis for mania than for depression, and supplemental antidepressant strategies may be necessary either intermittently or continuously.

Lithium maintenance is almost always indicated after a second episode of bipolar I disorder depression or mania. Lithium maintenance should be seriously considered after a first episode for adolescents or for persons who have a family history of bipolar I disorder, have poor support systems, had no precipitating factors for the first episode, had a serious first episode, are at high risk for suicide, are 30 years old or older, had a sudden onset of their first episode, had a first episode of mania, or are male. Lithium is also effective treatment for persons with severe cyclothymic disorder.

The wisdom of initiating maintenance therapy after a first manic episode is illustrated by several observations. First, each episode of mania increases the risk for subsequent episodes. Second, among people responsive to lithium, relapses are 28 times more likely to occur after lithium is discontinued. Third, case reports describe persons who were initially responsive to lithium, then stopped taking it and had a relapse, and were no longer responsive to lithium during subsequent episodes.

The response to lithium treatment is such that continued maintenance treatment is often associated with increasing efficacy and reduced mortality. It does not necessarily represent treatment failure, therefore, if an episode of depression or mania occurs after a relatively short period of lithium maintenance. However, lithium treatment alone may begin to lose its effectiveness after several years of successful use. If this occurs, then supplemental treatment with carbamazepine or valproate may be useful.

Maintenance lithium dosages often can be adjusted to achieve a serum or plasma concentration somewhat lower than that needed for the treatment of acute mania. If lithium use is to be discontinued, then the dosage should be slowly tapered. Abrupt discontinuation of lithium therapy is associated with an increased risk for rapid recurrence of manic or depressive episodes.

3. Dosage and clinical guidelines

a. Initial medical workup. Before the clinician administers lithium, a physician other than a psychiatrist should conduct a routine laboratory and physical examination. The laboratory examination should include measurement of the serum creatinine concentration (or the 24-hour urine creatinine concentration if the clinician has any reason to be concerned about renal function), an electrolyte screen, thyroid function tests (thyroid-stimulating hormone, tri-iodothyronine, and thyroxine), a complete blood cell count, an ECG, and a pregnancy test in women of childbearing age.

b. **Dosage recommendations.** In the United States, lithium formulations include 150-, 300-, and 600-mg regular-release lithium carbonate capsules (Eskalith, Lithonate); 300-mg regular-release lithium carbonate tablets (Lithotabs); 450-mg controlled-release lithium carbonate capsules (Eskalith CR); and lithium citrate syrup in a concentration of 8 mEq/5 mL.

The starting dosage for most adult persons is 300 mg of the regular-release formulation three times daily. The starting dosage in elderly persons or persons with renal impairment should be 300 mg once or twice daily. An eventual dosage of between 900 and 1,200 mg/day usually produces a therapeutic concentration of 0.6 to 1 mEq/L, and a dosage of 1,200 to 1,800 mg/day usually produces a therapeutic concentration of 0.8 to 1.2 mEq/L. Maintenance dosing can be given either in two or three divided doses of the regular-release formulation or in a single dose of the sustained-release formulation that is equivalent to the combined daily doses of the regular-release formulation. The use of divided doses reduces gastric upset and avoids single high-peak lithium concentrations.

c. **Serum and plasma concentrations.** The measurement of serum and plasma concentrations of lithium is a standard method of assessment, and these values serve as a basis for titration. Lithium concentrations should be determined routinely every 2 to 6 months, and promptly in persons who are suspected to be noncompliant with the prescribed dosage, exhibit signs of toxicity, or are undergoing a dosage adjustment.

The most common guidelines are 1.0 to 1.5 mEq/L for the treatment of acute mania and 0.4 to 0.8 mEq/L for maintenance treatment.

4. **Precautions and adverse reactions.** Fewer than 20% of persons taking lithium experience no adverse effects, and significant adverse effects are experienced by at least 30% of those taking lithium. The most common adverse effects of lithium treatment are gastric distress, weight gain, tremor, fatigue, and mild cognitive impairment.

5. **Drug interactions.** Lithium drug interactions are summarized in Table 25–12.

B. **Valproate.** Valproate is a first-line drug in the treatment of bipolar I disorder, at least equal in efficacy and safety to lithium. Available formulations include valproic acid (Depakene), a 1:1 mixture of valproic acid and sodium valproate (Depakote), and injectable sodium valproate (Depacon). Each of these is therapeutically equivalent because at physiologic pH, valproic acid dissociates into valproate ion.

1. **Pharmacological actions.** All valproate formulations are rapidly and completely absorbed after oral administration. The steady-state half-life of valproate is about 8 to 17 hours, and clinically effective plasma concentrations can usually be maintained with dosing once,

TABLE 25-12
CLINICAL INFORMATION FOR THE TRICYCLIC AND TETRACYCLIC DRUGS

Generic Name	Trade Name	Usual Adult Dosage Range (mg a day)
Imipramine	Tofranil	150–300[b]
Desipramine	Norpramin	150–300[b]
Trimipramine	Surmontil	150–200
Amitriptyline	Elavil	150–300[b]
Nortriptyline	Pamelor, Aventyl	50–150
Protriptyline	Vivactil	15–60
Amoxapine	Asendin	150–400
Doxepin	Adapin, Sinequan	150–300[b]
Maprotiline	Ludiomil	150–225
Clomipramine	Anafranil	150–250

[a] Exact range may vary among laboratories.
[b] Includes parent compound and desmethyl metabolite.

twice, or three or four times per day. Protein binding becomes saturated and concentrations of therapeutically effective free valproate increase at serum concentrations above 50 to 100 μg/mL.

2. Therapeutic efficacy

    a. Manic episodes. Valproate effectively controls manic symptoms in about two thirds of persons with acute mania. Valproate also reduces overall psychiatric symptoms and the need for supplemental doses of benzodiazepines or dopamine receptor agonists. Persons with mania usually respond 1 to 4 days after valproate serum concentrations rise above 50 μg/mL. With the use of gradual dosing strategies, this serum concentration can be achieved within 1 week of initiation of dosing, but newer, rapid oral loading strategies achieve therapeutic serum concentrations in 1 day and can control manic symptoms within 5 days. The short-term antimanic effects of valproate can be augmented with the addition of lithium, carbamazepine, or dopamine receptor agonists. SDAs and gabapentin (Neurontin) may also potentiate the effects of valproate, albeit less rapidly. Because of its more favorable profile of cognitive, dermatologic, thyroid, and renal adverse effects, valproate is preferred to lithium for the treatment of acute mania in children and elderly persons.

    b. Depressive episodes. Valproate alone is less effective for the short-term treatment of depressive episodes in bipolar I disorder than for the treatment of manic episodes. In patients with depressive symptoms, valproate is a more effective treatment for agitation than for dysphoria.

    c. Maintenance. Valproate is effective in the maintenance treatment of bipolar I disorder, with fewer, less severe, and shorter manic episodes noted. In direct comparisons, valproate is at least as effective as lithium and is better tolerated than lithium. In comparison with lithium, valproate may be particularly effective in persons with rapid-cycling and ultrarapid-cycling bipolar I disorder, dysphoric or mixed mania, and mania secondary to a general medical condition, and in persons who have comorbid substance abuse or panic attacks or who have not shown a completely favorable response to lithium treatment. The combination of valproate and lithium may be more effective than lithium alone.

In persons with bipolar I disorder, maintenance valproate treatment markedly reduces the frequency and severity of manic episodes, but it is only mildly to moderately effective in the prevention of depressive episodes.

The prophylactic effectiveness of valproate can be augmented by the addition of lithium, carbamazepine, dopamine receptor antagonists, SDAs, antidepressant drugs, gabapentin, or lamotrigine (Lamictal).

3. **Clinical guidelines**
   a. **Pretreatment evaluation.** Pretreatment evaluation should routinely include white blood cell and platelet counts, measurement of hepatic transaminase concentrations, and pregnancy testing, if applicable. Amylase and coagulation studies should be performed if baseline pancreatic disease or coagulopathy is suspected.
   b. **Dosage and administration.** Valproate is available in a number of formulations and dosages (Table 25–13). For treatment of acute mania, an oral loading strategy of 20 to 30 mg/kg per day can be used to accelerate control of symptoms. This regimen is usually well tolerated but can cause excessive sedation and tremor in elderly persons. Rapid stabilization of agitated behavior can be achieved with an intravenous infusion of valproate. If acute mania is absent, it is best to initiate the drug treatment gradually so as to minimize the common adverse effects of nausea, vomiting, and sedation. The dosage on the first day should be 250 mg administered with a meal. The dosage can be increased to 250 mg orally three times daily during the course of 3 to 6 days.

   Trough plasma concentrations can be assessed in the morning before the first daily dose of the drug is administered. Therapeutic plasma concentrations for the control of seizures range between 50 to 150 mg/mL, but concentrations up to 200 mg/mL are usually well tolerated. It is reasonable to use the same range for the treatment of mental disorders; most of the controlled studies have used 50 to 100 mg/mL.

TABLE 25–13
AVAILABLE PREPARATIONS AND TYPICAL DOSAGES OF MAOIs

Generic Name	Trade Name	Preparations	Usual Daily Dosage (mg)	Usual Maximum Daily Dosage (mg)
Isocarboxazid[a]	Marplan	10-mg tablets	20–40	60
Moclobemide[b]	Manerix	100, 150-mg tablets	300–600	600
Phenelzine	Nardil	15-mg tablets	30–60	90
Selegiline	Eldepryl, Atapryl	5-mg capsules, 5-mg tablets	10	30
Tranylcypromine	Parnate	10-mg tablets	20–60	60

[a] Available directly from the manufacturer.
[b] Not available in the United Stages.

Most persons attain therapeutic plasma concentrations on a dosage of between 1,200 and 1,500 mg/day administered in divided doses. Once symptoms are well controlled, the full daily dose can be taken at once before sleep.

c. **Laboratory monitoring.** White blood cell and platelet counts and hepatic transaminase concentrations should be determined 1 month after the initiation of therapy and every 6 to 24 months thereafter. However, because even frequent monitoring may not predict serious organ toxicity, it is prudent to emphasize the need for prompt evaluation of any illnesses when giving instructions to patients. Asymptomatic elevations of transaminase concentrations to up to three times the upper limit of normal are common and do not require any change in dosage.

4. **Precautions and adverse reactions.** Valproate treatment is generally well tolerated and safe, and valproate is less likely than lithium to be discontinued because of adverse effects. The most common adverse effects are nausea, vomiting, dyspepsia, and diarrhea. The gastrointestinal effects are generally most common during the first month of treatment, particularly if the dosage is increased rapidly. Unbuffered valproic acid is more likely than the enteric-coated "sprinkle" or the delayed-release divalproex formulations to cause gastrointestinal symptoms. Gastrointestinal symptoms may respond to histamine H_2 receptor antagonists. Other common adverse effects involve the nervous system (e.g., sedation, ataxia, dysarthria, and tremor). Valproate-induced tremor may respond well to treatment with β-adrenergic receptor antagonists or gabapentin. To treat the other neurological adverse effects, the valproate dosage must usually be lowered.

Weight gain is a common adverse effect, especially in long-term treatment, and can best be treated by recommending a combination of a reasonable diet and moderate exercise.

The two most serious adverse effects of valproate treatment involve the pancreas and liver. If symptoms of lethargy, malaise, anorexia, nausea and vomiting, edema, and abdominal pain occur in a person treated with valproate, the clinician must consider the possibility of severe hepatotoxicity. Rare cases of pancreatitis have been reported; they occur most often in the first 6 months of treatment, and the condition occasionally results in death.

C. **Carbamazepine.** Carbamazepine is effective for the treatment of acute mania and for the prophylactic treatment of bipolar I disorder. It is a first-line agent, along with lithium and valproic acid.

1. **Therapeutic efficacy.**

a. **Manic episodes.** The efficacy of carbamazepine in the treatment of acute mania is comparable with that of lithium and antipsychotics. Carbamazepine is also effective as a second-line agent to prevent both manic and depressive episodes in bipolar I disorder, after lithium and valproic acid.

b. **Depressive episodes.** Carbamazepine is an alternative drug for patients whose depressive episodes show a marked or rapid periodicity.

2. Clinical guidelines

a. **Dosage and administration.** Carbamazepine is available in 100- and 200-mg tablets and as a suspension containing 100 mg/5 mL. The usual starting dosage is 200 mg orally two times a day; however, with titration, three-times-a-day dosing is optimal. An extended-release version suitable for twice-a-day dosing is available in 100-, 200-, and 400-mg tablets. The dosage should be increased by no more than 200 mg/day every 2 to 4 days to minimize the occurrence of adverse effects.

b. **Blood concentrations.** The anticonvulsant blood concentration range of 4 to 12 mg/mL should be reached before it is determined that carbamazepine is not effective in the treatment of a mood disorder. The dosage necessary to achieve plasma concentrations in the usual therapeutic range varies from 400 to 1,600 mg/day, with a mean of about 1,000 mg/day.

3. Precautions and adverse reactions.

The rarest but most serious adverse effects of carbamazepine are blood dyscrasias, hepatitis, and exfoliative dermatitis. Otherwise, carbamazepine is relatively well tolerated by persons except for mild gastrointestinal and CNS effects that can be significantly reduced if the dosage is increased slowly and minimal effective plasma concentrations are maintained.

4. Drug interactions.

Principally because it induces several hepatic enzymes, carbamazepine may interact with many drugs (Table 25–14).

D. **Other anticonvulsants.** Initial experience with three newer anticonvulsants appears promising for the treatment of bipolar and disorders; however, data are limited at this time.

1. **Gabapentin**
2. **Lamotrigine**
3. **Topiramate (Topamax)**
4. **Oxcarbamazepine (Trileptal)**

VIII. Stimulants

A. **Sympathomimetics.** (Also called *analeptics* and *psychostimulants*.) The sympathomimetics are effective in the treatment of attention-deficit/hyperactivity disorder (ADHD). The first-line sympathomimetics are methylphenidate (Ritalin, Concerta), dextroamphetamine (Dexedrine), and a reformulation of existing dextroamphetamine and amphetamine (Adderall). Pemoline (Cylert) is now considered a second-line agent because of rare but potentially fatal hepatic toxicity.

1. **Pharmacological actions.** All the drugs are well absorbed from the gastrointestinal tract. Dextroamphetamine and the reformulation reach peak plasma concentrations in 2 to 3 hours and have a half-life of about 6 hours, so that once- or twice-daily dosing is necessary. Methylphenidate reaches peak plasma levels in 1 to 2 hours and has a short half-life of 2 to 3 hours, so that multiple daily dosing is necessary. A sustained-release formulation doubles the effective half-life of methylphenidate. A novel osmotic pump capsule (Concerta) may sustain the effects of methylphenidate for 12 hours.

TABLE 25-14
CARBAMAZEPINE-DRUG INTERACTIONS

Effect of Carbamazepine on Plasma Concentration of Concomitant Agents	Agents That May Affect Carbamazepine Plasma Concentrations
Carbamazepine may decrease drug plasma concentration of	*Agents that may increase carbamazepine plasma concentration*
Acetaminophen	Allopurinol
Alprazolam	Cimetidine
Amitriptyline	Clarithromycin
Bupropion	Danazol
Clomipramine	Diltiazem
Clonazepam	Erythromycin
Clozapine	Fluoxetine
Cyclosporine	Fluvoxamine
Desipramine	Gemfibrozil
Dicumarol	Isoniazid[a]
Doxepine	Itraconazole
Doxycycline	Ketoconazole
Ethosuximide	Lamotrigine
Felbamate	Loratidine
Fentanyl	Macrolides
Fluphenazine	Nefazodone
Haloperidol	Nicotinamide
Hormonal contraceptives	Propoxyphene
Imipramine	Troleandomycin
Lamotrigine	Valproate[a]
Methadone	Verapamil
Methsuximide	Viloxazine
Methylprednisolone	
Nimodipine	*Drug that may decrease carbamazepine plasma concentration*
Pancuronium	
Phensuximide	
Phenytoin	Carbazmazepine (autoinduction)
Primidone	Cisplatin
Theophylline	Doxorubicin HCl
Valproate	Felbamate
Warfarin	Phenobarbital
	Phenytoin
Carbamazepine may increase drug plasma concentrations of	Primidone
	Rifampin[b]
	Theophylline
Clomipramine	Valproate
Phenytoin	
Primidone	

[a] Increased concentration of the active 10,11-epoxide.
[b] Decreased concentration of carbamazepine and increased concentrations of the 10,11-epoxide.
Table by Carlos A. Zarate, Jr., M.D., and Mauricio Tohen, M.D., Dr.P.H.

2. **Therapeutic efficacy.** Sympathomimetics are effective about 75% of the time. Methylphenidate and dextroamphetamine are generally equally effective and work within 15 to 30 minutes. The drugs decrease hyperactivity, increase attentiveness, and reduce impulsivity. They may also reduce comorbid oppositional behaviors associated with ADHD. Many persons take these drugs throughout their schooling and beyond. In responsive persons, the use of a sympathomimetic may be a critical determinant of scholastic success. Sympathomimetics improve the core ADHD symptoms—hyperactivity, impulsivity, and inattentiveness—and permit improved social interactions with teachers, family, other adults, and peers.

The success of long-term treatment of ADHD with sympathomimetics, which are efficacious for most of the various constellations of ADHD symptoms present from childhood to adulthood, supports a model in which ADHD results from a genetically determined neurochemical imbalance that requires lifelong pharmacological management. A recent head-to-head comparison between medication and psychosocial approaches for the treatment of ADHD found clear benefit with medication but little improvement with nonpharmacological treatments.

3. **Clinical guidelines**

   a. **Pretreatment evaluation.** The pretreatment evaluation should include an assessment of the patient's cardiac function, with particular attention to the presence of hypertension or tachyarrhythmias. The clinician should also examine the patient for the presence of movement disorders (e.g., tics and dyskinesia) because these conditions can be exacerbated by the administration of sympathomimetics. If tics are present, many experts do not use sympathomimetics but instead choose clonidine (Catapres) or antidepressants. However, recent data indicate that sympathomimetics may cause only a mild increase in motor tics and may actually suppress vocal tics.

   Hepatic and renal function should be assessed, and dosages of sympathomimetics should be reduced if the patient's metabolism is impaired. In the case of pemoline, any elevation of liver enzymes is a compelling reason to discontinue the medication.

   b. **Dosage and administration.** The dosage ranges and the available preparations for sympathomimetics are presented in Table 25–15.

      (1) **Methylphenidate.** Methylphenidate is the agent most commonly used initially, at a dosage of 5 to 10 mg every 3 to 4 hours. The dosage may be increased to a maximum of 20 mg four times daily. Use of the 20-mg sustained-release formulation, to provide 6 hours of benefit and eliminate the need for dosing at school, is supported by many, but not all, experts, some of whom feel it is less effective than the immediate-release formulation. Experience with the osmotic pump formulation (18 to 54 mg/day) is extremely limited at this time.

      Children with ADHD can take immediate-release methylphenidate at 8 a.m. and 12 noon. The sustained-release preparation of methylphenidate may be taken once at 8 a.m. The starting dose of methylphenidate ranges from 2.5 mg (regular preparation) to 20 mg (sustained-release). If this is inadequate, the dosage may be increased to a maximum of 20 mg four times daily.

      (2) **Dextroamphetamine.** The dosage of dextroamphetamine is 2.5 to 40 mg/day (up to 0.5 mg/kg a day). Dextroamphetamine is about twice as potent as methylphenidate on a per-milligram basis and provides 6 to 8 hours of benefit.

      (3) **Treatment failures.** Seventy percent of nonresponders to one sympathomimetic may benefit from another. All the sympathomimetic drugs should be tried before the patient is switched to a drug of a different class.

TABLE 25–15
SYMPATHOMIMETICS COMMONLY USED IN PSYCHIATRY

Generic Name	Trade Name	Preparations	Initial Daily Dosage	Usual Daily Dosage for ADHD[a]	Usual Daily Dosage for Narcolepsy	Maximum Daily Dosage
Amphetamine–dextroamphetamine	Adderall	5-, 10-, 20-, 30-mg tablets	5–10 mg	20–30 mg	5–60 mg	Children: 40 mg Adults: 60 mg
Dextroamphetamine	Dexedrine, DextroStat	5-, 10-, 15-mg extended-release (ER) capsules; 5-, 10-mg tablets	5–10 mg	20–30 mg	5–60 mg	Children: 40 mg Adults: 60 mg
Modafinil	Provigil	100-, 200-mg tablets	100 mg	Not used	400 mg	400 mg
Methamphetamine	Desoxyn	5-mg tablets; 5-, 10-, 15-mg ER tablets	5–10 mg	20–25 mg	Not generally used	45 mg
Methylphenidate	Ritalin, Methidate, Methylin, Attenade, Concerta	5-, 10-, 20-mg tablets; 10-, 20-mg sustained-release (SR) tablets; 18-, 36-mg ER tablets	5–10 mg	5–60 mg	20–30 mg	Children: 80 mg Adults: 90 mg
Pemoline	Cylert	18.75-, 37.5-, 75-mg tablets; 37.5 chewable tablets	37.5 mg	56.25–75 mg	Not used	112.5 mg

[a] For children 6 years of age or older.

4. Precautions and adverse reactions. The most common adverse effects associated with amphetamine-like drugs are stomach pain, anxiety, irritability, insomnia, tachycardia, cardiac arrhythmias, and dysphoria. The treatment of common adverse effects in children with ADHD is usually straightforward (Table 25–16). The drugs may also increase the heart rate and blood pressure and cause palpitations.

Less common adverse effects include the induction of movement disorders (e.g., tics, Tourette's disorder–like symptoms, and dyskinesias), which are often self-limited over 7 to 10 days. If one of these movement disorders develops in a person taking a sympathomimetic, a correlation between the dosage of the medication and the severity of the disorder must be firmly established before the dosage is adjusted. Small to moderate dosages of sympathomimetics may be well tolerated without causing an increase in the frequency and severity of the tics. In severe cases, augmentation with risperidone is necessary.

Methylphenidate may worsen tics in one third of patients, who fall into two groups: those whose methylphenidate-induced tics resolve immediately after the dose has been metabolized, and a smaller group in whom methylphenidate appears to trigger tics that persist for several months but eventually resolve spontaneously.

The most limiting adverse effect of sympathomimetics is their association with psychological and physical dependence. Sympathomimetics may exacerbate glaucoma, hypertension, cardiovascular

TABLE 25–16
MANAGEMENT OF COMMON STIMULANT-INDUCED ADVERSE EFFECTS IN ATTENTION-DEFICIT/HYPERACTIVITY DISORDER

Adverse Effect	Management
Anorexia, nausea, weight loss	• Administer stimulant with meals. • Use calorie-enhanced supplements. Discourage forcing meals. • If using pemoline, check liver function tests.
Insomnia, nightmares	• Administer stimulants earlier in day. • Change to short-acting preparations. • Discontinue afternoon or evening dosing. • Consider adjunctive treatment (e.g., antihistamines, clonidine, antidepressants).
Dizziness	• Monitor blood pressure. • Encourage fluid intake. • Change to long-acting form.
Rebound phenomena	• Overlap stimulant dosing. • Change to long-acting preparation or combine long- and short-acting preparations. • Consider adjunctive or alternative treatment (e.g., clonidine, antidepressants).
Irritability	• Assess timing of phenomena (during peak or withdrawal phase). • Evaluate comorbid symptoms. • Reduce dose. • Consider adjunctive or alternative treatment (e.g., lithium, antidepressants, anticonvulsants).
Dysphoria, moodiness, agitation	• Consider comorbid diagnosis (e.g., mood disorder). • Reduce dose or change to long-acting preparation. • Consider adjunctive or alternative treatment (e.g., lithium, anticonvultants, antidepressants).

Adapted from Wilens TE, Biederman J. The stimulants. In: Shaffer D, ed. *The Psychiatric Clinics of North America: Pedriatic Psychopharmacology.* Philadelphia: Saunders, 1992, with permission.

disorders, hyperthyroidism, anxiety disorders, psychotic disorders, and seizure disorders.

High doses of sympathomimetics can cause dry mouth, pupillary dilation, bruxism, formication, excessive ebullience, restlessness, and emotional lability. The long-term use of a high dosage can cause a delusional disorder that is indistinguishable from paranoid schizophrenia.

Patients who have taken overdoses of sympathomimetics present with hypertension, tachycardia, hyperthermia, toxic psychosis, delirium, and occasionally seizures. Overdoses of sympathomimetics can also result in death, often caused by cardiac arrhythmias. Seizures can be treated with benzodiazepines, cardiac effects with β-adrenergic receptor antagonists, fever with cooling blankets, and delirium with dopamine receptor agonists.

B. Alternatives to sympathomimetics. Second- and third-line alternatives to sympathomimetics for ADHD include bupropion, venlafaxine, guanfacine (Tenex), clonidine, and tricyclic drugs.

Bupropion is an appropriate choice for persons with comorbid ADHD and depression or persons with comorbid ADHD, conduct disorder, or substance abuse.

IX. Cholinesterase inhibitors

A. Therapeutic efficacy. Donepezil (Aricept) and rivastigmine (Exelon) are among the few proven treatments for mild to moderate dementia of the Alzheimer's type. They reduce the intrasynaptic cleavage and inactivation of acetylcholine and thus potentiate cholinergic neurotransmission, which in turn tends to produce a modest improvement in memory and goal-directed thought. These drugs are considered most useful for persons with mild to moderate memory loss, who nevertheless still have enough preserved basal forebrain cholinergic neurons to benefit from an augmentation of cholinergic neurotransmission.

Donepezil is well tolerated and widely used. Rivastigmine appears more likely than donepezil to cause gastrointestinal and neuropsychiatric adverse effects. An older cholinesterase inhibitor, tacrine (Cognex), is currently very rarely used because of its potential for hepatotoxicity. Cholinesterase inhibitors have been coadministered with vitamin E and gingko biloba extract.

The cholinesterase inhibitors in long-term use slow the progression of memory loss and diminish apathy, depression, hallucinations, anxiety, euphoria, and purposeless motor behaviors. Functional autonomy is less well preserved. Some persons note immediate improvement in memory, mood, psychotic symptoms, and interpersonal skills. Others note little initial benefit but are able to retain their cognitive and adaptive faculties at a relatively stable level for many months. The use of cholinesterase inhibitors may delay or reduce the need for nursing home placement.

B. Clinical guidelines

1. Pretreatment evaluation. Before the initiation of treatment with cholinesterase inhibitors, potentially treatable causes of dementia should be ruled out, and the diagnosis of dementia of the Alzheimer's type should be established with a thorough neurological evaluation. Detailed neuropsychological testing can detect early signs of Alzheimer's disease. The psychiatric evaluation should focus on depression, anxiety, and psychosis.

   2. **Dosage and administration**

      a. **Donepezil.** Donepezil is available in 5-mg and 10-mg tablets. Treatment should be initiated with a dosage of 5 mg/day, taken at night. If well tolerated and of some discernible benefit after 4 weeks, the dosage should be increased to a maintenance level of 10 mg/day. Donepezil absorption is unaffected by meals.

      b. **Rivastigmine.** Rivastigmine is available in 1.5-, 3-, 4.5-, and 6-mg capsules. The recommended initial dosage is 1.5 mg twice daily for a minimum of 2 weeks, after which increases of 1.5 mg/day can be made at intervals of at least 2 weeks to a target dosage of 6 mg/day, taken in two equal doses. If tolerated, the dosage may be further titrated upward to a maximum of 6 mg twice daily. The risk for adverse gastrointestinal events can be reduced by taking rivastigmine with food.

C. **Precautions and adverse reactions**

   1. **Donepezil.** Donepezil is generally well tolerated at recommended dosages. Fewer than 3% of persons taking donepezil experience nausea, diarrhea, and vomiting. These mild symptoms are more common at the 10-mg than the 5-mg dose, and when present, they tend to resolve after 3 weeks of continued use. Donepezil may cause weight loss. Donepezil treatment has been infrequently associated with bradyarrhythmias, especially in persons with underlying cardiac disease. A small number of persons experience syncope.

   2. **Rivastigmine.** Rivastigmine is generally well tolerated, but recommended dosages may need to be scaled back in the initial period of treatment to limit gastrointestinal and CNS adverse effects. These mild symptoms are more common at dosages above 6 mg/day, and when present, they tend to resolve once the dosage is lowered.

      The most common adverse effects associated with rivastigmine are nausea (38% vs. 10% with placebo), vomiting (24% vs. 6% with placebo), dizziness (20% vs. 10% with placebo), headache (16% vs. 13% with placebo), diarrhea (16% vs. 9% with placebo), abdominal pain (12% vs. 7% with placebo), anorexia (12% vs. 4% with placebo), fatigue (7% vs. 5% with placebo), and somnolence (6% vs. 3% with placebo). Central and peripheral nervous system and psychiatric adverse effects also occur more frequently with rivastigmine than with placebo. Rivastigmine may cause weight loss, but it does not appear to cause hepatic, renal, hematologic, or electrolyte abnormalities.

X. **Other drugs**

   A. **α₂-Adrenergic agonists: clonidine and guanfacine.** Clonidine and guanfacine are used in psychiatry to control symptoms caused by withdrawal from opiates and opioids, treat Tourette's disorder, suppress agitation in posttraumatic stress disorder, and control aggressive or hyperactive behavior in children, especially those with autistic features.

The most common adverse effects associated with clonidine are dry mouth and eyes, fatigue, sedation, dizziness, nausea, hypotension, and constipation. A similar but milder adverse effect profile is seen with guanfacine, especially at dosages of 3 mg/day or more. Clonidine and guanfacine should not be taken by adults with blood pressure below 90/60 mm Hg or with cardiac arrhythmias, especially bradycardia. Clonidine in particular is associated with sedation, and tolerance does not usually develop to this adverse effect. Uncommon CNS adverse effects of clonidine include insomnia, anxiety, and depression; rare CNS adverse effects include vivid dreams, nightmares, and hallucinations. Fluid retention associated with clonidine treatment can be treated with diuretics.

B. β-Adrenergic receptor antagonists. β-Adrenergic receptor antagonists (e.g., propanolol [Inderal], pindolol [Visken]) are effective peripherally and centrally acting agents for the treatment of social phobia (e.g., performance anxiety), lithium-induced postural tremor, and neuroleptic-induced acute akathisia, and for the control of aggressive behavior.

The β-adrenergic receptor antagonists are contraindicated for use in people with asthma, insulin-dependent diabetes, congestive heart failure, significant vascular disease, persistent angina, and hyperthyroidism.

The most common adverse effects of β-adrenergic receptor antagonists are hypotension and bradycardia. Serious CNS adverse effects (e.g., agitation, confusion, and hallucinations) are rare.

C. Anticholinergics and amantadine (Symmetrel). In the clinical practice of psychiatry, the anticholinergic drugs are primarily used to treat medication-induced movement disorders, particularly neuroleptic-induced parkinsonism, neuroleptic-induced acute dystonia, and medication-induced postural tremor.

XI. ECT

A. Indications
1. **Major depressive disorder (any type)**
2. **Bipolar disorder—depression**
3. **Bipolar disorder—mania**
4. **Schizophrenia**
5. **Pregnancy**

B. Therapeutic efficacy
1. Does not cure any illness but can induce remissions in an acute episode.
2. Should be followed by other treatments.
3. Also may be used prophylactically to prevent recurrence.

C. Clinical guidelines
1. **Pretreatment evaluation**
   a. Pertinent history.
      (1) Hypertension.
      (2) Musculoskeletal injuries or osteoporosis.

(3) Reserpine or anticholinesterases.
(4) Lithium.
(5) Tricyclic antidepressants.
(6) Antipsychotics.
b. Drugs that raise the seizure threshold should be discontinued.
c. Preparing the patient.
(1) Informed consent.
(2) Alternative treatments.
(3) Adverse effects.
(4) Convalescent period.

2. Procedure
a. Medications.
(1) Anticholinergics.
(2) Anesthesia.
(a) Methohexital (Brevital).
(b) Ketamine (Ketalar) or etomidate (Amidate).
(c) Propofol (Diprivan).
(3) Muscle relaxants.
(a) Succinylcholine (Anectine).
(b) Curare.
b. Types of electrical stimuli.
(1) Sine wave.
(2) Brief pulse.
c. Electrode placement.
(1) Bilateral.
(2) Nondominant unilateral.
(3) Other.
d. Administering the stimulus.
(1) Check vital signs (temperature, cardiac rhythm, blood pressure, pulse).
(2) Apply electrodes and make sure treatment bed is not grounded.
(3) Clear patient's mouth, remove any hearing aids.
(4) Begin anesthesia (before muscle relaxants).
(5) Administer muscle relaxants.
(6) Ventilation.
(7) Apply bite block.
(8) Apply electrical stimulus.
(9) Induce a seizure that is therapeutic.
e. Monitoring.
(1) ECG.
(2) EEG.

D. Precautions and adverse effects
1. Relative contraindications. There are no absolute contraindications, but consider the following:
a. Fever.
b. Significant arrhythmias.
c. Extreme hypertension.
d. Coronary ischemia.

2. Adverse effects
   a. Cardiac.
   b. CNS.
   c. General.

For more detailed discussion of this topic, see Biological Therapies, Ch 35, p 2235, in CTP/VII.

26

Laboratory Tests and Brain Imaging in Psychiatry

I. General introduction

High rates of medical comorbidity in psychiatric patients, myriad psychiatric manifestations of medical disorders, and the required laboratory monitoring during psychopharmacological treatment make laboratory testing an integral part of psychiatric assessment and treatment.

Psychiatrists must be sensitive to the possibility of comorbid medical illness in their patients, particularly in elderly, chronically mentally ill, indigent, and substance-abusing populations. The possibility of occult medical illness must always be considered when patients present with psychiatric syndromes. Thyroid and adrenal disease may present as a psychotic or mood disorder, and cancer may present as depression. Table 26–1 lists medical conditions that can present with psychiatric symptoms. Each of these diagnoses can argue for a different set of laboratory or diagnostic tests. Laboratory testing is also used to monitor dosing, compliance, and toxic effects of various psychotropic medications (e.g., lithium and other mood stabilizers).

The initial evaluation must always include a thorough assessment of the prescribed and over-the-counter medications that the patient is taking. Many psychiatric syndromes can be of iatrogenic origin, caused by medications (e.g., depression by antihypertensives, delirium by anticholinergics, and psychosis by steroids). Often, if clinically possible, a washout of medications may aid the diagnosis.

II. Screening tests for medical illnesses

See Table 26–2.

A. Outpatients. Routine outpatient psychotherapy requires no specific tests, but a thorough medical history should be obtained and tests ordered if indicated. Suspected organicity warrants a neurological consultation.

B. Inpatients. Rule out organic causes for the psychiatric disorder. A thorough screening battery of laboratory tests administered on admission may detect a significant degree of morbidity. The routine admission workup includes the following:

1. Complete blood cell count with differential.
2. Complete blood chemistries (including measurements of electrolytes, glucose, calcium, and magnesium and tests of hepatic and renal function).
3. Thyroid function tests.
4. Rapid plasma reagent (RPR) or Venereal Disease Research Laboratory (VDRL) test.

TABLE 26–1
SOME MEDICAL CONDITIONS THAT MAY PRESENT WITH NEUROPSYCHIATRIC SYMPTOMS

Neurological
Cerebrovascular disorders (hemorrhage, infarction)
Head trauma (concussion, posttraumatic hematoma)
Epilepsy (especially complex partial seizures)
Narcolepsy
Brain neoplasms (primary or metastatic)
Normal-pressure hydrocephalus
Parkinson's disease
Multiple sclerosis
Huntington's disease
Dementia of the Alzheimer's type
Metachromatic leukodystrophy
Migraine

Endocrine
Hypothyroidism
Hyperthyroidism
Hypoadrenalism
Hyperadrenalism
Hypoparathyroidism
Hyperparathyroidism
Hypoglycemia
Hyperglycemia
Diabetes mellitus
Panhypopituitarism
Pheochromocytoma
Gonadotropic hormonal disturbances
Pregnancy

Metabolic and systemic
Fluid and electrolyte disturbances (e.g., syndrome of inappropriate antidiuretic hormone secretion (SIADH))
Hepatic encephalopathy
Uremia
Porphyria
Hepatolenticular degeneration (Wilson's disease)
Hypoxemia (chronic pulmonary disease)
Hypotension
Hypertensive encephalopathy

Toxic
Intoxication or withdrawal associated with drug or alcohol abuse
Adverse effects of prescribed and over-the-counter medications
Environmental toxins (volatile hydrocarbons, heavy metals, carbon monoxide, organophosphates)

Nutritional
Vitamin B_{12} deficiency (pernicious anemia)
Nicotinic acid deficiency (pellagra)
Folate deficiency (megaloblastic anemia)
Thiamine deficiency (Wernicke-Korsakoff syndrome)
Trace metal deficiency (zinc, magnesium)
Nonspecific malnutrition and dehydration

Infectious
AIDS
Neurosyphilis
Viral meningitides and encephalitides (e.g., herpes simplex)
Brain abscess
Viral hepatitis
Infectious mononucleosis
Tuberculosis
Systemic bacterial infections (especially pneumonia) and viremia
Streptococcal infections
Pediatric infection-triggered, autoimmune neuropsychiatric disorders

Autoimmune
Systemic lupus erythematosus

TABLE 26-1—*continued*

Neoplastic
  CNS primary and metastatic tumors
  Endocrine tumors
  Pancreatic carcinoma
  Paraneoplastic syndromes

Table adapted from Darrell G. Kirch, M.D.

5. Urinalysis.
6. Urine toxicology screen.
7. Electrocardiogram (ECG).
8. Chest roentgenography (for patients over age 35).
9. Plasma levels of any drugs being taken, if appropriate.

III. Psychiatric drugs

Before prescribing any psychotropic medication, take a detailed medical history, noting a previous response to specific drugs, a family response to specific drugs, allergic reactions, renal or hepatic disease, and glaucoma (for any drugs that have anticholinergic activity). In cases of impaired renal or hepatic function, a reduced dose of medication is often required. Tests of liver function and measurements of blood urea nitrogen and creatinine levels are useful in this regard.

   A. Benzodiazepines. No special tests are needed before benzodiazepines are prescribed, although liver function tests are often useful. These drugs are metabolized in the liver by either oxidation or conjugation. If hepatic function is impaired, the elimination half-life of benzodiazepines that are oxidized is increased, but the effect on benzodiazepines that are conjugated (oxazepam [Serax], lorazepam [Ativan], and temazepam [Restoril]) is less pronounced. Benzodiazepines also can precipitate porphyria.

   B. Antipsychotics. No special tests are needed, although it is good to obtain baseline values for liver function and a complete blood cell count. Antipsychotics are metabolized primarily in the liver, with metabolites excreted primarily in urine. Many metabolites are active. Peak plasma concentration usually is reached 2 to 3 hours after an oral dose. Elimination half-life is 12 to 30 hours but may be much longer. Steady state requires at least 1 week at a constant dose (months at a constant dose of depot antipsychotics). With the exception of clozapine (Clozaril), all antipsychotics acutely cause an elevation in serum prolactin (secondary to tuberoinfundibular activity). A normal prolactin level often indicates either noncompliance or nonabsorption. Side effects include leukocytosis, leukopenia, impaired platelet function, mild anemia (both aplastic and hemolytic), and agranulocytosis. Bone marrow and blood element side effects can occur abruptly, even when the dosage has remained constant. Low-potency antipsychotics are most likely to cause agranulocytosis, which is the most common bone marrow side effect. These agents may cause hepatocellular injury and intrahepatic biliary stasis (indicated by elevated total and direct bilirubin and elevated transaminases). They also

TABLE 26-2
PSYCHIATRIC INDICATIONS FOR DIAGNOSTIC TESTS

Test	Major Psychiatric Indications	Comments
Acid phosphatase	Cognitive/medical workup	Increased in prostate cancer, benign prostatic hypertrophy, excessive platelet destruction, bone disease
Adrenocorticotropic hormone (ACTH)	Cognitive/medical workup	Changed in steroid abuse; may be increased in seizures, psychoses, and Cushing's disease, and in response to stress
		Decreased in Addison's disease
Alanine aminotransferase (ALT)	Cognitive/medical workup	Increased in hepatitis, cirrhosis, liver metastases
		Decreased in pyridoxine (vitamin B_6) deficiency
	Cognitive/medical workup	Increased in dehydration
Albumin		Decreased in malnutrition, hepatic failure, burns, multiple myeloma, carcinomas
	Eating disorders	Increased in patients who abuse ipecac (e.g., bulimic patients), some patients with schizophrenia
Aldolase	Schizophrenia	
Alkaline phosphatase	Cognitive/medical workup Use of pscyhiatric medications	Increased in Paget's disease, hyperparathyroidism, hepatic disease, liver metastases, heart failure, phenothiazine use
		Decreased in pernicious anemia (vitamin B_{12} deficiency)
	Cognitive/medical workup	Increased in hepatic encephalopathy, liver failure, Reye's syndrome; increases with gastrointestinal hemorrhage and severe congestive heart failure
Ammonia, serum		
Amylase, serum	Eating disorders	May be increased in bulimia nervosa
Antinuclear antibodies	Cognitive/medical workup	Found in systemic lupus erythematosus (SLE) and drug-induced lupus (e.g., secondary to phenothiazines, anticonvulsants); SLE can be associated with delirium, psychosis, mood disorder
Aspartate aminotransferase (AST)	Cognitive/medical workup	Increased in heart failure, hepatic disease, pancreatitis, eclampsia, cerebral damage, alcoholism
		Decreased in pyridoxine (vitamin B_6) deficiency and terminal stages of liver disease
Bicarbonate, serum	Panic disorder	Decreased in hyperventilation syndrome, panic disorder, anabolic steroid abuse
	Eating disorders	May be elevated in patients with bulimia nervosa, in laxative abuse, psychogenic vomiting
Bilirubin	Cognitive/medical workup	Increased in hepatic disease
Blood urea nitrogen (BUN)	Delirium	Elevated in renal disease, dehydration
	Use of psychiatric medications	Elevations associated with lethargy, delirium
		If elevated, can increase toxic potential of psychiatric medications, especially lithium and amantadine (Symmetrel)

continued

TABLE 26–2—*continued*

Test	Major Psychiatric Indications	Comments
Bromide, serum	Dementia	Bromide intoxication can cause psychosis, hallucinations, delirium
	Psychosis	Part of dementia workup, especially when serum chloride is elevated
Caffeine level, serum	Anxiety/panic disorder	Evaluation of patients with suspected caffeinism
Calcium (Ca), serum	Cognitive/medical workup	Increased in hyperparathyroidism, bone metastases
	Mood disorders	Increase associated with delirium, depression, psychosis
	Psychosis	Decreased in hypoparathyroidism, renal failure
	Eating disorders	Decrease associated with depression, irritability, delirium, chronic laxative abuse
Carotid ultrasonography	Dementia	Occasionally included in dementia workup, especially to rule out multiinfarct dementia
		Primary value is in search for possible infarct causes
Catecholamines, urinary and plasma	Panic attacks Anxiety	Elevated in pheochromocytoma
Cerebrospinal fluid (CSF)	Cognitive/medical workup	Increased protein and cells in infection, positive VDRL in neurosyphilis, bloody CSF in hemorrhagic conditions
Ceruloplasmin, serum; copper, serum	Cognitive/medical workup	Low in Wilson's disease (hepatolenticular disease)
Chloride (Cl), serum	Eating disorders	Decreased in patients with bulimia and psychogenic vomiting
	Panic disorder	Mild elevation in hyperventilation syndrome, panic disorder
Cholecystokinin (CCK)	Eating disorders	Compared with controls, blunted in bulimic patients after eating meal (may normalize after treatment with antidepressants)
CO_2 inhalation; sodium bicarbonate infusion	Anxiety/panic attacks	Panic attacks produced in subgroup of patients
Coombs' test, direct and indirect	Hemolytic anemias secondary to psychiatric medications	Evaluation of drug-induced hemolytic anemias, such as those secondary to chlorpromazine, phenytoin, levodopa, and methyldopa
Copper, urine	Cognitive/medical workup	Elevated in Wilson's disease
Cortisol (hydrocortisone)	Cognitive/medical workup Mood disorders	Excessive level may indicate Cushing's disease associated with anxiety, depression, and a variety of other conditions
Creatine phosphokinase (CPK)	Use of antipsychotic agents Use of restraints Substance abuse	Increased in neuroleptic malignant syndrome, intramuscular injection rhabdomyolysis (secondary to substance abuse), patients in restraint, patients experiencing dystonic reactions; asymptomatic elevation with use of antipsychotic drugs
Creatinine, serum	Cognitive/medical workup	Elevated in renal disease (*see* BUN)
Dopamine (DA) (levodopa stimulation of dopamine)	Depression	Inhibits prolactin Test used to assess functional integrity of dopaminergic system, which is impaired in Parkinson's disease, depression

TABLE 26-2—continued

Test	Major Psychiatric Indications	Comments
Doppler ultrasonograpy	Impotence Cognitive/medical workup	Carotid occlusion, transient ischemic attack (TIA), reduced penile blood flow in impotence
Echocardiogram (ECG)	Panic disorder	Among patients with panic disorder, 10 to 40% show mitral valve prolapse
Electroencephalogram (EEG)	Cognitive/medical workup	Seizures, brain death, lesions; shortened rapid eye movement (REM) latency in depression High-voltage activity in stupor, low-voltage fast activity in excitement, functional nonorganic cases (e.g., dissociative states); alpha activity present in the background, which responds to auditory and visual stimuli Biphasic or triphasic slow bursts seen in dementia of Creutzfeldt-Jacob disease
Epstein-Barr virus (EBV); cytomeglovirus (CMV)	Cognitive/medical workup	Part of herpesvirus group EBV Is causative agent for infectious mononucleosis, which can present with depression, fatigue, and personality change
	Anxiety	CMV can produce anxiety, confusion, mood disorders
	Mood disorders	EBV may be associated with chronic mononucleosis-like syndrome associated with chronic depression and fatigue
Eythrocyte sedimentation rate (ESR)	Cognitive/medical workup	An increase in ESR represents a nonspecific test of infectious, inflammatory, autoimmune, or malignant disease; sometimes recommended in the evaluation of anorexia nervosa
Estrogen	Mood disorder	Decreased in menopausal depression and premenstrual syndrome; variable changes in anxiety
Ferritin, serum	Cognitive/medical workup	Most sensitive test for iron deficiency
Folate (folic acid), serum	Alcohol abuse	Usually measured with vitamin B_{12} deficiencies associated with psychosis, paranoia, fatigue, agitation, dementia, delirium
	Use of specific medications	Associated with alcoholism, use of phenytoin, oral contraceptives, estrogen
Follicle-stimulating hormone (FSH)	Depression	High normal in anorexia nervosa, higher values in postmenopausal women; low levels in patients with panhypopituitarism
Glucose, fasting blood (FBS)	Panic attacks Anxiety Delirium Depression	Very high FBS associated with delirium Very low FBS associated with delirium, agitation, panic attacks, anxiety, depression
Glutamyl transaminase, serum	Alcohol abuse	Increase in alcohol abuse, cirrhosis, liver disease
Gonadotropin-releasing hormone (GnRH)	Cognitive/medical workup	Decrease in schizophrenia; increase in anorexia; variable in depression, anxiety

continued

TABLE 26–2—*continued*

Test	Major Psychiatric Indications	Comments
Growth hormone (GH)	Depression Anxiety Schizophrenia	Blunted GH responses to insulin-induced hypoglycemia in depressed patients; increased GH responses to dopamine agonist challenge in schizophrenic patients; increased in some cases of anorexia
Hematocrit (Hct); hemoglobin (Hb)	Cognitive/medical workup	Assessment of anemia (anemia may be associated with depression and psychosis)
Hepatitis A viral antigen (HAAg)	Mood disorders Cognitive/medical workup	Less severe, better prognosis than hepatitis B; may present with anorexia, depression
Hepatitis B surface antigen (HBsAg); hepatitis B core antigen (HBcAg)	Mood disorders Cognitive/medical workup	Active hepatitis B infection indicates greater degree of infectivity and progression to chronic liver disease May present with depression
Holter monitor	Panic disorder	Evaluation of panic-disordered patients with palpitations and other cardiac symptoms
Human immunodeficiency virus (HIV)	Cognitive/medical workup	CNS involvement; AIDS dementia, organic personality disorder, organic mood disorder, acute psychosis
17-Hydroxycorticosteroid	Depression	Deviations detect hyperadrenocorticalism, which can be associated with major depression Increased in steroid abuse
5-Hydroxyindoleacetic acid (5-HIAA)	Depression Suicide Violence	Decrease in CSF in aggressive or violent patients with suicidal or homicidal impulses May be indicator of decreased impulse control and predictor of suicide
Iron, serum	Cognitive/medical workup	Iron-deficiency anemia
Lactate dehydrogenase (LDH)	Cognitive/medical workup	Increased in myocardial infarction, pulmonary infarction, hepatic disease, renal infarction, seizures, cerebral damage, megaloblastic (pernicious) anemia, factitious elevations secondary to rough handling of blood specimen tube
Lupus anticoagulant (LA)	Use of phenothiazines	An antiphospholipid antibody, which has been described in some patients using phenothiazines, especially chlorpromazine; often associated with elevated PTT; associated with anticardiolipin antibodies
Lupus erythematosus (LE) test	Depression Psychosis Delirium Dementia	Positive test associated with systemic LE, which may present with various psychiatric disturbances, such as psychosis, depression, delirium, dementia; also tested with antinuclear antibody (ANA) and anti-DNA antibody tests
Luteinizing hormone (LH)	Depression	Low in patients with panhypopituitarism; decrease associated with depression

TABLE 26-2—*continued*

Test	Major Psychiatric Indications	Comments
Magnesium, serum	Alcohol abuse Cognitive/medical workup	Decreased in alcoholism; low levels associated with agitation, delirium, seizures
Monoamine oxidase (MAO), platelet	Depression	Low in depression; has been used to monitor MAO inhibitor therapy
MCV (mean corpuscular volume) (average volume of a red blood cell)	Alcohol abuse	Elevated in alcoholism and vitamin B_{12} and folate deficiency
Melatonin	Seasonal affective disorder	Produced by light and pineal gland and decreased in seasonal affective disorder
Metal (heavy) intoxication (serum or urinary)	Cognitive/medical workup	Lead—apathy, irritability, anorexia, confusion Mercury—psychosis, fatigue, apathy, decreased memory, emotional lability, "mad hatter" Manganese—manganese madness, Parkinson-like syndrome Aluminum—dementia Arsenic—fatigue, blackouts, hair loss
3-Methoxy-4-hydroxyphenylglycol (MHPG)	Depression Anxiety	Most useful in research; decreases in urine may indicate decreases centrally; may predict response to certain antidepressants
Myoglobin, urine	Phenothiazine use Substance abuse Use of restraints	Increased in neuroleptic malignant syndrome; in phencyclidine (PCP), cocaine, or lysergic acid diethylamide (LSD) intoxication; and in patients in restraints
Nicotine	Anxiety Nicotine addiction	Anxiety, smoking
Nocturnal penile tumescence	Impotence	Quantification of penile circumference changes, penile rigidity, frequency of penile tumescence Evaluation of erectile function during sleep Erections associated with REM sleep Helpful in differentiation between organic and functional causes of impotence
Parathyroid hormone (parathormone)	Anxiety	Low level causes hypocalcemia and anxiety
	Cognitive/medical workup	Dysregulation associated with wide variety of organic mental disorders
Partial thromboplastin time (PTT)	Treatment with antipsychotics, heparin	Monitor anticoagulant therapy; increased in presence of lupus anticoagulant and anticardiolipin antibodies
Phosphorus, serum	Cognitive/medical workup Panic disorder	Increased in renal failure, diabetic acidosis hypoparathyroidism, hypervitaminosis D; decreased in cirrhosis, hypokalemia, hyperparathyroidism, panic attacks, hyperventilation syndrome

continued

TABLE 26–2—*continued*

Test	Major Psychiatric Indications	Comments
Platelet count	Use of psychotropic medications	Decreased by certain psychotropic medications (carbamazepine, clozapine, phenothiazines)
Porphobilinogen (PBG) Porphyria-synthesizing enzyme	Cognitive/medical workup Psychosis Cognitive/medical workup	Increased in acute porphyria Acute neuropsychiatric disorder can occur in acute porphyria attack, which may be precipitated by barbiturates, imipramine
Potassium (K), serum	Cognitive/medical workup Eating disorders	Increased in hyperkalemic acidosis; increase associated with anxiety in cardiac arrhythmia Decreased in cirrhosis, metabolic alkalosis, laxative abuse, diuretic abuse; decrease is common in bulimic patients and in psychogenic vomiting, anabolic steroid abuse
Prolactin, serum	Use of antipsychotic medications	Antipsychotics, by decreasing dopamine, increase prolactin synthesis and release, especially in women
	Cocaine use	Elevated prolactin levels may be seen secondary to cocaine withdrawal
	Pseudoseizures	Lack of prolactin rise after seizure suggests pseudoseizure
Protein, total serum	Cognitive/medical workup	Increased in multiple myeloma, myxedema, lupus Decreased in cirrhosis, malnutrition, overhydration
	Use of psychotropic medications	Low serum protein can result in greater sensitivity to conventional doses of protein-bound medications (lithium is not protein-bound)
Prothrombin time (PT)	Cognitive/medical workup	Elevated in significant liver damage (cirrhosis)
Reticulocyte count (estimate of red blood cell production in bone marrow)	Cognitive/medical workup	Low in megaloblastic or iron-deficiency anemia and anemia of chronic disease
	Use of carbamazepine	Must be monitored in patient taking carbamazepine
Salicylate, serum	Organic hallucinosis Suicide attempts	Toxic levels may be seen in suicide attempts; may also cause organic hallucinosis with high levels
Sodium (Na), serum	Cognitive/medical workup	Decreased with water intoxication, syndrome of inappropriate secretion of antidiuretic hormone (SIADH) Decreased in hypoadrenalism, myxedema, congestive heart failure, diarrhea, polydipsia, use of carbamazepine, anabolic steroids
	Use of lithium	Low levels associated with greater sensitivity to conventional dose of lithium
Testosterone, serum	Impotence	Increase in anabolic steroid abuse May be decreased in organic workup of impotence

TABLE 26–2—*continued*

Test	Major Psychiatric Indications	Comments
	Inhibited sexual desire	Decrease may be seen with inhibited sexual desire
		Follow-up of sex offenders treated with medroxyprogesterone
		Decreased with medroxyprogesterone treatment
Thyroid function tests	Cognitive/medical workup Depression	Detection of hypothyroidism or hyperthyroidism
		Abnormalities can be associated with depression, anxiety, psychosis, dementia, delirium, lithium treatment
Urinalysis	Cognitive/medical workup Pretreatment workup of lithium Drug screening	Provides clues to cause of various cognitive disorders (assessing general apperance, pH, specific gravity, bilirubin, glucose, blood, ketones, protein); specific gravity may be affected by lithium
Urinary creatinine	Cognitive/medical workup	Increased in renal failure, dehydration
	Substance abuse Lithium use	Part of pretreatment workup for lithium; sometimes used in follow-up evaluations of patients treated with lithium
Venereal Disease Research Laboratory (VDRL)	Syphilis	Positive (high titers) in secondary syphilis (may be positive or negative in primary syphilis); rapid plasma reagent (RPR) test also used
		Low titers (or negative) in tertiary syphilis
Vitamin A, serum	Depression Delirium	Hypervitaminosis A is associated with a variety of mental status changes, headache
Vitamin B$_{12}$, serum	Cognitive/medical workup	Part of workup of megaloblastic anemia and dementia
	Dementia	B$_{12}$ deficiency associated with psychosis, paranoia, fatigue, agitation, dementia, delirium
	Mood disorder	Often associated with chronic alcohol abuse
White blood cell (WBC) count	Use of psychiatric medications	Leukopenia and agranulocytosis associated with certain psychotropic medications, such as phenothiazines, carbamazepine, clozapine
		Leukocytosis associated with lithium and neuroleptic malignant syndrome

Table by Richard B. Rosse, M.D., Lynn H. Deutsch, D.O., and Stephen J. Deutsch, M.D., Ph.D.

can cause electrocardiographic changes (not as frequently as with tricyclic antidepressants), including a prolonged QT interval; flattened, inverted, or bifid T waves; and U waves. Dose–plasma concentration relations differ widely among patients.

1. Antipsychotic levels
   a. In general, the plasma level does not correlate with the clinical response.

b. High plasma levels possibly correlate with toxic side effects (especially with chlorpromazine [Thorazine] and haloperidol [Haldol]).

c. Minimum therapeutic levels may be determined in the future but have been difficult to establish because of wide individual variation.

d. Radioreceptor assays measure serum dopamine blockage activity and can account for active metabolites, but a correlation with brain dopamine blockage is unclear.

e. No relation is known between antipsychotic levels and tardive dyskinesia.

2. **Conclusions**

a. Generally useful only to detect noncompliance or nonabsorption (but prolactin levels can also help).

b. May be useful in identifying nonresponders. Table 26–3 lists therapeutic and toxic blood levels for various drugs.

c. Adverse effects. Other side effects include hypotension, sedation, lowering of the seizure threshold, anticholinergic effects, tremor, dystonia, cogwheel rigidity, rigidity without cogwheeling, akathisia, akinesia, perioral tremor (rabbit syndrome), and tardive dyskinesia.

C. **Cyclic antidepressants.** A baseline ECG and follow-up ECGs at least annually are needed. Heart block is a relative contraindication. Baseline liver function tests and complete blood cell count are useful. Thyroid function tests are also necessary because thyroid disease may present as depression, and antidepressants can have synergistic effects with thyroxine. Side effects include bone marrow depression; neurological (especially anticholinergic), hepatic, gastrointestinal, and dermatologic effects; platelet dysfunction and other blood element effects; and a lowered seizure threshold. A common and possibly dangerous side effect is orthostatic hypotension, to which no tolerance develops. Nortriptyline (Pamelor, Aventyl) is less likely to cause hypotension than imipramine (Tofranil), desipramine (Norpramin), and amitriptyline (Elavil). Congestive heart failure considerably increases the risk for hypotension. Patients with congestive heart failure in whom hypotension develops while they are taking tricyclic antidepressants should be treated with nortriptyline. Toxic ECG changes include a prolonged PR interval (>0.2 s),

TABLE 26–3
THERAPEUTIC AND TOXIC PLASMA CONCENTRATIONS

Drug	Therapeutic Range	Toxic Levels
Amitriptyline	>120 ng/mL (but studies differ)	500 ng/mL
Bupropion	20–75 ng/mL	—
Carbamazepine	8–12 μg/mL	15 μg/mL
Clomipramine	Max 1,000 ng/mL	—
Desipramine	>125 ng/mL	500 ng/mL
Doxepin	150–250 ng/mL	—
Imipramine	>200–250 ng/mL	500 ng/mL
Lithium	0.6–1.2 mEq/L for maintenance 1.0–1.5 mEq/L for acute mania	1.5–2 mEq/L
Nortriptyline	Therapeutic window 50–150 ng/mL	500 ng/mL
Valproic acid	50–100 μg/mL	200 μg/mL

prolonged QRS interval (>0.12 s), prolonged QT interval (more than one third of R-R interval), sinus tachycardia (often secondary to hypotension), and heart block of all kinds (more likely in patients with preexisting conduction defects—the site of the effect is thought to be the intraventricular bundle). At therapeutic levels, tricyclic antidepressants usually suppress arrhythmias, including premature ventricular contractions, bigeminy, and ventricular tachycardia, by a quinidine-like effect.

1. **Tricyclic levels**—should be routinely obtained when imipramine, desipramine, or nortriptyline are used to treat depression. Levels must also include the measurement of active metabolites:

    imipramine → desipramine

    amitriptyline → nortriptyline

    These assays are difficult to perform and interpret, and measure extremely low concentrations. Active metabolites can contaminate the results. Reported data have been collected only for inpatients with nondelusional endogenous depression.

2. All tricyclic agents show complete gastrointestinal absorption, a high degree of tissue and plasma protein binding, a large volume of distribution, hepatic metabolism with prominent first-pass effect, and a plasma level that correlates directly with the brain level at steady state.

    a. **Imipramine (Tofranil).**

    (1) Favorable response correlates linearly with plasma level between 200 and 250 ng (of imipramine plus desipramine) per mL.

    (2) Some patients may respond at a lower level.

    (3) At levels above 250 ng/mL, no improved favorable response is noted, and side effects increase.

    b. **Nortriptyline (Pamelor).**

    (1) Therapeutic window (therapeutic range) is between 50 and 150 ng/mL.

    (2) Response rate decreases at levels above 150 ng/mL.

    c. **Desipramine (Norpramin).** Levels above 125 ng/mL correlate with a higher percentage of favorable responses.

    d. **Amitriptyline (Elavil).** Different studies show conflicting results.

3. Some patients are unusually poor metabolizers of tricyclic antidepressants and may have levels as high as 2,000 ng/mL while taking normal doses. These patients may show a favorable response only at these extremely high levels, but they must be monitored very closely for cardiac side effects. Patients with levels above 1,000 ng/mL are generally at risk for cardiotoxicity. Other patients have been reported with extremely high plasma levels at normal dosages who do not respond until the level is maintained somewhere between the usual therapeutic dosage and their extremely high levels.

4. Procedure—draw a blood specimen 10 to 14 hours after the most recent dose. Usually, this is in the morning after a bedtime dose. The patient must have been on a stable daily dose for at least 5 days. Use an appropriate specimen container.

5. Indications.
   a. Routine for patients receiving imipramine, desipramine, or nortriptyline.
   b. Poor response at a normal dose.
   c. High-risk patient for whom lowest possible therapeutic level should be maintained.

D. Monoamine oxidase inhibitors (MAOIs). Record the normal blood pressure and follow blood pressure during treatment because MAOIs can cause hypertensive crisis if a tyramine-restricted diet is not followed. MAOIs also often cause orthostatic hypotension (a direct drug side effect unrelated to diet). Baseline thyroid function tests are recommended. Relatively devoid of other side effects, although some patients may have insomnia or become irritable. May induce mania. A test used in both research and current clinical practice involves correlating the therapeutic response with the degree of platelet MAO inhibition.

E. Mood stabilizers—see Chapter 25, Psychopharmacology and Other Biological Therapies, for laboratory testing requirements for lithium, valproic acid (Depakene), and carbamazepine (Tegretol).

IV. Endocrine stimulation techniques

A. Dexamethasone suppression test (DST)

1. **Procedure**
   a. Give 1 mg of dexamethasone orally at 11 p.m.
   b. Measure plasma cortisol at 4 p.m. and 11 p.m. the next day (may also take 8 p.m. sample).
   c. Any plasma cortisol level above 5 μg/dL is abnormal (although the normal range should be adjusted according to the local assay so that 95% of normals are within the normal range).
   d. Baseline plasma cortisol level may be helpful.

2. **Indications**
   a. To help confirm a diagnostic impression of major depressive disorder. Not routinely used because it is unreliable. Abnormal results may confirm need for somatic treatment.
   b. To follow a depressed nonsuppressor through treatment of depression.
   c. To differentiate major depression from minor dysphoria.
   d. Some evidence indicates that depressed nonsuppressors are more likely to respond positively to treatment with electroconvulsive therapy or tricyclic antidepressants.
   e. Proposed utility in predicting outcome of treatment, but DST result may normalize before depression resolves.
   f. Proposed utility in predicting relapse in patients who are persistent nonsuppressors or whose DST results revert to abnormal.
   g. Possible utility in differentiating delusional from nondelusional depression.
   h. Highly abnormal plasma cortisol levels ($>$10 μg/dL) are more significant than mildly elevated levels.

TABLE 26–4
CAUSES OF FALSE-POSITIVE OR NEGATIVE RESULTS ON THE DEXAMETHASONE SUPPRESSION TEST

False-Positives	False-Negatives
Cushing's syndrome	Addison's disease
Weight loss or malnutrition	Hypopituitarism
Obesity	Slow dexamethasone metabolism
Bulimia nervosa	Drugs
Pregnancy	Synthetic corticosteroids
Alcohol abuse and withdrawal	Indomethacin
Anorexia nervosa	High doses of benzodiazepines
Temporal lobe epilepsy	High doses of cyproheptadine
Dementia	
Diabetes mellitus	
Infection	
Trauma	
Recent surgery	
Advanced age	
Fever	
Carcinoma	
Renal or cardiac failure	
Renovascular hypertension	
Cerebrovascular disorder	
Antipsychotic withdrawal	
Tricyclic withdrawal	
Drugs	
High doses of estrogens	
Narcotics	
Sedative-hypnotics	
Anticonvulsants	

Adapted from Darrell G. Kirch, M.D.

      i. False-positive results (Table 26–4).

      j. Sensitivity of DST is 45% in major depression, 70% in psychotic depressive disorders.

      k. Specificity of DST is 90% in comparison with controls, 77% in comparison with other psychiatric diagnoses overall.

B. Thyrotropin-releasing hormone stimulation test.   Used to help diagnose hypothyroidism.

  1. Procedure

     a. At 8 a.m., after an overnight fast, have the patient lie down and warn of a possible urge to urinate after the injection.

     b. Measure baseline levels of thyroid-stimulating hormone, tri-iodothyronine (T_3), thyroxine (T_4), and T_3 resin uptake.

     c. Inject 500 μg of thyroid-releasing hormone intravenously.

     d. Measure thyroid-stimulating hormone levels at 15, 30, 60, and 90 minutes.

  2. Indications

     a. Marginally abnormal thyroid test results or suspicion of subclinical hypothyroidism.

     b. Suspected lithium-induced hypothyroidism.

     c. Detection of patient who may require adjuvant 1:0 liothyronine (Cytomel) with tricyclic antidepressant.

d. Detection of incipient hypothyroidism, of which depression is often the first symptom. Grade 3 hypothyroidism is defined as normal thyroid function test result with abnormal thyrotropin-releasing hormone stimulation test result.

e. Eight percent of all depressed patients have some thyroid disease.

3. Results

a. If thyroid-stimulating hormone level changes by the following values:

(1) More than 35 μIU/mL, positive.

(2) Between 20 and 35 μIU/mL, early hypothyroidism.

(3) Less than 7 μIU/mL, blunted (may correlate with diagnosis of depression).

b. Peak thyroid-stimulating hormone level should be about double the baseline value in normals (i.e., 7 to 20 μIU/mL).

c. Does not distinguish well between hypothalamic and pituitary disease.

C. Provocation of panic attacks with sodium lactate

1. Indications

a. Possible diagnosis of panic disorder.

b. Lactate-provoked panic attack confirms presence of panic attacks.

c. Up to 72% of patients with panic attacks will have a lactate-provoked attack.

d. Has been used to induce flashbacks in patients with posttraumatic stress disorder.

2. Procedure. Infuse 0.5-M racemic sodium lactate (total of 10 mL/kg of body weight) during a 20-minute period or until panic occurs.

3. Note physiologic changes resulting from lactate infusion. Include hemodilution, metabolic alkalosis (metabolized to bicarbonate), hypocalcemia (calcium bound to lactate), and hypophosphatemia (due to increased glomerular filtration rate).

4. Comments

a. Effect is a direct peripheral response to lactate or metabolism of lactate.

b. Simple hyperventilation has not been as sensitive in inducing panic attacks.

c. Lactate-induced panic is not blocked by peripheral beta blockers but is inhibited by alprazolam (Xanax) and tricyclic antidepressants.

d. Inhalation of carbon dioxide precipitates panic attacks, but the mechanism is thought to be central and related to CNS concentrations of carbon dioxide, which possibly stimulates the locus ceruleus (carbon dioxide crosses the blood–brain barrier, whereas bicarbonate does not).

e. Lactate crosses the blood–brain barrier through an easily saturated active transport system.

f. L-Lactate is metabolized to pyruvate.

V. Electrophysiology

A. EEG

1. First clinical application was by the psychiatrist Hans Berger in 1929.
2. Measures voltages between electrodes placed on skin.
3. Provides gross description of electrical activity of CNS neurons.
4. Each person's EEG is unique, like a fingerprint.
5. For decades, researchers have attempted to correlate specific psychiatric conditions with characteristic EEG changes but have been unsuccessful.
6. EEG changes with age.
7. Normal EEG pattern does not rule out seizure disorder or medical disease; yield is higher in sleep-deprived subjects and with placement of nasopharyngeal leads.
8. Indications.
   a. General cognitive and medical workup; evaluation of delirium and dementia.
   b. Part of routine workup for any first-break psychosis.
   c. Can help diagnose some seizure disorders (e.g., epilepsy).
      (1) Grand mal seizures—onset characterized by epileptic recruiting rhythm of rhythmic, synchronous high-amplitude spikes between 8 and 12 Hz (cycles per second). After 15 to 30 seconds, spikes may become grouped and separated by slow waves (correlation with clonic phase). Finally, a quiescent phase of low-amplitude delta (slow) waves occurs.
      (2) Petit mal seizures—sudden onset of bilaterally synchronous generalized spike-and-wave pattern with high-amplitude and characteristic 3-Hz frequency.
   d. Helpful in diagnosing space-occupying lesions and vascular lesions of the CNS and encephalopathies, among others.
   e. Can detect characteristic changes caused by specific drugs.
   f. EEG exquisitely sensitive to drug changes.
   g. Diagnosis of brain death.
9. EEG waves.
   a. Beta, 14 to 30 Hz.
   b. Alpha, 8 to 13 Hz.
   c. Theta, 4 to 7 Hz.
   d. Delta, 0.5 to 3 Hz.

B. Polysomnography

1. Records EEG during sleep; often used with ECG, electrooculography (EOG), electromyography (EMG), chest expansion, and recordings of penile tumescence, blood oxygen saturation, body movement, body temperature, galvanic skin response (GSR), and gastric acid levels.
2. Indications—to assist in the diagnosis of the following:
   a. Sleep disorders—insomnias, hypersomnias, parasomnias, sleep apnea, nocturnal myoclonus, and sleep-related bruxism.

b. Childhood sleep-related disorders—enuresis, somnambulism (sleepwalking), and sleep terror disorder (pavor nocturnus).

c. Other conditions—erectile disorder, seizure disorders, migraine and other vascular headaches, substance abuse, gastroesophageal reflux, and major depressive disorder.

d. Comments.

(1) Rapid eye movement (REM) latency correlates with major depressive disorder; degree of decreased REM latency correlates with degree of depression.

(2) Shortened REM latency as a diagnostic test for major depressive disorder seems to be slightly more sensitive than DST.

(3) Use with DST or thyroid-releasing hormone stimulation test can improve sensitivity. Preliminary data indicate that depressed DST nonsuppressors are extremely likely to have shortened REM latency.

3. Polysomnographic findings in major depressive disorder.

a. Most depressed patients (80–85%) exhibit hyposomnia.

b. In depressed patients, slow-wave (delta-wave) sleep is decreased and sleep stages III and IV are shorter.

c. In depressed patients, the time between onset of sleep and onset of the first REM period (REM latency) is shorter.

d. In depressed patients, a greater proportion of REM sleep takes place early in the night (opposite true for nondepressed controls).

e. More REMs during the entire night (REM density) have been observed in depressed patients than in nondepressed controls.

C. Evoked potentials

1. Evoked potentials are brain electrical activity elicited by stimuli.

2. Visual, auditory, and somatosensory evoked potentials can detect abnormalities of peripheral and central neural conduction.

3. Can differentiate some functional complaints from organic complaints (e.g., studies with visual evoked potentials can be used to evaluate hysterical blindness).

4. Can be useful for detecting underlying neurological illness (e.g., demyelinating disorder).

VI. Drug-assisted interview

Common use of amobarbital (Amytal)—a barbiturate with a medium half-life of 8 to 42 hours—led to popular name, *Amytal interview.*

A. Diagnostic indications.
Catatonia; supposed conversion disorder; unexplained muteness; differentiating functional from organic stupors (organic conditions should worsen, and functional conditions should improve because of decreased anxiety).

B. Therapeutic indications.
As an interview aid for patients with disorders of repression and dissociation.

1. Abreaction of posttraumatic stress disorder.

2. Recovery of memory in dissociative amnesia and fugue.

3. Recovery of function in conversion disorder.

C. Procedure
1. Have patient recline in an environment in which cardiopulmonary resuscitation is readily available should hypotension or respiratory depression develop.
2. Explain to patient that medication should help him or her to relax and feel like talking.
3. Insert a narrow-bore needle into a peripheral vein.
4. Inject 5% solution of sodium amobarbital (500 mg dissolved in 10 mL of sterile water) at a rate no faster than 1 mL/min (50 mg/min).
5. Begin interview by discussing neutral topics. Often, it is helpful to prompt the patient with known facts about his or her life.
6. Continue infusion until either sustained lateral nystagmus or drowsiness is noted.
7. To maintain level of narcosis, continue infusion at a rate of 0.5 to 1.0 mL/5 min (25 to 50 mg/5 min).
8. Have the patient recline for at least 15 minutes after the interview is terminated and until the patient can walk without supervision.
9. Use the same method every time to avoid dosage errors.

D. Contraindications
1. Upper respiratory infection or inflammation.
2. Severe hepatic or renal impairment.
3. Hypotension.
4. History of porphyria.
5. Barbiturate addiction.

E. Diazepam.   Many clinicians use intravenous or oral diazepam (Valium) to conduct a drug-assisted interview.

VII. Brain imaging
A. Computed tomography (CT)
1. Clinical indications—dementia or depression, general cognitive and medical workup, and routine workup for any first-break psychosis.
2. Research.
   a. Differentiating subtypes of Alzheimer's disease.
   b. Cerebral atrophy in alcohol abusers.
   c. Cerebral atrophy in benzodiazepine abusers.
   d. Cortical and cerebellar atrophy in schizophrenia.
   e. Increased ventricle size in schizophrenia.

B. Magnetic resonance imaging (MRI). Formerly called *nuclear magnetic resonance.*
1. Measures radio frequencies emitted by different elements in the brain following application of an external magnetic field and produces slice images.
2. Measures structure, not function.
3. Technique has been available to other sciences for 30 years.
4. Provides much higher resolution than CT, particularly in gray matter.
5. No radiation involved; minimal or no risk to patients from strong magnetic fields.

6. Can image deep midline structures well.
7. Does not actually measure tissue density; measures density of particular nucleus being studied.
8. A major problem is the time needed to make a scan (5 to 40 minutes).
9. May offer information about cell function in the future, but stronger magnetic fields are needed.
10. The ideal technique for evaluating multiple sclerosis and other demyelinating diseases.

C. Positron emission tomography (PET)

1. Positron emitters (e.g., carbon 11 or fluorine 18) are used to label glucose, amino acids, neurotransmitter precursors, and many other molecules (particularly high-affinity ligands), which are used to measure receptor densities.
2. Can follow the distribution and fate of these molecules.
3. Produces slice images, as CT does.
4. Labeled antipsychotics can map out location and density of dopamine receptors.
5. Dopamine receptors have been shown to decrease with age (through PET).
6. Can assess regional brain function and blood flow.
7. 2-Deoxyglucose (a glucose analogue) is absorbed into cells as easily as glucose but is not metabolized. Can be used to measure regional glucose uptake.
8. Measures brain function and physiology.
9. Potential for increasing our understanding of brain function and sites of action of drugs.
10. Research.
   a. Usually compares laterality, anteroposterior gradients, and cortical-to-subcortical gradients.
   b. Findings reported in schizophrenia.
      (1) Cortical hypofrontality (also found in depressed patients).
      (2) Steeper subcortical-to-cortical gradient.
      (3) Uptake decreased in left compared with right cortex.
      (4) Higher rate of activity in left temporal lobe.
      (5) Lower rate of metabolism in left basal ganglia.
      (6) Higher density of dopamine receptors (replicated studies needed).
      (7) Greater increase in metabolism in anterior brain regions in response to unpleasant stimuli, but this finding is not specific to patients with schizophrenia.

D. Brain electrical activity mapping (BEAM)

1. Topographic imaging of EEG and evoked potentials.
2. Shows areas of varying electrical activity in the brain through scalp electrodes.
3. New data-processing techniques produce new ways of visualizing massive quantities of data produced by EEG and evoked potentials.
4. Each point on the map is given a numeric value representing its electrical activity.

   5. Each value is computed by linear interpolation among the three nearest electrodes.
   6. Some preliminary results show differences in schizophrenic patients. Evoked potentials differ spatially and temporally; asymmetric beta-wave activity is increased in certain regions; delta-wave activity is increased, most prominently in the frontal lobes.

E. Regional cerebral blood flow (rCBF)
   1. Yields a two-dimensional cortical image representing blood flow to different brain areas.
   2. Blood flow is believed to correlate directly with neuronal activity.
   3. Xenon 133 (radioisotope that emits low-energy gamma rays) is inhaled. Crosses blood–brain barrier freely but is inert.
   4. Detectors measure rate at which xenon 133 is cleared from specific brain areas and compare with calculated control to obtain a mean transit time for the tracer.
      a. Gray matter—clears quickly.
      b. White matter—clears slowly.
   5. rCBF may have great potential in studying diseases that involve a decrease in the amount of brain tissue (e.g., dementia, ischemia, atrophy).
   6. Highly susceptible to transient artifacts (e.g., anxiety, hyperventilation, low carbon dioxide pressure, high rate of CBF).
   7. Test is fast, equipment relatively inexpensive.
   8. Low levels of radiation.
   9. Compared with PET, spatial resolution less but temporal resolution better.
   10. Preliminary data show that in schizophrenic patients, CBF in the dorsolateral frontal lobe may be decreased and CBF in the left hemisphere may be increased during activation (e.g., when subjected to the Wisconsin Card Sorting Test).
   11. No differences have been found in resting schizophrenic patients.
   12. Still under development.

F. Single photon emission computed tomography (SPECT)
   1. Adaptation of rCBF techniques to obtain slice tomograms rather than two-dimensional surface images.
   2. Presently can obtain tomograms 2, 6, and 10 cm above and parallel to the canthomeatal line.
   3. Aids in diagnosis of Alzheimer's disease. Typically shows decrease in bilateral temporoparietal perfusion in Alzheimer's disease and single perfusion defects or multiple areas of hypoperfusion in vascular dementia.

G. Functional MRI (fMRI)
   1. May provide functional brain images with clarity of MRI.
   2. fMRI can be correlated with high-resolution three-dimensional MRI.
   3. Schizophrenic patients show less frontal activation and more left temporal activation during a word fluency task in comparison with controls.
   4. Used in research clinical settings in other disorders (e.g., panic disorder, phobias, and substance-related disorders).

H. Magnetic resonance spectroscopy (MRS)

1. Uses powerful magnetic fields to evaluate brain function and metabolism.
2. Provides information regarding brain intracellular pH and phospholipid, carbohydrate, protein, and high-energy phosphate metabolism.
3. Can provide information about lithium and fluorinated psychopharmacological agents.
4. Has detected decreased adenosine triphosphate and inorganic orthophosphate levels, suggestive of dorsal prefrontal hypoactivity, in schizophrenic patients in comparison with controls.
5. Further use in research is expected with refinements in technique.

I. Magnetoencephalography

1. Research tool.
2. Uses conventional and computerized EEG data.
3. Detects magnetic fields associated with neuronal electrical activity in cortical and deep brain structures.
4. Noninvasive with no radiation exposure.

VIII. Biochemical markers

Many potential biochemical markers, including neurotransmitters and their metabolites, may help in the diagnosis and treatment of psychiatric disorders. Research in this area is still evolving.

A. Monoamines

1. Plasma homovanillic acid (pHVA), a major dopamine metabolite, may have value in identifying schizophrenic patients who respond to antipsychotics.
2. 3-Methoxy-4-hydroxyphenylglycol (MHPG) is a norepinephrine metabolite.
3. 5-Hydroxyindoleacetic acid is associated with suicidal behavior, aggression, poor impulse control, and depression. Elevated levels may be associated with anxious, obsessional, and inhibited behaviors.

B. Alzheimer's disease

1. Apolipoprotein E allele—associated with increased risk for Alzheimer's disease. Reduced glucose metabolism noted on PET in some asymptomatic middle-aged persons, similar to findings in Alzheimer's patients.
2. Neural thread protein—reported to be increased in patients with Alzheimer's disease. CSF neural thread protein is marketed as a diagnostic test.
3. Other potential CSF tests include CSF tau (increased), CSF amyloid (decreased), ratio of CSF albumin to serum albumin (normal in Alzheimer's disease, elevated in vascular dementia), and inflammatory markers (e.g., CSF acute-phase reactive proteins). The gene for the amyloid precursor protein is considered to be possible etiologic significance, but further research is needed.

TABLE 26-5
DRUGS OF ABUSE THAT CAN BE TESTED IN URINE

Drug	Length of Time Detected in Urine
Alcohol	7–12 hours
Amphetamine	48 hours
Barbiturate	24 hours (short-acting)
	3 weeks (long-acting)
Benzodiazepine	3 days
Cocaine	6–8 hours (metabolites 2–4 days)
Codeine	48 hours
Heroin	36–72 hours
Marijuana (tetrahydrocannabinol)	3 days–4 weeks (depending on use)
Methadone	3 days
Methaqualone	7 days
Morphine	48–72 hours
Phencyclidine	8 days
Propoxyphene	6–48 hours

TABLE 26-6
LABORATORY DIAGNOSTIC TESTS OF POTENTIAL RELEVANCE TO THE PSYCHIATRIC PATIENT

Hematology
 Complete blood cell (CBC) count[a]
 Sedimentation rate
 Prothrombin time, partial thromboplastin time

Chemistry
 Serum electrolytes[a]
 Blood glucose[a]
 Blood urea nitrogen (BUN)[a]
 Serum creatinine[a]
 Serum calcium[a]
 Serum phosphorus
 Serum magnesium
 Total protein
 Serum protein electrophoresis
 Serum albumin
 Liver enzymes
 Creatine phosphokinase (CPK)
 Alkaline phosphatase
 Blood ammonia nitrogen (plasma ammonia)
 Serum bilirubin
 Thyroid function tests
  Thyroxine (T_4)[a]
  Triiodothyronine (T_3)
  Thyroid-stimulating hormone (TSH)
 Serum B_{12} and folate
 Plasma cortisol levels
 Blood alcohol
 Drug screen (or specific illicit drug level)
 Medication blood levels
 Serum caffeine
 Erythrocyte uroporphyrinogen-1-synthetase
 Serum copper and ceruloplasmin
 Serum amylase
 Serum lipase

Serology
 Screening test for syphilis (VDRL or RPR)[a]
 Human immunodeficiency virus (HIV) serology
 Hepatitis screens
 Lupus erythematosus (LE) cell preparation
 Serum antinuclear antibodies (ANA)
 Lupus anticoagulant
 Anticardiolipin antibodies (ACA)
 Antithyroid antibodies

Urine tests
 Urinalysis
 Urine screens for illicit drug use[a]
 Urinary uroporphyrins, porphobilinogen, and
  Δ-aminolevulinic acid
 Urinary catecholamines
 Urine copper and ceruloplasmin, heavy metals
 Urine myoglobin
 Urinary free cortisol (UFC)

Stool tests
 Occult blood
 Tests for suspected laxative abuse

Radiologic procedures
 Chest roentgenography
 Skull roentgenography
 Computed tomography (CT) of the brain
 Magnetic resonance imaging (MRI) of the brain
 Single-photon emission computed tomography
  (SPECT)
 Positron emission tomography (PET)

Other procedures
 Lumbar puncture
 Electrocardiogram (ECG)
 Electroencephalogram (EEG) and other
  electrophysiologic studies (e.g., brainstem
  evoked potential)
 Polysomnography
 Pupillometry
 Pulse oximetry
 Arterial blood gases
 Pregnancy tests in potentially childbearing
  women
 Dexamethasone suppression test (DST)
 Corticotropin-releasing hormone (CRH)
  stimulation test
 Thyrotropin-releasing hormone (TRH) stimulation
  test
 Tuberculosis tests
 Blood lead levels
 Genetic testing

[a] Although no complete consensus exists as to which tests should be included in a routine screening battery for a psychiatric patient, these tests may be included in such a screen.
Table by Richard B. Rosse, M.D., Lynn H. Deutsch, D.O., and Stephen Deutsch, M.D., Ph.D.

TABLE 26–7
CONVERSION FACTORS

1 gram (g)	=	1,000 milligrams (mg)
1 milligram (mg)	=	1,000 micrograms (μg)
1 microgram (μg)	=	1,000 nanograms (ng)
Blood concentrations:		
1 microgram per milliliter (mL)	=	100 micrograms per deciliter (dL)
	=	1 milligram per liter (L)
	=	1,000 nanograms per milliliter
100 milligrams per deciliter	=	0.1 gram per deciliter
	=	1,000 milligrams (1 gram) per liter
	=	1.0 milligram per milliliter

IX. Other laboratory tests

Drugs of abuse that can be tested in urine are listed in Table 26–5.

The laboratory tests listed in Table 26–6 are applied in clinical and research psychiatry. The reader is directed to a standard textbook of medicine for laboratory values. Always know the normal values of the particular laboratory performing the test because values vary from one laboratory to another. Two types of units of measurement currently are in use—the customary and the Système International (SI) units. The latter, now the more commonly accepted, comprise an international language of measurement calculated by multiplying the conventional unit by a number factor being adopted by many laboratories. The SI measurement system uses *moles* as the basic unit for the amount of a substance, *kilograms* for its mass, and *meters* for its length. Conversion factors are listed on Table 26–7.

For more detailed discussion of this topic, see Diagnosis and Psychiatry Examination of the Psychiatric Patient, Ch 7, p 652, in CTP/VII.

27

Medication-Induced Movement Disorders

I. General introduction

The typical antipsychotic drugs are associated with a number of uncomfortable and potentially serious neurological adverse effects. The drugs act by blocking the binding of dopamine to the dopamine receptors involved in the control of both voluntary and involuntary movements. The newer antipsychotics, the serotonin-dopamine antagonists, block binding to dopamine receptors to a much lesser degree and are less likely to produce such syndromes. The movement disorders include (1) neuroleptic-induced parkinsonism, (2) neuroleptic-induced acute dystonia, (3) neuroleptic-induced acute akathisia, (4) neuroleptic-induced tardive dyskinesia, (5) neuroleptic malignant syndrome, and (6) medication-induced postural tremor.

II. Neuroleptic-induced parkinsonism

A. Diagnosis, signs, and symptoms. Symptoms include muscle stiffness (lead pipe rigidity), cogwheel rigidity, shuffling gait, stooped posture, and drooling. The pill-rolling tremor of idiopathic parkinsonism is rare, but a regular, coarse tremor similar to essential tremor may be present. A focal, perioral tremor, sometimes referred to as *rabbit syndrome,* is another parkinsonian effect seen with antipsychotics, although perioral tremor is more likely than other tremors to occur late in the course of treatment.

B. Epidemiology. Parkinsonian adverse effects occur in about 15% of patients who are treated with antipsychotics, usually within 5 to 90 days of the initiation of treatment. Women are affected about twice as often as men, and the disorder can occur at all ages, although it is most common after age 40.

C. Etiology. Caused by blockade of dopaminergic transmission in the nigrostriatal tract. All antipsychotics can cause the symptoms, especially high-potency drugs with low levels of anticholinergic activity (e.g., trifluoperazine [Stelazine]). Chlorpromazine [Thorazine] and thioridazine [Mellaril] are not likely to be involved. The newer, atypical antipsychotics (e.g., risperidone [Risperdal]) are less likely to cause parkinsonism.

D. Differential diagnosis. Includes idiopathic parkinsonism, other organic causes of parkinsonism, and depression, which can also be associated with parkinsonian symptoms.

E. Treatment. Can be treated with anticholinergic agents, amantadine (Symmetrel), or diphenhydramine (Benadryl) (Table 27–1). Anticholinergics should be withdrawn after 4 to 6 weeks to assess whether toler-

TABLE 27–1
DRUG TREATMENT OF EXTRAPYRAMIDAL DISORDERS

Generic Name	Trade Name	Usual Daily Dosage	Indications
Anticholinergics			
Benztropine	Cogentin	PO 0.5–2 mg tid; IM or IV 1–2 mg	Acute dystonia, parkinsonism, akinesia, akathisia
Biperiden	Akineton	PO 2–6 mg tid; IM or IV 2 mg	
Procyclidine	Kemadrin	PO 2.5–5 mg bid-qid	
Trihexyphenidyl	Artane, Tremin	PO 2–5 mg tid	
Orphenadrine	Norflex, Dispal	PO 50–100 mg bid-qid; IV 60 mg	Rabbit syndrome
Antihistamine			
Diphenhydramine	Benadryl	PO 25 mg qid; IM or IV 25 mg	Acute dystonia, parkinsonism, akinesia, rabbit syndrome
Amantadine	Symmetrel	PO 100–200 mg bid	Parkinsonism, akinesia rabbit syndrome
β-Adrenergic antagonist			
Propranolol	Inderal	PO 20–40 mg tid	Akathisia, tremor
α-Adrenergic antagonist			
Clonidine	Catapres	PO 0.1 mg tid	Akathisia
Benzodiazepines			
Clonazepam	Klonopin	PO 1 mg bid	Akathisia, acute dystonia
Lorazepam	Ativan	PO 1 mg tid	
Buspirone	BuSpar	PO 20–40 mg qid	Tardive dyskinesia
Vitamin E	—	PO 1,200–1,600 IU/d	Tardive dyskinesia

PO, oral; IM, intramuscular; IV, intravenous; qd, per day; bid, twice a day; tid, three times a day; qid; four times a day.

ance to the parkinsonian effects has developed; about half of patients with neuroleptic-induced parkinsonism require continued treatment. Even after the antipsychotics are withdrawn, parkinsonian symptoms may last for up to 2 weeks and even up to 3 months in elderly patients. With such patients, the clinician may continue the anticholinergic drug after the antipsychotic has been stopped until the parkinsonian symptoms resolve completely.

III. Neuroleptic-induced acute dystonia

A. Diagnosis, signs, and symptoms. Dystonic movements result from a slow, muscular contraction or spasm than can result in an involuntary movement. Dystonia can involve the neck (spasmodic torticollis or retrocollis), jaw (forced closing resulting in a dislocation of the jaw or trismus), tongue (protrusions, twisting), or entire body (opisthotonos). Involvement of the eyes can result in an oculogyric crisis, characterized by upward lateral movement of the eyes. Other dystonias include blepharospasm and glossopharyngeal dystonia; the latter results in dysarthria, dysphagia, and even difficulty in breathing, which can cause cyanosis. Children are particularly likely to evidence opisthotonos, scoliosis, lordosis, and writhing movements. Dystonia can be painful and frightening and often results in noncompliance with future drug treatment regimens.

B. Epidemiology. About 10% of all patients experience dystonia as an adverse effect of antipsychotics, usually in the first few hours or days of treatment. Dystonia is most common in young men (<40 years old) but can occur at any age in either sex.

C. Etiology. Although it is most common with intramuscular doses of high-potency antipsychotics, dystonia can occur with any antipsychotic. It is least common with thioridazine and is uncommon with risperidone. The mechanism of action is thought to be dopaminergic hyperactivity in the basal ganglia that occurs when CNS levels of the antipsychotic drug begin to fall between doses.

D. Differential diagnosis. Includes seizures and tardive dyskinesia.

E. Course and prognosis. Dystonia can fluctuate spontaneously and respond to reassurance, so that the clinician acquires the false impression that the movement is hysterical or completely under conscious control.

F. Treatment. Prophylaxis with anticholinergics or related drugs (Table 27–1) usually prevents dystonia, although the risks of prophylactic treatment weigh against that benefit. Treatment with intramuscular anticholinergics or intravenous or intramuscular diphenhydramine (50 mg) almost always relieves the symptoms. Diazepam (Valium) (10 mg intravenously), amobarbital (Amytal), caffeine sodium benzoate, and hypnosis have also been reported to be effective. Although tolerance for the adverse effect usually develops, it is sometimes prudent to change the antipsychotic if the patient is particularly concerned that the reaction may recur.

IV. Neuroleptic-induced acute akathisia

A. Diagnosis, signs, and symptoms. Akathisia is a subjective feeling of muscular discomfort that can cause the patient to be agitated, pace relentlessly, alternately sit and stand in rapid succession, and feel generally dysphoric. The symptoms are primarily motor and cannot be controlled by the patient at will. Akathisia can appear at any time during treatment. Once akathisia is recognized and diagnosed, the antipsychotic dose should be reduced to the minimal effective level.

B. Treatment. Treatment can be attempted with anticholinergics or amantadine, although these drugs are not particularly effective for akathisia. Drugs that may be more effective include propranolol (Inderal) (30 to 120 mg/day), benzodiazepines, and clonidine (Catapres). In some cases of akathisia, no treatment seems to be effective.

V. Neuroleptic-induced tardive dyskinesia

A. Diagnosis, signs, and symptoms. Tardive dyskinesia is a delayed effect of antipsychotics; it rarely occurs until after 6 months of treatment. The disorder consists of abnormal, involuntary, irregular choreoathetoid movements of the muscles of the head, limbs, and trunk. The severity of the movements ranges from minimal—often missed by patients and their families—to grossly incapacitating. Perioral movements are the most common and include darting, twisting, and protruding movements of the tongue, chewing and lateral jaw movements, lip puckering, and facial grimacing. Finger movements and hand clenching are also common. Torticollis, retrocollis, trunk twisting, and pelvic thrusting occur in severe cases. Respiratory dyskinesia has also been reported. Dyskinesia is exacerbated by stress and disappears during sleep.

B. **Epidemiology.** Tardive dyskinesia develops in about 10–20% of patients who are treated for more than a year. About 15–20% of patients undergoing long-term hospitalization have tardive dyskinesia. Women are more likely to be affected than men. Children, patients who are more than 50 years of age, and patients with brain damage or mood disorders are also at high risk.

C. **Course and prognosis.** Between 5% and 40% of all cases of tardive dyskinesia eventually remit, and between 50% and 90% of all mild cases remit. However, tardive dyskinesia is less likely to remit in elderly patients than in young patients.

D. **Treatment.** The three basic approaches to tardive dyskinesia are prevention, diagnosis, and management. Prevention is best achieved by using antipsychotic medications only when clearly indicated and in the lowest effective doses. The new antipsychotics (e.g., risperidone) are associated with less tardive dyskinesia than the old antipsychotics. Patients who are receiving antipsychotics should be examined regularly for the appearance of abnormal movements, preferably with the use of a standardized rating scale (Table 27–2).

TABLE 27–2
ABNORMAL INVOLUNTARY MOVEMENT SCALE (AIMS) EXAMINATION PROCEDURE

Patient Identification	Date
Rated by	

Either before or after completing the examination procedure, observe the patient unobtrusively at rest (e.g., in waiting room).

The chair to be used in this examination should be a hard, firm one without arms.

After observing the patient, rate him or her on a scale of 0 (none), 1 (minimal), 2 (mild), 3 (moderate), and 4 (severe) according to the severity of the symptoms.

Ask the patient whether there is anything in his or her mouth (i.e., gum, candy, etc.) and, if so, to remove it.

Ask the patient about the current condition of his or her teeth. Ask patient if he or she wears dentures. Do teeth or dentures bother patient now?

Ask patient whether he or she notices any movement in mouth, face, hands, or feet. If yes, ask patient to describe and indicate to what extent they currently bother patient or interfere with his or her activities.

0 1 2 3 4 Have patient sit in chair with hands on knees, legs slightly apart, and feet flat on floor. (Look at entire body for movement while in this position.)

0 1 2 3 4 Ask patient to sit with hands hanging unsupported. If male, between legs, if female and wearing a dress, hanging over knees. (Observe hands and other body areas.)

0 1 2 3 4 Ask patient to open mouth. (Observe tongue at rest within mouth.) Do this twice.

0 1 2 3 4 Ask patient to protrude tongue. (Observe abnormalities of tongue movement.) Do this twice.

0 1 2 3 4 Ask the patient to tap thumb, with each finger, as rapidly as possible for 10 to 15 seconds: separately with right hand, then with left hand. (Observe facial and leg movements.)

0 1 2 3 4 Flex and extend patient's left and right arms. (One at a time.)

0 1 2 3 4 Ask patient to stand up. (Observe in profile. Observe all body areas again, hips included.)

0 1 2 3 4 [a] Ask patient to extend both arms outstretched in front with palms down. (Observe trunk, legs, and mouth.)

0 1 2 3 4 [a] Have patient walk a few paces, turn, and walk back to chair. (Observe hands and gait.) Do this twice.

[a] Activated movements.

Once tardive dyskinesia is recognized, the clinician should consider reducing the dose of the antipsychotic or even stopping the medication altogether. Alternatively, the clinician may switch the patient to clozapine or to one of the new dopamine receptor antagonists, such as risperidone. In patients who cannot continue taking any antipsychotic medication, lithium, carbamazepine (Tegretol), or benzodiazepines may effectively reduce the symptoms of both the movement disorder and the psychosis.

VI. Neuroleptic malignant syndrome

A. Diagnosis, signs, and symptoms. Neuroleptic malignant syndrome is a life-threatening complication that can occur anytime during the course of antipsychotic treatment. The motor and behavioral symptoms include muscular rigidity and dystonia, akinesia, mutism, obtundation, and agitation. The autonomic symptoms include hyperpyrexia (up to 107°F), sweating, and increased pulse and blood pressure. Laboratory findings include an increased white blood cell count and increased levels of creatinine phosphokinase, liver enzymes, plasma myoglobin, and myoglobinuria, occasionally associated with renal failure.

B. Epidemiology. Men are affected more frequently than women, and young patients are affected more commonly than elderly patients. The mortality rate can reach 20–30% or even higher when depot antipsychotic medications are involved.

C. Pathophysiology. Unknown.

D. Course and prognosis. The symptoms usually evolve over 24 to 72 hours, and the untreated syndrome lasts 10 to 14 days. The diagnosis is often missed in the early stages, and the withdrawal or agitation may mistakenly be considered to reflect an exacerbation of the psychosis.

E. Treatment. The first step in treatment is immediate discontinuation of antipsychotic drugs; medical support to cool the patient; monitoring of vital signs, electrolytes, fluid balance, and renal output; and symptomatic treatment of fevers. Antiparkinsonian medications may reduce some of the muscle rigidity. Dantrolene (Dantrium), a skeletal muscle relaxant (0.8 to 2.5 mg/kg every 6 hours, up to a total dosage of 10 mg/day), may be useful in the treatment of the disorder. Once the patient can take oral medications, the dantrolene can be given in dosages of 100 to 200 mg/day. Bromocriptine (20 to 30 mg/day in four divided doses) or perhaps amantadine can be added to the regimen. Treatment should usually be continued for 5 to 10 days. When antipsychotic treatment is restarted, the clinician should consider switching to a low-potency drug or one of the new serotonin-dopamine antagonists (e.g., clozapine), although neuroleptic malignant syndrome has also been reported to be associated with these newer drugs.

VII. Medication-induced postural tremor

A. Diagnosis, signs, and symptoms. Tremor is a rhythmic alteration in movement that is usually faster than one beat per second.

B. Epidemiology. Typically, tremors decrease during periods of relaxation and sleep and increase with stress or anxiety.

TABLE 27–3
DRUG INDUCED CENTRAL HYPERTHERMIC SYNDROMES[a]

Condition (and Mechanism)	Common Drug Causes	Frequent Symptoms	Possible Treatment[b]	Clinical Course
Hyperthermia (↓ heat dissipation) (↑ heat production)	Atropine, lidocaine, meperidine NSAID toxicity, pheochromocytoma, thyrotoxicosis	Hyperthermia, diaphoresis, malaise	Acetaminophen per rectum (325 mg every 4 hours), diazepam oral or per rectum (5 mg every 8 hours) for febrile seizures	Benign, febrile seizures in children
Malignant hyperthermia (↑ heat production)	NMJ blockers (succinylcholine), halothane	Hyperthermia, **muscle rigidity, arrhythmias,** ischemia,[c] hypotension, **rhabdomyolysis;** disseminated intravascular coagulation	Dantrolene sodium (1–2 mg/ kg/min IV infusion)[d]	Familial, 10% mortality if untreated
Tricyclic overdose (↑ heat production)	Tricyclic antidepressants, cocaine	Hyperthermia, confusion, visual hallucinations, agitation, **hyperreflexia, muscle relaxation, anticholinergic effects** (dry skin, pupil dilation), arrhythmias	Sodium bicarbonate (1 mEq/kg IV bolus) if arrhythmias are present, physostigmine (1–3 mg IV) with cardiac monitoring	Fatalities have occurred if untreated
Autonomic hyperreflexia (↑ heat production)	CNS stimulants (amphetamines)	Hyperthermia excitement, **hyperreflexia**	Trimethaphan (0.3–7 mg/minute IV infusion)	Reversible
Lethal catatonia (↓ heat dissipation)	Lead poisoning	Hyperthermia, intense anxiety, **destructive behavior, psychosis**	Lorazepam (1–2 mg IV every 4 hours), antipsychotics may be contraindicated	High mortality if untreated
Neuroleptic malignant syndrome (mixed: hypothalamic, ↓ heat dissipation, ↑ heat production)	Antipsychotics (neuroleptics), methyldopa, reserpine	Hyperthermia, **muscle rigidity, diaphoresis (60%),** leukocytosis, delirium, **rhabdomyolysis, elevated CPK,** autonomic deregulation, **extrapyramidal symptoms**	**Bromocriptine (2–10 mg every 8 hours orally or nasogastric tube),** lisuride (0.02–0.1 mg/hour IV infusion), carbidopa-levodopa (Sinemet) (25/100) PO every 8 hours), dantrolene sodium (0.3–1 mg/kg IV every 6 hours)	Rapid onset, 20% mortality if untreated

[a] Boldface indicates features that may be used to distinguish one syndrome from another. NSAID, nonsteroidal antiinflammatory drugs; MAOI, monoamine oxidase inhibitors; NMJ, neuromuscular junction; CNS, central nervous system; CPK, creatine phosphokinase; IV, intravenously.
[b] Gastric lavage and supportive measures, including cooling, are required in most cases.
[c] Oxygen consumption increases by 7% for every 1°F up in body temperature.
[d] Has been associated with idiosyncratic hepatocellular injury, as well as severe hypotension in one case.
From Theoharides TC, Harris RS, Weckstein D. Neuroleptic malignant-like syndrome due to cyclobenzaprine? (letter). *J Clin Psychopharmacol* 1995;15:80, with permission.

C. Etiology.   Whereas all the above diagnoses specifically include an association with a neuroleptic, a range of psychiatric medications can produce tremor—most notably lithium, antidepressants, and valproate (Depakene).

D. Treatment.   The treatment involves four principles.

1. The lowest possible dose of the psychiatric drug should be taken.
2. Patients should minimize caffeine consumption.
3. The psychiatric drug should be taken at bedtime to minimize the amount of daytime tremor.
4. β-Adrenergic receptor antagonists (e.g., propranolol [Inderal]) can be given to treat drug-induced tremors.

VIII. Hyperthermic syndromes

All the medication-induced movement disorders may be associated with hyperthermia. Table 27–3 lists the various conditions associated with hyperthermia.

For more detailed discussion of this topic, see Neuropsychiatric Aspects of Movement Disorders, Section 2.6, p 285; Schizophrenia: Somatic Treatment, Section 12.8, p 1197; Medication-induced Movement Disorders, Section 31.4, p 2265; and Dopamine Receptor Antagonists (Typical Antipsychotics), Section 31.17, p 2356, in CTP/VII.

28

Legal and Ethical Issues

I. Introduction

Forensic psychiatrists evaluate cases and testify in court about legal matters such as competency, involuntary hospitalization, criminal responsibility, and malpractice litigation, among many other issues. In these situations, no rule of confidentiality applies. The primary goal is to make an accurate diagnosis of the patient's disorder. Only in special cases is there the goal of improving or curing mental or emotional dysfunction.

Because laws and regulations regarding the mentally ill change rapidly as new legislation is passed or new cases are decided, practitioners should seek legal advice when uncertainty in psychiatric situations raises legal issues.

II. Legal issues in psychiatry

A. Psychiatrists and the courts. Psychiatrists in court can act as two kinds of witnesses.

1. **Witness of fact.** The psychiatrist's role is the same as that of an ordinary witness. Any psychiatrist at any level of training can fulfill this role.

2. **Expert witness.** The term *expert witness* indicates acceptance by the court and by advocates of both sides in a case that the psychiatrist is qualified to perform expert functions; it is independent of a clinician's actual or presumed expertise in a given area. An expert witness may draw conclusions from data and thereby render an opinion. Experts play a role in determining the standard of care and the reasonable practice of psychiatry.

3. **Direct examination and cross-examination.** In court, the psychiatrist undergoes both direct examination and cross-examination under oath.

   a. Direct examination. The first questioning of the psychiatrist by the attorney for the party on whose behalf the witness is called; it generally consists of open-ended questions that require narrative answers.

   b. Cross-examination. The questioning of a witness by the attorney for the opposing party; it usually involves long, possibly leading questions that require a "yes" or "no" answer.

4. **Court-mandated evaluations.** Judges ask clinicians to act as consultants to the court; clinical information may have to be revealed to the court, so that clinicians do not have the same confidential relationship with their patients as they have in private practice. They are under an ethical obligation so to inform their patients at the outset of an examination and to make sure that the patients understand that confidentiality does not exist and that a report will be made of the interview.

5. **Evaluation of witnesses' credibility.** A trial judge may grant a psychiatric examination requested by one of the parties to the action. Psychiatrists cannot testify regarding whether someone is telling the truth, but they can discuss personality or psychological factors affecting the way information is reported.

B. **Informed consent.** Proper informed consent requires that a patient be informed about a particular treatment, alternative treatments, and their potential risks and benefits; that the patient understands this information; and that the patient freely and knowingly gives consent. The psychiatrist should document the patient's consent, preferably with a signed form.

1. **Consent form.** A written document outlining a patient's consent to a proposed procedure or treatment plan. It should include a fair explanation of procedures and their purposes, including the following: (1) identification of procedures that are experimental; (2) discomfort and risks to be expected; (3) disclosure of alternative procedures that may be advantageous; (4) an offer to answer any inquiries concerning the procedures; and (5) instructions that the patient is free to withdraw consent and discontinue participation at any time without prejudice.

2. **Exceptions to the rules of informed consent**

   a. **Emergencies.** Usually defined in terms of imminent physical danger to the patient or others.

   b. **Therapeutic privilege.** Information that in the opinion of the psychiatrist would harm the patient or be antitherapeutic and that may be withheld on those grounds.

C. **Confidentiality.** The therapeutic relationship gives rise to a legal and ethical duty of confidentiality, which requires the physician to hold secret all information revealed by a patient. Breach of confidentiality can result in an action for damages for defamation, invasion of privacy, or breach of contract.

D. **Exceptions to the duty of confidentiality**

1. **Duty to warn.** The most important exception to confidentiality is the duty to warn, which requires psychotherapists to warn potential victims of their patient's expressed intention to harm the victim (Tarasoff I, 1974). In 1976, the Tarasoff II decision broadened the original ruling by requiring the therapist to take some action in the face of a threat of harm to another (the duty to protect).

2. **Release of information.** A patient must consent to disclosure of information in his or her record before the psychiatrist can release that information. The actual physical record is the legal property of the psychiatrist or the institution; however, the patient has the legal right to his or her psychiatric records. The psychiatrist may claim therapeutic privilege as noted above, but disclosure must then be made to a representative of the patient, usually the patient's lawyer or advocate, according to the particular law of the state.

3. **Third-party payers and supervision.** To provide coverage, an insurance carrier must be able to obtain information with which it can assess the administration and costs of various programs. The therapist in

training may breach a patient's confidence by discussing the case with a supervisor. It is acceptable for psychiatrists-in-training to advise their patients that they are being supervised.

4. **Discussion about patients.** Psychiatrists have an obligation not to disclose identifiable patient information (and, perhaps, any descriptive patient information) without appropriate informed consent.

5. **Child abuse.** All states now legally require that psychiatrists, among others, who believe that a child has been the victim of physical or sexual abuse make an immediate report to an appropriate agency. Confidentiality is limited on the ground that potential or actual harm to vulnerable children outweighs the value of confidentiality in a psychiatric setting.

6. **Disclosure to safeguard.** A physician must report to the authorities in situations specifically required by law. Such mandatory reporting would include, for example, a patient with epilepsy who is operating a motor vehicle, a patient abusing a child, or a patient engaging in sexual activity with a child.

7. **Testimonial privilege.** Privilege protects the patient's right to privacy and belongs to the patient. The psychiatrist may not reveal information about patients against their will.

   Some exceptions to the doctrine of testimonial privilege are (1) hospitalization proceedings, (2) court-ordered examinations (military or civilian), (3) child custody hearings, and (4) malpractice claims. Psychiatrists and other physicians do not legally enjoy the same privilege that exists between client and attorney, priest and churchgoer, and husband and wife.

E. **Laws governing hospitalization.** The power of the state (society) to confine an individual (legally known as commitment) is based on two separate concepts: (1) the police power of the state to protect society for society's benefit, and (2) the parens patriae power of the state, in which the needs of the individual are of concern. The issue here is the need for treatment.

   1. **Types of admissions procedures.** Patients may be admitted to a psychiatric hospital in one of four ways.

      a. **Informal**—entry into and release from the hospital may be requested orally. The patient may leave at any time, even against medical advice.

      b. **Voluntary**—written application for admission with limitations placed on release (to allow for conversion into involuntary admission).

      c. **Involuntary**—if patients are a danger to themselves (suicidal) or others (homicidal), they may be admitted to a hospital after a friend or relative applies for admission and two physicians confirm the need for hospitalization.

      d. **Emergency**—a temporary form of involuntary commitment for patients who are senile, confused, or unable to make their own decisions. In an emergency admission, the patient cannot be hospitalized against his or her will for more than 15 days.

2. **Involuntary discharge.** Under a variety of circumstances, patients may have to be discharged from a hospital against their will—if they have broken a major hospital rule intentionally, refused treatment, or been restored to health but still wish to remain hospitalized.
   a. **Abandonment as cause of action.** The potential pitfall of involuntary discharge or involuntary termination is the charge of abandonment; clinicians should exercise special care in such charged situations.
   b. **Ending the relationship.** An involuntary discharge entails all the pain of the usual process of terminating therapy with far less opportunity for healing, growth, and gaining perspective. The clinician directly opposes the patient's proclaimed wishes and thereby severely strains the therapeutic alliance. Consultation and documentation of the rationale for the action are two safeguards against liability. Termination does not mean abandonment when a transfer of services is made in good faith through an appropriate referral to another hospital or therapist. The clinician is not obliged to accept any patient back into treatment.
   c. **Emergencies.** The one circumstance in which clinicians cannot terminate patients is a state of emergency (e.g., if the patient attacks a therapist or another patient). The therapist cannot terminate the patient's care until the emergency situation has been resolved.
3. **Criteria for commitment.** Although specific criteria for commitment under the various categories differ across states, all require mental illness, dangerousness to self or others, need for care and treatment, or lack of judgment to care for oneself.
4. **Procedural safeguards.** Specific procedural safeguards for meeting the requirements of due process vary among states. These include (1) application requirements, (2) physician's evaluation, (3) patient's advocate, (4) judicial review, (5) limits on retention, and (6) notice of rights.
5. **Right to treatment.** The right of an involuntarily committed patient to active treatment has been enunciated by lower federal courts and enacted in some state statutes.

    The principal case, *Wyatt v. Stickney* (1971), set the pattern of reform by requiring treatment in addition to hospitalization. It also required specific changes in the operations of institutions and their programs, including changes in physical conditions, staffing, and quality of treatment provided.

    In the case of *Donaldson v. O'Connor* (1976), the United States Supreme Court held that an involuntarily committed person who is not dangerous and who can survive by himself or herself with help must be released from the hospital.
6. **Right to refuse treatment.** One of the most controversial legal issues in the practice of psychiatry today is the right to refuse treatment. The issue arises when the patient's competence to make the necessary decisions is in question.
   a. **Status of the patient**—only involuntary patients may be treated against their will.

    b. Who decides? In the past, the treating psychiatrist had the prerogative simply to order treatment (e.g. medication) in the face of a patient's objection. Subsequently, procedures were developed to obtain a second or third opinion from a psychiatrist in the facility (a so-called administrative review). That is still the extent of the process in many states.

  7. Involuntary outpatient commitment. This procedure, which has been adopted in a number of states, requires regular mandated outpatient visits for treatment and permits the immediate hospitalization of an outpatient who does not comply with medical treatment. As such, it has been found to be a useful alternative to hospitalization and allows for treatment in the community.

F. Civil rights of patients. Thanks to several clinical, public, and legal movements, criteria for the civil rights of people who are mentally ill, apart from their rights as patients, have been both established and affirmed.

  1. Least restrictive alternative. Patients have the right to receive the least restrictive means of treatment for the requisite clinical effect.

  2. Visitation rights. Patients have the right to receive visitors at reasonable hours (customary hospital visiting hours). A patient's attorney, private physician, and members of the clergy have unrestricted access to the patient, including the right to privacy in their discussions. Allowance must be made for the possibility that a patient's clinical condition may not permit visits.

  3. Communication rights. Patients should have access to free and open communication with the outside world by telephone or mail; this right varies regionally.

  4. Privacy rights. Patients have the right to privacy, confidentiality, private bathroom and shower space, secure storage space for clothing and other belongings, and adequate floor space per person. They also have the right to wear their own clothes and carry their own money.

  5. Economic rights. Psychiatric patients generally are permitted to manage their own financial affairs. If the patient works in the institution, the requirement is that they be paid.

G. Seclusion and restraint. *Seclusion* refers to placing and keeping an inpatient in a special room for the purpose of containing a clinical situation that may result in a state of emergency. *Restraint* involves measures designed to confine a patient's bodily movements, such as the use of leather cuffs and anklets or straitjackets. The doctrine of the least restrictive alternative is used (i.e., seclusion should be used only when no less restrictive alternative is available).

H. Malpractice

  1. Definition. *Malpractice* can be broadly defined as occurrences in a professional practice that result in injury to a patient and are the consequence of a psychiatrist's lack of care or skill. The psychiatrist need not have intended to harm the patient.

  2. Four Ds. Four elements must be proved in a malpractice case.

    a. Duty—a standard of care; a requirement to exercise a particular degree of skill and care. The duty is predicated on the existence of a professional (i.e., doctor–patient) relationship. The physician does not have a duty to cure. The standard of care is usually national rather than local.

   b. **Dereliction**—a failure to exercise such care (i.e., a breach of duty). Dereliction may be a consequence of carelessness, incompetence, inappropriate treatment, or failure to obtain the proper consent.

   c. **Direct causation**—a direct, or proximate, causal relationship between dereliction of duty and damage to a patient. Sometimes phrased as "but for" the dereliction of duty, the damage would not have occurred.

   d. **Damages**—some specific damage or injury to the patient must be proved.

3. **Common causes of malpractice lawsuits in psychiatry**

   a. **Suicide**—the suicide of a psychiatric patient often raises the question of malpractice and is the most common basis for malpractice lawsuits in psychiatry. For that reason, careful documentation of the treatment of a suicidal patient is necessary.

   b. **Improper somatic therapy**—the negligent administration of medications or electroconvulsive therapy is the second most frequent basis for malpractice suits in psychiatry. Tardive dyskinesia as an adverse effect of pharmacotherapy and fractures as an adverse effect of electroconvulsive therapy are some concerns.

   c. **Negligent diagnosis**—although this is a relatively rare basis for a lawsuit, it may be used when a psychiatrist fails to assess properly a patient's dangerousness to others.

   d. **Sexual activity with a patient**—an area of increasing concern, it is now a crime in a number of states. Sexual activity with a patient has been deemed unethical in the ethical annotations of the American Psychiatric Association and has been determined to be a breach of contract as well as a form of malpractice.

   e. **Informed consent**—the alleged failure of a psychiatrist to obtain proper informed consent is often the basis of a malpractice lawsuit.

4. **Preventing liability**

   a. Clinicians should provide only the care they are qualified to offer.

   b. The decision-making process, the clinician's rationale for treatment, and an evaluation of the costs and benefits should all be documented.

   c. Consultations help guard against liability because they provide a second opinion and allow the clinician to obtain information about the peer group's standard of practice.

III. Legal issues in child and adolescent psychiatry

   A. **Involuntary commitment of minors.** In a landmark decision, *Parham v. J.R.* (1979), the Supreme Court held that minors may be involuntarily committed to a psychiatric facility by their parents or guardians. The Court said that parents should "retain a substantial if not dominant role" in the commitment decision. However, although minors may be involuntarily committed to a psychiatric facility by their parents or guardians, such civil commitment of juveniles now requires various procedural safeguards.

The Supreme Court held that the civil commitment of juveniles requires constitutional safeguards, including the right to counsel. Once juveniles are committed, housing and treatment must be adequate. The Supreme Court has ruled that inadequate housing or lack of treatment for committed juveniles is unconstitutional.

B. Consent of minors.   The principles of informed consent apply, except that the issue of competence turns on the state's legal definition of what constitutes a minor for the particular issue involved.

An emancipated minor is usually one who is married or financially independent. For particular situations, usually related to contracts, the emancipated minor is treated as an adult.

C. Custody.   The increasing divorce rate has led to a substantial increase in the number of cases of contested custody.

In cases of disputed custody, the almost universally accepted criterion is "the best interest of the child." In that context, the task of the psychiatrist is to provide an expert opinion and supporting data regarding which party should be granted custody to best serve the interests of the child.

The mental disability of a parent can lead to the transfer of custody to the other parent or to a public agency. When the mental disability is chronic and the parent is incapacitated, a procedure for the termination of parental rights may result. That also is the case when evidence of child abuse is pervasive. In the Gault decision (1967), the Supreme Court held that a juvenile also has constitutional rights to due process and procedural safeguards (e.g., counsel, jury, trials).

IV. Psychiatry and civil law

A. Mental competence.   Psychiatrists often are called on to give an opinion about a person's psychological capacity or competence to perform certain civil and legal functions (e.g., make a will, manage his or her financial affairs).

Competence is context-related (i.e., the ability to perform a certain function for a particular legal purpose). It is especially important to emphasize that incompetence in one area does not imply incompetence in any or all areas. A person may have a mental disorder and still be competent.

B. Contracts.   When a party to an otherwise legal contract is mentally ill and the illness directly and adversely affects the person's ability to understand what he or she is doing (called **contractual capacity**), the law may void the contract.

The psychiatrist must evaluate the condition of the party seeking to void the contract at the time that the contract was supposedly entered into. The psychiatrist must then render an opinion as to whether the psychological condition of the party caused an incapacity to understand the important aspects or ramifications of the contract.

C. Wills.   The criteria concerning wills (called *testamentary capacity*) are whether, when the will was made, the testator was capable of knowing without prompting (1) the nature of the act, (2) the nature and extent of his or her property, and (3) the natural objects of his or her bounty and their claims on him or her (e.g., heirs, relatives, family members).

The mental health of the testator also will indicate whether he or she was in such a condition as to be subject to undue influence.

D. Marriage. A marriage may be void or voidable if one of the parties was incapacitated because of mental illness such that he or she could not reasonably understand the nature and consequences of the transaction (i.e., consent).

E. Guardianship. Guardianship involves a court proceeding for the appointment of a guardian in case of a formal adjudication of incompetence. The criterion is whether, by reason of mental illness, a person can manage his or her own affairs.

F. Durable power of attorney. Permits people to make provisions for their own anticipated loss of decision-making capacity. It permits the advance selection of a substitute decision maker.

G. Competence to inform. Involves a patient's interaction with a clinician. A clinician explains to the patient the value of being honest with the clinician and then determines whether the patient is competent to weigh the risks and benefits of withholding information about suicidal or homicidal intent.

V. Psychiatry and criminal law

A. Competence to stand trial. At any point in the criminal justice process, the psychiatrist may be called on to assess a defendant's present competence to be arraigned, be tried, enter a plea, be sentenced, or be executed. The criteria for competence to be tried are whether, in the presence of a mental disorder, the defendant (1) understands the charges against him or her and (2) can assist in his or her defense.

The Supreme Court has set forth a number of further standards. In the case of *Dusky v. U.S.* (1960), the Court held that the criteria for competence to stand trial require more than a mere orientation and some recall of the event. The defendant must be able to consult with his or her lawyer "with a reasonable degree of rational understanding" and have a "rational as well as factual understanding of the proceedings against him." In *Pate v. Robinson* (1966), the Court held that the psychiatric examination for competence to stand trial is a constitutional right. Finally, in *Jackson v. Indiana* (1972), the Court held that a permanently incompetent person (in that case, a mentally retarded, deaf, and mute person) must be discharged from the criminal justice system.

B. Competence to be executed. Requirement for competence rests on three general principles: (1) A person's awareness of what is happening is supposed to heighten the retributive element of the punishment. (2) A competent person who is about to be executed is believed to be in the best position to make whatever peace is appropriate for his or her religious beliefs, including confession and absolution. (3) A competent person who is about to be executed preserves, until the end, the possibility of recalling a forgotten detail of the events or the crime that may prove exonerating. It is unethical for any clinician to participate in state-mandated executions; a physician's duty to preserve life transcends all other competing requirements.

C. **Criminal responsibility (the insanity defense).**   The legal issues of competence to stand trial and criminal responsibility (the insanity defense) are different in a number of respects and must not be confused. In contrast to competence to stand trial, the question of criminal responsibility involves a time in the past during which the criminal act was committed. The outcomes are different; finding of incompetence to stand trial usually only delays the legal proceedings, whereas a successful insanity plea results in exculpation in the form of a verdict of not guilty by reason of insanity. The underlying philosophical principles are different; competence to stand trial involves the integrity of the judicial process, whereas criminal responsibility relates to moral blameworthiness. In contrast to the criteria for competence to stand trial, the criteria for criminal responsibility involve two separate aspects—whether, at the time of the act, as a consequence of mental disorder, the defendant (1) did not know what he or she was doing or that it was wrong (a cognitive test) or (2) could not conform his or her conduct to the requirements of the law (a volitional test).

1. **M'Naghten rule.** The most famous set of criteria for the insanity defense were developed by the House of Lords after the defendant was exculpated in the M'Naghten case (England, 1843). The M'Naghten rule states that the defendant is to be acquitted if "at the time of the committing of the act, the party accused was laboring under such a defect of reason, from disease of the mind, as not to know the nature of the act he was doing, or, if he did know it, that he did not know he was doing what was wrong." The M'Naghten rule, therefore, is a cognitive test.

2. **Irresistible impulse.** In 1922, a committee of jurists suggested broadening the concept of insanity in criminal cases to include the irresistible impulse test, which rules that a person charged with a criminal offense is not responsible for an act that was committed under an impulse that the person was unable to resist because of mental illness. The court grants an impulse to be irresistible only when it can be determined that the accused would have committed the act even if a policeman had been at the elbow of the accused.

3. **ALI rule.** The American Law Institute (ALI) incorporates both a cognitive and a volitional test in its model penal code. The ALI rule has been adopted in a substantial number of states. The criterion for legal insanity set forth in the rule is that "a person is not responsible for criminal conduct if at the time of such conduct he lacks substantial capacity either to appreciate the criminality (wrongfulness) of his conduct (the cognitive prong) or to conform his conduct to the requirements of the law (the volitional prong)."

   To prevent the inclusion of antisocial behavior, the ALI rule adds, "As used in this article, the terms 'mental disease or defect' do not include an abnormality manifested only by repeated criminal or otherwise antisocial conduct."

   The ALI rule was used in the John Hinckley case (1983). Hinckley's acquittal raised a storm of protest. It seemed clear that the jury had decided that although Hinckley knew what he was doing when he attempted to murder President Ronald Reagan, he could not control him-

TABLE 28–1
ETHICAL QUESTIONS AND ANSWERS

Topic	Question	Answer
Abandonment	How can psychiatrists avoid being charged with patient abandonment upon retirement?	Retiring psychiatrists are not abandoning patients if they provide their patients with sufficient notice and make every reasonable effort to find follow-up care for the patients.
	Is it ethical to provide only outpatient care to a seriously ill patient, who may require hospitalization?	This could constitute abandonment unless the outpatient practitioner or agency arranges for their patients to receive inpatient care from another provider.
Bequests	A dying patient bequeaths his or her estate to his or her treating psychiatrist. Is this ethical?	No. Accepting the bequest seems improper and exploitational of the therapeutic relationship. However, it may be ethical to accept a token bequest from a decreased patient who named his or her psychiatrist in the will without that psychiatrist's knowledge.
Competency	Is it ethical for psychiatrists to perform vaginal exams? Hospital physicals?	Psychiatrists may provide nonpsychiatric medical procedures if they are competent to do so and if the procedures do not preclude effective psychiatric treatment by distorting the transference. Pelvic exams carry a high risk of distorting the transference and would be better performed by another clinician.
	Can ethics committees review issues of physician competency?	Yes. Incompetency is an ethical issue.
Confidentiality	Must confidentiality be maintained after the death of a patient?	Yes. Ethically, confidences survive a patient's death. Exceptions include protecting others from imminent harm or proper legal compulsions.
	Is it ethical to release information about a patient to an insurance company?	Yes, if the information provided is limited to that which is needed to process the insurance claim.
	Can a videotaped segment of a therapy session be used at a workshop for professionals?	Yes, if informed, uncoerced consent has been obtained, anonymity maintained, the audience is advised that editing makes this an incomplete session, and the patient knows the purpose of the videotape.
	Should a physician report mere suspicion of child abuse in a state requiring reporting of child abuse?	No. A physician must make several assessments before deciding whether to report suspected abuse. One must consider whether abuse is ongoing, whether abuse is responsive to treatment, and whether reporting will cause potential harm. Check specific statues. Make safety for potential victims the top priority.
Conflict of interest	Is there a potential ethical conflict if a psychiatrist has both psychotherapeutic and administrative duties in dealing with students or trainees?	Yes. You must define your role in advance to the trainees or students. Administrative opinions should be obtained from a psychiatrist who is not involved in a treatment relationship with the trainee or student.
Diagnosis without examination	Is it ethical to offer a diagnosis based only upon review of records to determine, for insurance purposes, if suicide was the result of the illness?	Yes.

continued

TABLE 28-1—*continued*

Topic	Question	Answer
	Is it ethical for a supervising psychiatrist to sign a diagnosis on an insurance form for services provided by a supervisee when the psychiatrist has not examined the patient?	Yes, if the psychiatrist ensures that proper care is given and the insurance form clearly indicates the role of supervisor and supervisee.
Exploitation (also see Bequests)	What constitutes exploitation of the therapeutic relationship?	Exploitation occurs when the psychiatrist uses the therapeutic relationship for personal gain. This includes adopting or hiring a patient as well as sexual or financial relationships.
Fee splitting	What is fee splitting?	Fee splitting occurs when one physician pays another for a patient referral. This would also apply to lawyers giving a forensic psychiatrist referrals in exchange for a percentage of the fee. Fee splitting may occur in an office setting if the psychiatrist takes a percentage of his or her office-mates' fees for supervision or expenses. Costs for such items or services must be arranged separately. Otherwise, it would appear that the office owner could benefit from referring patients to a colleague in the office. Fee splitting is illegal.
Informed consent	Is it ethical to refuse to divulge information about a patient who has agreed to give this information to those requesting it?	No. It is the patient's decision, not the therapist's.
	Is informed consent needed when presenting or writing about case material?	Not if the patient is aware of the supervisory/teaching process and confidentiality is preserved.
Moonlighting	Can psychiatric residents ethically "moonlight"?	They can if their duties are not beyond their ability, if they are properly supervised, and if the moonlighting does not interfere with their residency training.
Reporting	Should psychiatrists expose or report unethical behavior of a colleague or colleagues? Can a spouse bring an ethical complaint?	Psychiatrists are obligated to report colleagues' unethical behavior. A spouse with knowledge of unethical behavior can bring an ethical complaint as well.
Research	How can ethical research be performed with subjects who cannot give informed consent?	Consent can be given by a legal guardian or via a living will. Incompetent persons have the right to withdraw from the research project at any time.
Retirement	See Abandonment.	
Supervision	What are the ethical requirements when a psychiatrist supervises other mental health professionals?	The psychiatrist must spend sufficient time to ensure that proper care is given and that the supervisee is not providing services that are outside the scope of their training. It is ethical to charge a fee for supervision.
Taping and recording	Can videotapes of patient interviews be used for training purposes on a national level (e.g., workshops, board exam preparation)?	Appropriate and explicit informed consent must be obtained. The purpose and scope of exposure of the tape must be emphasized in addition to the resulting loss of confidentiality.

Table by Eugene Rubin, M.D. Adapted from American Psychiatric Association: *Opinions of the Ethics Committee on the Principles of Medical Ethics with Annotation Especially Applicable to Psychiatry.* Washington, DC: American Psychiatric Association, 1995.

self, so they acquitted him by means of the volitional prong of the test. In response to powerful political demands, both the American Psychiatric Association and the American Bar Association recommended a return to the M'Naghten rule (i.e., the cognitive test only). The American Medical Association went so far as to recommend abolishing the insanity defense altogether.

VI. Ethical issues in psychiatry

See Table 28–1.

For more detailed discussion of this topic, see Forensic Child and Adolescent Psychiatry, Sec 49.12, p 2938; Ethical Issues in Child and Adolescent Psychiatry, Sec 49.13, p 2942; Forensic Issues, Sec 51.6b, p 3150; Ethical Issues, Sec 51.6c, p 3158; and Ethics and Forensic Psychiatry, Ch 54, p 3272, in CTP/VII.

Index

Page numbers followed by *t* indicate tabular material.

B

Baclofen
  as cause of depression, 140*t*
  as cause of mania, 140*t*
Barbiturates, 90
  antipsychotic drug interactions, 352*t*
  as cause of depression, 140*t*
  for dementia, 41
  in male sexual dysfunction, 192*t*
  neuropsychiatric side effects with HIV, 65*t*
  psychoactive drug-related conditions and
    treatments, 85*t*
  urine testing for, 405*t*
BDI. *See* Beck Depression Inventory
BEAM. *See* Brain electrical activity mapping
Beck, Aaron, 136
Beck Depression Inventory (BDI), 136–137
Behavior
  in mania, 131
  normal, in children, 276*t*–277*t*
  with pain disorder, 173
Behavioral and psychological symptoms of
    dementia (BPSD), 307
Behavior modification, for separation anxiety
    disorder, 303
Behavior therapy, 327–328. *See also* cognitive-
    behavioral therapy
  for anxiety disorders, 164
  aversion therapy, 327
  for bipolar disorders, 148
  for borderline personality disorder, 251
  clinical applications, 328*t*
  for dependent personality disorder, 258
  for depression, 145
  dialectical, 332
  flooding, 328
  for kleptomania, 221
  for mental retardation in children, 285
  positive reinforcement and, 327
  for pyromania, 221
  for schizophrenia, 114
  systematic desensitization, 327–328
  token economy, 327
Belladonna alkaloids, psychoactive drug-related
    conditions and treatments, 85*t*
Benadryl. *See* Diphenhydramine
Benaphetamine, characteristics, 338*t*
Bender-Gestalt test, for anxiety, 158
Benzene, psychoactive drug-related conditions and
    treatments, 85*t*
Benzisoxazole, for schizophrenia, 112*t*
Benzodiazepines, 90, 341–343
  for acute anxiety, 339
  adverse effects, 358
  for anxiety disorders, 161–162, 161*t*
  for avoidant personality disorder, 257
  as cause of depression, 140*t*
  characteristics, 338*t*
  for children, 287*t*
  for chronic anxiety, 339
  contraindications, 41
  for conversion disorder, 172
  for delirium, 37
  dependence, 342–343
  duration of action, 342, 342*t*

  for extrapyramidal disorders, 408*t*
  guidelines for treatment of withdrawal, 91*t*
  half-lives, doses, and preparations, 340*t*
  indications, 341
  for insomnia, 341
  for intermittent explosive disorder, 221
  laboratory testing and, 386
  for neuroleptic-induced acute akathisia, 409
  for neuroleptic-induced tardive dyskinesia, 411
  neuropsychiatric side effects with HIV, 65*t*
  pharmacological effects, 341*t*
  potency, 341
  prevalence of use, 89*t*
  for psychiatric emergency, 269*t*
  psychoactive drug-related conditions and
    treatments, 85*t*
  for serotonin syndrome, 360
  for trichotillomania, 221
  urine testing for, 405*t*
  for violence, 267
  withdrawal symptoms, 342–343, 342*t*
Benzphetamine (Didrex), for obesity, 207*t*
Benztropine (Cogentin), for extrapyramidal
    disorders, 408*t*
Benzydamine, as cause of depression, 140*t*
Bequests, 423*t*
Bereavement, 30, 222. *See also* Grief
  complications, 322*t*
  mood disorders and, 139
  in patients and children, 321*t*
Beta-blockers. *See* β-Adrenergic antagonists
Bethanidine, as cause of depression, 140*t*
Bicarbonate, serum test, 387*t*
Bilirubin test, 387*t*
Binge-eating disorder, classification in DSM-IV-
    TR, 31
Binswanger's disease, 46
Bioavailability, definition, 336
Biochemical markers, 404–406. *See also*
    Alzheimer's disease; Monoamine oxidase
    inhibitors
Biofeedback, 333*t*, 334
  for trichotillomania, 221
Biogenic amines, in mood disorders, 134–135
Biological factors
  in adjustment disorders, 222
  in anorexia nervosa, 201
  in anxiety, 157
  in bulimia nervosa, 203
  in conversion disorder, 170
  delusional disorder and, 120
  in gender identity disorders, 197
  in mood disorders, 134–136
  in obesity, 205
  with pain disorder, 173
Biperiden (Akineton)
  drug interactions, 348
  for extrapyramidal disorders, 408*t*
Bipolar disorders. *See also* Bipolar I disorder;
    Bipolar II disorder; Cyclothymic disorder;
    Hypomanic episode; Mania; Manic
    episode; Mood disorders
  classification in DSM-IV-TR, 27–28
  delusional disorder and, 121
  diagnosis, signs, and symptoms, 133–134

About the Authors

BENJAMIN JAMES SADOCK, M.D., is the Menas S. Gregory Professor of Psychiatry and Vice Chairman of the Department of Psychiatry at the New York University (NYU) School of Medicine. He is a graduate of Union College, received his M.D. degree from New York Medical College, and completed his internship at Albany Hospital. He completed his residency at Bellevue Psychiatric Hospital and then entered the military service, where he served as Acting Chief of Neuropsychiatry at Sheppard Air Force Base in Texas. He has held faculty and teaching appointments at Southwestern Medical School and Parkland Hospital in Dallas and at New York Medical College, St. Luke's Hospital, the New York State Psychiatric Institute, and Metropolitan Hospital in New York City. Dr. Sadock joined the faculty of the NYU School of Medicine in 1980 and served in various positions: Director of Medical Student Education in Psychiatry, Co-Director of the Residency Training Program in Psychiatry, and Director of Graduate Medical Education. Currently, Dr. Sadock is Director of Student Mental Health Services, Psychiatric Consultant to the Admissions Committee, and Co-Director of Continuing Education in Psychiatry at the NYU School of Medicine. He is on the staff of Bellevue Hospital and Tisch Hospital and is a Consultant Psychiatrist at Lenox Hill Hospital. Dr. Sadock is a Diplomate of the American Board of Psychiatry and Neurology and served as Assistant and Associate Examiner for the Board for more than a decade. He is a Fellow of the American Psychiatric Association, a Fellow of the American College of Physicians, a Fellow of the New York Academy of Medicine, and a member of Alpha Omega Alpha Honor Society. He is active in numerous psychiatric organizations and is president and founder of the NYU-Bellevue Psychiatric Society. Dr. Sadock was a member of the National Committee in Continuing Education in Psychiatry of the American Psychiatric Association, served on the Ad Hoc Committee on Sex Therapy Clinics of the American Medical Association, was a Delegate to the Conference on Recertification of the American Board of Medical Specialists, and was a representative of the American Psychiatric Association Task Force on the National Board of Medical Examiners and the American Board of Psychiatry and Neurology. In 1985, he received the Academic Achievement Award from New York Medical College and was appointed a Faculty Scholar at NYU School of Medicine in 2000. He is the author or editor of more than 100 publications and a book reviewer for psychiatric journals, and he lectures on a broad range of topics in general psychiatry. Dr. Sadock maintains a private practice for diagnostic consultations, psychotherapy, and pharmacotherapy. He has been married to Virginia Alcott Sadock, M.D., a clinical professor of psychiatry at NYU School of Medicine, since completing his residency. Dr. Sadock enjoys opera, skiing, and traveling and is an enthusiastic fly fisherman.

VIRGINIA ALCOTT SADOCK, M.D., joined the faculty of the New York University (NYU) School of Medicine in 1980, where she is currently a Clinical Professor of Psychiatry. She is an Attending Psychiatrist at Tisch Hospital and Bellevue Hospital. She is Director of the Program in Human Sexuality and Sex Therapy at the NYU Medical Center, one of the largest treatment and training programs of its kind in the United States. She is the author of more than 50 articles and chapters on sexual behavior and was the developmental editor of *The Sexual Experience,* one of the first major textbooks on human sexuality, published by Williams & Wilkins. She serves as a referee and book reviewer for several medical journals, including the *American Journal of Psychiatry* and the *Journal of the American Medical Association.* She has long been interested in the role of women in medicine and psychiatry and was a founder of the Committee on Women in Psychiatry of the New York County District Branch of the American Psychiatric Association. She is active in academic matters, has served as an Assistant and Associate Examiner for the American Board of Psychiatry and Neurology for more than 15 years, and was also a member of the Test Committee in Psychiatry for both the American Board of Psychiatry and the Psychiatric Knowledge and Self-Assessment Program (PKSAP) of the American Psychiatric Association. She has chaired the Committee on Public Relations of the New York County District Branch of the American Psychiatric Association and has participated in the National Medical Television Network series *Women in Medicine* and the Emmy Award-winning PBS television documentary *Women and Depression.* She has been Vice-President of the Society of Sex Therapy and Research and a regional council member of the American Association of Sex Education Counselors and Therapists, and she is currently President of the Alumni Association of Sex Therapists. She lectures extensively both in this country and abroad on sexual dysfunction, relational problems, and depression and anxiety disorders. She is a Fellow of the American Psychiatric Association, a Fellow of the New York Academy of Medicine, and a Diplomate of the American Board of Psychiatry and Neurology. Dr. Sadock is a graduate of Bennington College, received her M.D. degree from New York Medical College, and trained in psychiatry at Metropolitan Hospital. She lives in Manhattan with her husband, Dr. Benjamin Sadock, where she maintains an active psychiatric practice that includes individual psychotherapy, couples and marital therapy, sex therapy, psychiatric consultation, and pharmacotherapy. She and her husband have two children, James and Victoria, both emergency physicians. In her leisure time, Dr. Sadock enjoys theater, film, reading fiction, and travel.

DSM-IV-TR Classification

NOS, not otherwise specified.

An *x* appearing in a diagnostic code indicates that a specific code number is required.

An ellipsis (. . .) is used in the names of certain disorders to indicate that the name of a specific mental disorder or general medical condition should be inserted when the name when recording (e.g., 293.0 Delirium due to hypothyroidism).

If criteria are currently met, one of the following severity specifiers may be noted after the diagnosis:
> Mild
> Moderate
> Severe

If criteria are no longer met, one of the following specifiers may be noted:
> In partial remission
> In full remission
> Prior history

> **Disorders Usually First Diagnosed in Infancy, Childhood, or Adolescence**

MENTAL RETARDATION
Note: *These are coded on Axis II.*

317	Mild mental retardation
318.0	Moderate mental retardation
318.1	Severe mental retardation
318.2	Profound mental retardation
319	Mental retardation, severity unspecified

LEARNING DISORDERS
315.00	Reading disorder
315.1	Mathematics disorder
315.2	Disorder of written expression
315.9	Learning disorder NOS

MOTOR SKILLS DISORDER
315.4	Developmental coordination disorder

COMMUNICATION DISORDERS
315.31	Expressive language disorder
315.32	Mixed receptive-expressive language disorder
315.39	Phonological disorder
307.0	Stuttering
307.9	Communication disorder NOS

PERVASIVE DEVELOPMENTAL DISORDERS
299.00	Autistic disorder
299.80	Rett's disorder
299.10	Childhood disintegrative disorder
299.80	Asperger's disorder
299.80	Pervasive developmental disorder NOS

ATTENTION-DEFICIT AND DISRUPTIVE BEHAVIOR DISORDERS
314.xx	Attention-deficit/hyperactivity disorder
.01	Combined type
.00	Predominantly inattentive type
.01	Predominantly hyperactive-impulsive type
314.9	Attention-deficit/hyperactivity disorder NOS
312.xx	Conduct disorder
.81	Childhood-onset type
.82	Adolescent-onset type
.89	Unspecified onset
313.81	Oppositional defiant disorder
312.9	Disruptive behavior disorder NOS

FEEDING AND EATING DISORDERS OF INFANCY OR EARLY CHILDHOOD
307.52	Pica
307.53	Rumination disorder
307.59	Feeding disorder of infancy or early childhood

TIC DISORDERS
307.23	Tourette's disorder
307.22	Chronic motor or vocal tic disorder
307.21	Transient tic disorder (115)
	Specify if: single episode/recurrent
307.20	Tic disorder NOS

ELIMINATION DISORDERS
——.—	Encopresis
787.6	With constipation and overflow incontinence
307.7	Without constipation and overflow incontinence
307.6	Enuresis (not due to a general medical condition)
	Specify type: nocturnal only/diurnal only/nocturnal and diurnal

OTHER DISORDERS OF INFANCY, CHILDHOOD, OR ADOLESCENCE
309.21	Separation anxiety disorder
	Specify if: early onset
313.23	Selective mutism
313.89	Reactive attachment disorder of infancy or early childhood
	Specify type: inhibited type/disinhibited type
307.3	Stereotypic movement disorder
	Specify if: with self-injurious behavior
313.9	Disorder of infancy, childhood, or adolescence NOS

Delirium, Dementia, and Amnestic and Other Cognitive Disorders

---

DELIRIUM

293.0   Delirium due to . . . *[indicate the general medical condition]*
——.—   Substance intoxication delirium *(refer to Substance-Related Disorders for substance-specific codes)*
——.—   Substance withdrawal delirium *(refer to Substance-Related Disorders for substance-specific codes)*
——.—   Delirium due to multiple etiologies *(code each of the specific etiologies)*
780.09   Delirium NOS

DEMENTIA

294.xx   Dementia of the Alzheimer's type, with early onset *(also code 331.0 Alzheimer's disease on Axis III)*
.10   Without behavioral disturbance
.11   With behavioral disturbance
294.xx   Dementia of the Alzheimer's type, with late onset *(also code 331.0 Alzheimer's disease on Axis III)*
.10   Without behavioral disturbance
.11   With behavioral disturbance
290.xx   Vascular dementia
.40   Uncomplicated
.41   With delirium
.42   With delusions
.43   With depressed mood
Specify if: with behavioral disturbance

Code presence or absence of a behavioral disturbance in the fifth digit for dementia due to a general medical condition:

0 = Without behavioral disturbance
1 = With behavioral disturbance

294.1x   Dementia due to HIV disease *(also code 042 HIV on Axis III)*
294.1x   Dementia due to head trauma *(also code 854.00 head injury on Axis III)*
294.1x   Dementia due to Parkinson's disease *(also code 332.0 Parkinson's disease on Axis III)*
294.1x   Dementia due to Huntington's disease *(also code 333.4 Huntington's disease on Axis III)*
294.1x   Dementia due to Pick's disease *(also code 331.1 Pick's disease on Axis III)*
294.1x   Dementia due to Creutzfeldt-Jakob disease *(also code 046.1 Creutzfeldt-Jakob disease on Axis III)*

294.1x   Dementia due to . . . *[indicate the general medical condition not listed above] (also code the general medical condition on Axis III)*
——.—   Substance-induced persisting dementia *(refer to Substance-Related Disorders for substance-specific codes)*
——.—   Dementia due to multiple etiologies *(code each of the specific etiologies)*
294.8   Dementia NOS

AMNESTIC DISORDERS

294.0   Amnestic disorder due to . . . *[indicate the general medical condition]* *Specify if:* transient/chronic
——.—   Substance-induced persisting amnestic disorder *(refer to Substance-Related Disorders for substance-specific codes)*
294.8   Amnestic disorder NOS

OTHER COGNITIVE DISORDERS

294.9   Cognitive disorder NOS

Mental Disorders Due to a General Medical Condition Not Elsewhere Classified

---

293.89   Catatonic disorder due to . . . *[indicate the general medical condition]*
310.1   Personality change due to . . . *[indicate the general medical condition]* *Specify type:* labile type/disinhibited type/aggressive type/apathetic type/paranoid type/other type/combined type/unspecified type
293.9   Mental disorder NOS due to . . . *[indicate the general medical condition]*

Substance-Related Disorders

The following specifiers apply to substance dependence as noted:

ᵃ With physiological dependence/without physiological dependence
ᵇ Early full remission/early partial remission/sustained full remission/sustained partial remission
ᶜ In a controlled environment
ᵈ On agonist therapy

The following specifiers apply to substance-induced disorders as noted:

ᴵ With onset during intoxication/ᵂWith onset during withdrawal

ALCOHOL-RELATED DISORDERS

Alcohol Use Disorders
303.90   Alcohol dependence[a,b,c]
305.00   Alcohol abuse

Alcohol-Induced Disorders
303.00   Alcohol intoxication
291.81   Alcohol withdrawal
        Specify if: with perceptual
        disturbances
291.0   Alcohol intoxication delirium
291.0   Alcohol withdrawal delirium
291.2   Alcohol-induced persisting dementia
291.1   Alcohol-induced persisting amnestic
        disorder
291.x   Alcohol-induced psychotic disorder
   .5   With delusions[I,W]
   .3   With hallucinations[I,W]
291.89   Alcohol-induced mood disorder[I,W]
291.89   Alcohol-induced anxiety disorder[I,W]
291.89   Alcohol-induced sexual dysfunction[I]
291.89   Alcohol-induced sleep disorder[I,W]
291.9   Alcohol-related disorder NOS

AMPHETAMINE- (OR AMPHETAMINE-LIKE)–RELATED DISORDERS

Amphetamine Use Disorders
304.40   Amphetamine dependence[a,b,c]
305.70   Amphetamine abuse

Amphetamine-Induced Disorders
292.89   Amphetamine intoxication
        Specify if: with perceptual
        disturbances
292.0   Amphetamine withdrawal
292.81   Amphetamine intoxication delirium
292.xx   Amphetamine-induced psychotic
        disorder
   .11   With delusions[I]
   .12   With hallucinations[I]
292.84   Amphetamine-induced mood
        disorder[I,W]
292.89   Amphetamine-induced anxiety
        disorder[I]
292.89   Amphetamine-induced sexual
        dysfunction[I]
292.89   Amphetamine-induced sleep
        disorder[I,W]
292.9   Amphetamine-related disorder NOS

CAFFEINE-RELATED DISORDERS

Caffeine-Induced Disorders
305.90   Caffeine intoxication
292.89   Caffeine-induced anxiety disorder[I]
292.89   Caffeine-induced sleep disorder[I]
292.9   Caffeine-related disorder NOS

CANNABIS-RELATED DISORDERS

Cannabis Use Disorders
304.30   Cannabis dependence[a,b,c]
305.20   Cannabis abuse

Cannabis-Induced Disorders
292.89   Cannabis intoxication
        Specify if: with perceptual
        disturbances
292.81   Cannabis intoxication delirium
292.xx   Cannabis-induced psychotic
        disorder
   .11   With delusions[I]
   .12   With hallucinations[I]
292.89   Cannabis-induced anxiety disorder
292.9   Cannabis-related disorder NOS

COCAINE-RELATED DISORDERS

Cocaine Use Disorders
304.20   Cocaine dependence[a,b,c]
305.60   Cocaine abuse

Cocaine-Induced Disorders
292.89   Cocaine intoxication
        Specify if: with perceptual
        disturbances
292.0   Cocaine withdrawal
292.81   Cocaine intoxication delirium
292.xx   Cocaine-induced psychotic disorder
   .11   With delusions[I]
   .12   With hallucinations[I]
292.84   Cocaine-induced mood disorder[I,W]
292.89   Cocaine-induced anxiety disorder[I,W]
292.89   Cocaine-induced sexual
        dysfunction[I]
292.89   Cocaine-induced sleep disorder[I,W]
292.9   Cocaine-related disorder NOS

HALLUCINOGEN-RELATED DISORDERS

Hallucinogen Use Disorders
304.50   Hallucinogen dependence[b,c]
305.30   Hallucinogen abuse

Hallucinogen-Induced Disorders
292.89   Hallucinogen intoxication
292.89   Hallucinogen persisting perception
        disorder (flashbacks)
292.81   Hallucinogen intoxication delirium
292.xx   Hallucinogen-induced psychotic
        disorder
   .11   With delusions[I]
   .12   With hallucinations[I]
292.84   Hallucinogen-induced mood
        disorder[I]
292.89   Hallucinogen-induced anxiety
        disorder[I]
292.9   Hallucinogen-related disorder NOS

INHALANT-RELATED DISORDERS

Inhalant Use Disorders
304.60   Inhalant dependence[b,c]
305.90   Inhalant abuse

Inhalant-Induced Disorders
292.89   Inhalant intoxication
292.81   Inhalant intoxication delirium
292.82   Inhalant-induced persisting
        dementia

292.xx	Inhalant-induced psychotic disorder
.11	With delusions[I]
.12	With hallucinations[I]
292.84	Inhalant-induced mood disorder[I]
292.89	Inhalant-induced anxiety disorder[I]
292.9	Inhalant-related disorder NOS

NICOTINE-RELATED DISORDERS

Nicotine Use Disorder
305.1	Nicotine dependence[a,b]

Nicotine-Induced Disorder
292.0	Nicotine withdrawal
292.9	Nicotine-related disorder NOS

OPIOID-RELATED DISORDERS

Opioid Use Disorders
304.00	Opioid dependence[a,b,c,d]
305.50	Opioid abuse

Opioid-Induced Disorders
292.89	Opioid intoxication
	Specify if: with perceptual disturbances
292.0	Opioid withdrawal
292.81	Opioid intoxication delirium
292.xx	Opioid-induced psychotic disorder
.11	With delusions[I]
.12	With hallucinations[I]
292.84	Opioid-induced mood disorder[I]
292.89	Opioid-induced sexual dysfunction[I]
292.89	Opioid-induced sleep disorder[I,W]
292.9	Opioid-related disorder NOS

PHENCYCLIDINE- (OR PHENCYCLIDINE-LIKE)–RELATED DISORDERS

Phencyclidine Use Disorders
304.60	Phencyclidine dependence[b,c]
305.90	Phencyclidine abuse

Phencyclidine-Induced Disorders
292.89	Phencyclidine intoxication
	Specify if: with perceptual disturbances
292.81	Phencyclidine intoxication delirium
292.xx	Phencyclidine-induced psychotic disorder
.11	With delusions[I]
.12	With hallucinations[I]
292.84	Phencyclidine-induced mood disorder[I]
292.89	Phencyclidine-induced anxiety disorder[I]
292.9	Phencyclidine-related disorder NOS

SEDATIVE-, HYPNOTIC-, OR ANXIOLYTIC-RELATED DISORDERS

Sedative, Hypnotic, or Anxiolytic Use Disorders
304.10	Sedative, hypnotic, or anxiolytic dependence[a,b,c]

305.40	Sedative, hypnotic, or anxiolytic abuse

Sedative-, Hypnotic-, or Anxiolytic-Induced Disorders
292.89	Sedative, hypnotic, or anxiolytic intoxication
292.0	Sedative, hypnotic, or anxiolytic withdrawal
	Specify if: with perceptual disturbances
292.81	Sedative, hypnotic, or anxiolytic intoxication delirium
292.81	Sedative, hypnotic, or anxiolytic withdrawal delirium
292.82	Sedative-, hypnotic-, or anxiolytic-induced persisting dementia
292.83	Sedative-, hypnotic-, or anxiolytic-induced persisting amnestic disorder
292.xx	Sedative-, hypnotic-, or anxiolytic-induced psychotic disorder
.11	With delusions[I,W]
.12	With hallucinations[I,W]
292.84	Sedative-, hypnotic-, or anxiolytic-induced mood disorder[I,W]
292.89	Sedative-, hypnotic-, or anxiolytic-induced anxiety disorder[W]
292.89	Sedative-, hypnotic-, or anxiolytic-induced sexual dysfunction[I]
292.89	Sedative-, hypnotic-, or anxiolytic-induced sleep disorder[I,W]
292.9	Sedative-, hypnotic-, or anxiolytic-related disorder NOS

POLYSUBSTANCE-RELATED DISORDER
304.80	Polysubstance dependence[a,b,c,d]

OTHER (OR UNKNOWN) SUBSTANCE-RELATED DISORDERS

Other (or Unknown) Substance Use Disorders
304.90	Other (or unknown) substance dependence[a,b,c,d]
305.90	Other (or unknown) substance abuse

Other (or Unknown) Substance-Induced Disorders
292.89	Other (or unknown) substance intoxication
	Specify if: with perceptual disturbances
292.0	Other (or unknown) substance withdrawal
	Specify if: with perceptual disturbances
292.81	Other (or unknown) substance-induced delirium
292.82	Other (or unknown) substance-induced persisting dementia
292.83	Other (or unknown) substance-induced persisting amnestic disorder

292.xx	Other (or unknown) substance-induced psychotic disorder
.11	With delusions[I,W]
.12	With hallucinations[I,W]
292.84	Other (or unknown) substance-induced mood disorder[I,W]
292.89	Other (or unknown) substance-induced anxiety disorder[I,W]
292.89	Other (or unknown) substance-induced sexual dysfunction[I]
292.89	Other (or unknown) substance-induced sleep disorder[I,W]
292.9	Other (or unknown) substance-related disorder NOS

Schizophrenia and Other Psychotic Disorders

295.xx   Schizophrenia

The following classification of longitudinal course applies to all subtypes of schizophrenia:

Episodic with interepisode residual symptoms (*specify if:* with prominent negative symptoms)/episodic with no interepisode residual symptoms

Continuous (*specify if:* with prominent negative symptoms)

Single episode in partial remission (*specify if:* with prominent negative symptoms)/single episode in full remission

Other or unspecified pattern

.30	Paranoid type
.10	Disorganized type
.20	Catatonic type
.90	Undifferentiated type
.60	Residual type
295.40	Schizophreniform disorder
	Specify if: without good prognostic features/with good prognostic features
295.70	Schizoaffective disorder
	Specify if: bipolar type/depressive type
297.1	Delusional disorder
	Specify if: erotomanic type/grandiose type/jealous type/persecutory type/somatic type/mixed type/unspecified type
298.8	Brief psychotic disorder
	Specify if: with marked stressor(s)/without marked stressor(s)/with postpartum onset
297.3	Shared psychotic disorder
293.xx	Psychotic disorder due to . . . *[indicate the general medical condition]*
.81	With delusions
.82	With hallucinations
——.—	Substance-induced psychotic disorder (*refer to*

Substance-Related Disorders for substance-specific codes)
Specify if: with onset during intoxication/with onset during withdrawal

298.9   Psychotic Disorder NOS

Mood Disorders
Code current state of major depressive disorder or bipolar I disorder in fifth digit:

1 = Mild
2 = Moderate
3 = Severe without psychotic features
4 = Severe with psychotic features
   Specify: mood-congruent psychotic features/mood-incongruent psychotic features
5 = In partial remission
6 = In full remission
0 = Unspecified

The following specifiers apply (for current or most recent episode) to mood disorders as noted:

[a]Severity/psychotic/remission specifiers/[b]Chronic/[c]With catatonic features/[d]With melancholic features/[e]With atypical features/[f]With postpartum onset

The following specifiers apply to mood disorders as noted:

[g]With or without full interepisode recovery/[h]With seasonal pattern/[i]With rapid cycling

DEPRESSIVE DISORDERS

296.xx	Major depressive disorder
.2x	Single episode[a,b,c,d,e,f]
.3x	Recurrent[a,b,c,d,e,f,g,h]
300.4	Dysthymic disorder
	Specify if: early onset/late onset
	Specify if: with atypical features
311	Depressive disorder NOS

BIPOLAR DISORDERS

296.xx	Bipolar I disorder
.0x	Single manic episode[a,c,f]
	Specify if: mixed
.40	Most recent episode hypomanic[g,h,i]
.4x	Most recent episode manic[a,c,f,g,h,i]
.6x	Most recent episode mixed[a,c,f,g,h,i]
.5x	Most recent episode depressed[a,b,c,d,e,f,g,h,i]
.7	Most recent episode unspecified[g,h,i]
296.89	Bipolar II disorder[a,b,c,d,e,f,g,h,i]
	Specify (current or most recent episode): hypomanic/depressed
301.13	Cyclothymic disorder
296.80	Bipolar disorder NOS
293.83	Mood disorder due to . . . *[indicate the general medical condition]*
	Specify type: with depressive features/with major depressive-like

episode/with manic features/with mixed features

———.— Substance-induced mood disorder *(refer to Substance-Related Disorders for substance-specific codes)* *Specify type:* with depressive features/with manic features/with mixed features *Specify if:* with onset during intoxication/with onset during withdrawal

296.90 Mood disorder NOS

Anxiety Disorders

300.01 Panic disorder without agoraphobia
300.21 Panic disorder with agoraphobia
300.22 Agoraphobia without history of panic disorder
300.29 Specific phobia
Specify type: animal type/natural environment type/blood-injection-injury type/situational type/other type
300.23 Social phobia
Specify if: generalized
300.3 Obsessive-compulsive disorder
Specify if: with poor insight
309.81 Posttraumatic stress disorder
Specify if: acute/chronic
Specify if: with delayed onset
308.3 Acute stress disorder
300.02 Generalized anxiety disorder
293.84 Anxiety disorder due to . . .
[Indicate the general medical condition]
Specify if: with generalized anxiety/with panic attacks/with obsessive-compulsive symptoms
———.— Substance-induced anxiety disorder *(refer to Substance-Related Disorders for substance-specific codes)* *Specify if:* with generalized anxiety/with panic attacks/with obsessive-compulsive symptoms/with phobic symptoms *Specify if:* with onset during intoxication/with onset during withdrawal
300.00 Anxiety disorder NOS

Somatoform Disorders

300.81 Somatization disorder
300.82 Undifferentiated somatoform disorder
300.11 Conversion disorder
Specify type: with motor symptom or deficit/with sensory symptom or deficit/with seizures or convulsions/with mixed presentation
307.xx Pain disorder

.80 Associated with psychological factors
.89 Associated with both psychological factors and a general medical condition
Specify if: acute/chronic
300.7 Hypochondriasis
Specify if: with poor insight
300.7 Body dysmorphic disorder
300.82 Somatoform disorder NOS

Factitious Disorders

300.xx Factitious disorder
.16 With predominantly psychological signs and symptoms
.19 With predominantly physical signs and symptoms
.19 With combined psychological and physical signs and symptoms
300.19 Factitious disorder NOS

Dissociative Disorders

300.12 Dissociative amnesia
300.13 Dissociative fugue
300.14 Dissociative identity disorder
300.6 Depersonalization disorder
300.15 Dissociative disorder NOS

Sexual and Gender Identity Disorders

SEXUAL DYSFUNCTIONS
The following specifiers apply to all primary sexual dysfunctions:
Lifelong type/acquired type
Generalized type/situational type
Due to psychological factors/due to combined factors

Sexual Desire Disorders
302.71 Hypoactive sexual desire disorder
302.79 Sexual aversion disorder

Sexual Arousal Disorders
302.72 Female sexual arousal disorder
302.72 Male erectile disorder

Orgasmic Disorders
302.73 Female orgasmic disorder
302.74 Male orgasmic disorder
302.75 Premature ejaculation

Sexual Pain Disorders
302.76 Dyspareunia (not due to a general medical condition)
306.51 Vaginismus (not due to a general medical condition)

Sexual Dysfunction Due to a General Medical Condition
625.8 Female hypoactive sexual desire disorder due to . . . *[indicate the general medical condition]*

608.89   Male hypoactive sexual desire disorder due to . . . *[indicate the general medical condition]*
607.84   Male erectile disorder due to . . . *[indicate the general medical condition]*
625.0   Female dyspareunia due to . . . *[indicate the general medical condition]*
608.89   Male dyspareunia due to . . . *[indicate the general medical condition]*
625.8   Other female sexual dysfunction due to . . . *[indicate the general medical condition]*
608.89   Other male sexual dysfunction due to . . . *[indicate the general medical condition]*
——.—   Substance-induced sexual dysfunction *(refer to Substance-Related Disorders for substance-specific codes)*
Specify if: with impaired desire/with impaired arousal/with impaired orgasm/with sexual pain
Specify if: with onset during intoxication
302.70   Sexual dysfunction NOS

PARAPHILIAS
302.4   Exhibitionism
302.81   Fetishism
302.89   Frotteurism
302.2   Pedophilia
Specify if: sexually attracted to males/sexually attracted to females/sexually attracted to both
Specify if: limited to incest
Specify type: exclusive type/nonexclusive type
302.83   Sexual masochism
302.84   Sexual sadism
302.3   Transvestic fetishism
Specify if: with gender dysphoria
302.82   Voyeurism
302.9   Paraphilia NOS

GENDER IDENTITY DISORDERS
302.xx   Gender identity disorder
.6   in children
.85   in adolescents or adults
Specify if: sexually attracted to males/sexually attracted to females/sexually attracted to both/sexually attracted to neither
302.6   Gender identity disorder NOS
302.9   Sexual disorder NOS

Eating Disorders

307.1   Anorexia nervosa
Specify type: restricting type; binge-eating/purging type

307.51   Bulimia nervosa
Specify type: Purging type/nonpurging type
307.50   Eating disorder NOS

Sleep Disorders

PRIMARY SLEEP DISORDERS

Dyssomnias
307.42   Primary insomnia
307.44   Primary hypersomnia
Specify if: recurrent
347   Narcolepsy
780.59   Breathing-related sleep disorder
307.45   Circadian rhythm sleep disorder
Specify type: delayed sleep phase type/jet lag type/shift work type/unspecified type
307.47   Dyssomnia NOS

Parasomnias
307.47   Nightmare disorder
307.46   Sleep terror disorder
307.46   Sleepwalking disorder
307.47   Parasomnia NOS

SLEEP DISORDERS RELATED TO ANOTHER MENTAL DISORDER
307.42   Insomnia related to . . . *[indicate the Axis I or Axis II disorder]*
307.44   Hypersomnia related to . . . *[indicate the Axis I or Axis II disorder]*

OTHER SLEEP DISORDERS
780.xx   Sleep disorder due to . . . *[indicate the general medical condition]*
.52   Insomnia type
.54   Hypersomnia type
.59   Parasomnia type
.59   Mixed type
——.—   Substance-induced sleep disorder *(refer to Substance-Related Disorders for substance-specific codes)*
Specify type: insomnia type/hypersomnia type/parasomnia type/mixed type
Specify if: with onset during intoxication/with onset during withdrawal

Impulse-Control Disorders Not Elsewhere Classified

312.34   Intermittent explosive disorder
312.32   Kleptomania
312.33   Pyromania
312.31   Pathological gambling
312.39   Trichotillomania
312.30   Impulse-control disorder NOS

Adjustment Disorders

309.xx	Adjustment disorder
.0	With depressed mood
.24	With anxiety
.28	With mixed anxiety and depressed mood
.3	With disturbance of conduct
.4	With mixed disturbance of emotions and conduct
.9	Unspecified
	Specify if: acute/chronic

Personality Disorders

Note: *These are coded on Axis II.*

301.0	Paranoid personality disorder
301.20	Schizoid personality disorder
301.22	Schizotypal personality disorder
301.7	Antisocial personality disorder
301.83	Borderline personality disorder
301.50	Histrionic personality disorder
301.81	Narcissistic personality disorder
301.82	Avoidant personality disorder
301.6	Dependent personality disorder
301.4	Obsessive-compulsive personality disorder
301.9	Personality disorder NOS

Other Conditions That May Be a Focus of Clinical Attention

PSYCHOLOGICAL FACTORS AFFECTING MEDICAL CONDITION

| 316 | . . . [specified psychological factor] affecting . . . [indicate the general medical condition] |

Choose name based on nature of factors:

Mental disorder affecting medical condition

Psychological symptoms affecting medical condition

Personality traits or coping style affecting medical condition

Maladaptive health behaviors affecting medical condition

Stress-related physiologic response affecting medical condition

Other or unspecified psychological factors affecting medical condition

MEDICATION-INDUCED MOVEMENT DISORDERS

332.1	Neuroleptic-induced parkinsonism
333.92	Neuroleptic malignant syndrome
333.7	Neuroleptic-induced acute dystonia
333.99	Neuroleptic-induced acute akathisia
333.82	Neuroleptic-induced tardive dyskinesia

| 333.1 | Medication-induced postural tremor |
| 333.90 | Medication-induced movement disorder NOS |

OTHER MEDICATION-INDUCED DISORDER

| 995.2 | Adverse effects of medication NOS |

RELATIONAL PROBLEMS

V61.9	Relational problem related to a mental disorder or general medical condition
V61.20	Parent–child relational problem
V61.10	Partner relational problem
V61.8	Sibling relational problem
V62.81	Relational problem NOS

PROBLEMS RELATED TO ABUSE OR NEGLECT

V61.21	Physical abuse of child *(code 995.54 if focus of attention is on victim)*
V61.21	Sexual abuse of child *(code 995.53 if focus of attention is on victim)*
V61.21	Neglect of child *(code 995.52 if focus of attention is on victim)*
——.—	Physical abuse of adult
V61.12	(if by partner)
V62.83	(if by person other than partner) *(code 995.81 if focus of attention is on victim)*
——.—	Sexual abuse of adult
V61.12	(if by partner)
V62.83	(if by person other than partner) *(code 995.83 if focus of attention is on victim)*

ADDITIONAL CONDITIONS THAT MAY BE A FOCUS OF CLINICAL ATTENTION

V15.81	Noncompliance with treatment
V65.2	Malingering
V71.01	Adult antisocial behavior
V71.02	Child or adolescent antisocial behavior
V62.89	Borderline intellectual functioning **Note:** *This is coded on Axis II.*
780.9	Age-related cognitive decline
V62.82	Bereavement
V62.3	Academic problem
V62.2	Occupational problem
313.82	Identity problem
V62.89	Religious or spiritual problem
V62.4	Acculturation problem
V62.89	Phase-of-life problem

Additional Codes

300.9	Unspecified mental disorder (nonpsychotic)
V71.09	No diagnosis or condition on Axis I
799.9	Diagnosis or condition deferred on Axis II
V71.09	No diagnosis on Axis II
799.9	Diagnosis deferred on Axis II

Multiaxial System

Axis I   Clinical disorders
          Other conditions that may be a
          focus of clinical attention

Axis II   Personality disorders, Mental
          retardation
Axis III General medical conditions
Axis IV   Psychosocial and environmental
          problems
Axis V   Global assessment of functioning